Text Mining Techniques for Healthcare Provider Quality Determination:

Methods for Rank Comparisons

Patricia Cerrito
University of Louisville, USA

A volume in the Advances in Data Mining
and Database Management (ADMDM)
Book Series

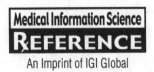

Medical Information Science
REFERENCE
An Imprint of IGI Global

Director of Editorial Content:	Kristin Klinger
Senior Managing Editor:	Jamie Snavely
Assistant Managing Editor:	Michael Brehm
Publishing Assistant:	Sean Woznicki
Typesetter:	Sean Woznicki
Cover Design:	Lisa Tosheff

Published in the United States of America by
Medical Information Science Reference (an imprint of IGI Global)
701 E. Chocolate Avenue
Hershey PA 17033
Tel: 717-533-8845
Fax: 717-533-8661
E-mail: cust@igi-global.com
Web site: http://www.igi-global.com

Library of Congress Cataloging-in-Publication Data

Cerrito, Patricia B.
 Text mining techniques for healthcare provider quality determination : methods for rank comparisons / by Patricia Cerrito.
    p. cm.
 Summary: "This book discusses defining a patient severity index for risk adjustments and comparison of patient outcomes to assess quality factors"--Provided by publisher.
 Includes bibliographical references and index.
 ISBN 978-1-60566-752-2 (hardcover) -- ISBN 978-1-60566-753-9 (ebook) 1. Outcome assessment (Medical care) 2. Data mining. 3. Medical care--Evaluation. I. Title.
 R853.O87C47 2010
 610.28'9--dc22
                                                    2009006954

This book is published in the IGI Global book series Advances in Data Mining and Database Management (ADMDM) (ISSN: 2327-1981; eISSN: 2327-199X)

British Cataloguing in Publication Data
A Cataloguing in Publication record for this book is available from the British Library.

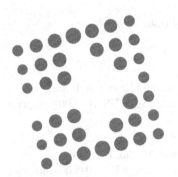

Advances in Data Mining and Database Management (ADMDM) Book Series

David Taniar
Monash University, Australia

ISSN: 2327-1981
EISSN: 2327-199X

MISSION

With the large amounts of information available to businesses in today's digital world, there is a need for methods and research on managing and analyzing the information that is collected and stored. IT professionals, software engineers, and business administrators, along with many other researchers and academics, have made the fields of data mining and database management into ones of increasing importance as the digital world expands. The **Advances in Data Mining & Database Management (ADMDM) Book Series** aims to bring together research in both fields in order to become a resource for those involved in either field.

COVERAGE

- Cluster Analysis
- Customer Analytics
- Data Mining
- Data Quality
- Data Warehousing
- Database Security
- Database Testing
- Decision Support Systems
- Enterprise Systems
- Text Mining

IGI Global is currently accepting manuscripts for publication within this series. To submit a proposal for a volume in this series, please contact our Acquisition Editors at Acquisitions@igi-global.com or visit: http://www.igi-global.com/publish/.

Titles in this Series

For a list of additional titles in this series, please visit: www.igi-global.com

Data Mining in Dynamic Social Networks and Fuzzy Systems
Vishal Bhatnagar (Ambedkar Institute of Advanced Communication Technologies and Research, India)
Information Science Reference • copyright 2013 • 412pp • H/C (ISBN: 9781466642133) • US $195.00 (our price)

Ethical Data Mining Applications for Socio-Economic Development
Hakikur Rahman (University of Minho, Portugal) and Isabel Ramos (University of Minho, Portugal)
Information Science Reference • copyright 2013 • 359pp • H/C (ISBN: 9781466640788) • US $195.00 (our price)

Design, Performance, and Analysis of Innovative Information Retrieval
Zhongyu (Joan) Lu (University of Huddersfield, UK)
Information Science Reference • copyright 2013 • 508pp • H/C (ISBN: 9781466619753) • US $195.00 (our price)

XML Data Mining Models, Methods, and Applications
Andrea Tagarelli (University of Calabria, Italy)
Information Science Reference • copyright 2012 • 538pp • H/C (ISBN: 9781613503560) • US $195.00 (our price)

Graph Data Management Techniques and Applications
Sherif Sakr (University of New South Wales, Australia) and Eric Pardede (LaTrobe University, Australia)
Information Science Reference • copyright 2012 • 502pp • H/C (ISBN: 9781613500538) • US $195.00 (our price)

Advanced Database Query Systems Techniques, Applications and Technologies
Li Yan (Northeastern University, China) and Zongmin Ma (Northeastern University, China)
Information Science Reference • copyright 2011 • 410pp • H/C (ISBN: 9781609604752) • US $180.00 (our price)

Knowledge Discovery Practices and Emerging Applications of Data Mining Trends and New Domains
A.V. Senthil Kumar (CMS College of Science and Commerce, India)
Information Science Reference • copyright 2011 • 414pp • H/C (ISBN: 9781609600679) • US $180.00 (our price)

Data Mining in Public and Private Sectors Organizational and Government Applications
Antti Syvajarvi (University of Lapland, Finland) and Jari Stenvall (Tampere University, Finland)
Information Science Reference • copyright 2010 • 448pp • H/C (ISBN: 9781605669069) • US $180.00 (our price)

Text Mining Techniques for Healthcare Provider Quality Determination Methods for Rank Comparisons
Patricia Cerrito (University of Louisville, USA)
Medical Information Science Reference • copyright 2010 • 410pp • H/C (ISBN: 9781605667522) • US $245.00 (our price)

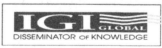

www.igi-global.com

701 E. Chocolate Ave., Hershey, PA 17033
Order online at www.igi-global.com or call 717-533-8845 x100
To place a standing order for titles released in this series, contact: cust@igi-global.com
Mon-Fri 8:00 am - 5:00 pm (est) or fax 24 hours a day 717-533-8661

I dedicate this book to my family, my beloved husband, John, and to my children, Nicholas, Brandon, Christopher, Maria, and Kevin. It is because of them that I embarked on the study of health outcomes.

I also wish to dedicate this book to my students, who became as fascinated with the study of health outcomes and data mining as I have been, and who have always strived to extract meaningful results from the data.

Table of Contents

Preface

The quest for quality in healthcare has led to attempts to develop models to determine which providers have the highest quality in healthcare, with the best outcomes for patients. However, it is not possible to compare providers directly without knowing something about the patients treated. A patient with diabetes, kidney failure, and congestive heart failure is very sick. If such a patient were to also get a serious infection, that patient will have a higher risk of death compared to a patient with a broken leg. Therefore, we must find a way to compare the severity of patients. We need to be able to identify which patients are sicker compared to others; this is difficult to do. Is a patient with congestive heart failure more or less sick compared to patients with liver or lung cancer? Once we can define a patient severity index, we need to use it to rank the quality of care across providers. We also need to be able to define what a high quality of care actually means.

We can examine patients for each separate procedure or reason for hospitalization. For example, we can look at all patients who are admitted for cardiovascular bypass surgery. However, many of these patients also have co-morbidities such as cancer and diabetes. Is it more or less risky to perform bypass surgery on a patient with diabetes, or on a patient with cancer? How does a patient rank with high cholesterol and blood pressure, but no other specific co-morbid problems? What if that patient also has asthma?

In addition, since there are so many different patient problems, it becomes extremely difficult to consider them all. If we only consider some of them, how do we choose which ones to consider and which ones to omit? Suppose we omit some patient conditions that turn out to have a high risk of mortality? Moreover, if we only use some conditions, and some providers (but not others) know which conditions are used to rank quality, do those providers have an advantage compared to those who do not know the model? They can focus on just the conditions in the model instead of having to look at all patient conditions. It becomes easier to show that a provider has more severe patients if that provider knows what conditions to record to define severity.

The purpose of this book is to discuss the general practice of defining a patient severity index. Such an index serves several purposes, amongst them to make risk adjustments to compare patient outcomes across multiple providers with the intent of ranking the providers in terms of quality. Another use is to determine which patients will need more care because of the severity of illness. As a specific example, a severity index can determine which patients are most at risk for infection while in the hospital to determine which patients might benefit from prophylactic treatment. It extends the work of an earlier text, Risk Adjustment, edited by Lisa Iezzoni in 2003 (Chicago, Hospital Administration Press). This book focuses on how severity indices are generally defined. We also examine the consequences of the models, and we investigate the general assumptions required to perform standard severity adjustment. Because the assumptions are rarely satisfied, other methods should be used that can investigate the model assumptions, and that can be used when standard assumptions are not valid. We will also look at how the severity index is used to rank the quality of providers. We examine whether these rankings are valid and reliable.

Chapter 1 gives a general introduction to the patient severity indices, and also a general introduction to the healthcare datasets that will be used throughout the book. We also give a brief introduction to SAS Enterprise Miner®, which is used throughout the book to examine the data. We do assume that the reader is familiar with basic SAS coding. If not, we suggest that you study The Little SAS Book: A Primer, 3rd Edition by Lora D. Delwiche and Susan J. Slaughter or The Little SAS Book for Enterprise Guide 4.1 by the same authors. Both books are available through SAS Press, Inc. The SAS software is the most versatile for investigating the complex data needed to define patient severity indices.

Because of the size of the datasets used to define patient severity, traditional statistical methods are not equipped to analyze the data. Therefore, we will introduce data mining techniques that have been developed in marketing and networking to investigate large databases. Data mining is a general term that is used to represent several steps when working with data. The primary outcome is not to test hypotheses; it is to make decisions that can be used in healthcare to improve care while simultaneously reducing the cost of care. In this book, we will demonstrate why data mining techniques are superior to traditional statistics when using the large datasets typically used to define patient severity indices.

Chapter 2 demonstrates the use of data visualization, especially kernel density estimation. Data visualizations, including the standard graphs, are invaluable when extracting knowledge about the data. We are concerned with the entire population distribution and not just with comparing averages. Because we are usually dealing with heterogeneous populations, we cannot assume that the population is normally distributed. Therefore, we need a technique that can provide an estimate of that distribution, and can model outcomes from such populations.

Chapter 3 discusses several statistical methods that are the primary techniques currently used to investigate health outcomes, including linear and logistic regression. In addition, it examines model assumptions for regression, especially the Central Limit Theorem. In contrast, Chapter 4 discusses the data mining technique of predictive modeling. It demonstrates how predictive modeling encompasses the more standard techniques of linear and logistic regression, but expands options to improve the potential of decision making from the data. Predictive modeling uses many different diagnostic tools to determine the effectiveness of the model.

Chapters 5, 6, and 7 discuss the patient severity indices defined by the Charlson Index, the All Patient Refined DRG, and resource utilization. All three of these indices suffer from a lack of uniformity when information is entered by different providers. For this reason, some providers can take advantage of the methodology to improve their quality rankings without actually improving the quality of care. The Charlson Index is publicly available and can be calculated given patient diagnosis codes. The other two coding methods are proprietary and not as readily available. However, we can examine the results of these severity measures.

Chapter 8 shows a novel method of text mining to define an improved patient severity index; one that can be validated using patient outcomes since it is defined independently from the outcomes. Moreover, it is not susceptible to the "gaming" that results from the variability in the terms of the coding mechanisms. Providers cannot take advantage of this variability to improve their standing. We can discover who is shifting patients into a higher severity category.

Chapter 9 demonstrates how to use patient claims data to define a severity index. It is more complicated to use since different providers use different coding methods. Hospitals generally use ICD9 codes; physicians use CPT or HCPCS codes. These coding methods are not equivalent. In particular, HCPCS codes can document more detail compared to ICD9 codes.

Chapter 10 examines the recent development of using reimbursements to reward providers who rank high using quality measures that in turn depend upon patient severity indices. We examine the data to determine whether those providers who game the system can be identified through an analysis of billing data. We also investigate the ability of these indices to determine whether infections are nosocomial (meaning hospital acquired), or community acquired. Providers are changing policy and will no longer reimburse providers for nosocomial infection.

Both Chapters 8 and 10 discuss in detail the issue of nosocomial infection. Currently, most risk adjustment methods focus upon patient mortality only without considering complications, errors, and infections. However, infection is also a major concern; patients want to know that a hospital stay will not make them sick. There is a problem of under-reporting nosocomial infection, so there needs to be a way to identify which infection is nosocomial versus community acquired. We also want to be able to anticipate problems, especially since providers will now be required to pay for the treatment of such infections. The ability to prevent infections by giving those at high prophylactic treatment is important, and can be examined using the same billing information now used to define patient severity indices.

Throughout this book, we will rely on public data readily available. In particular, the Medical Expenditure Panel Survey collects data on all household and individual usage of healthcare, including physician visits, inpatient and outpatient care, and medications. Costs, and the payer(s) of these costs are also available in the data. The National Inpatient Sample requires a small fee, but is also readily available for analysis purposes. Both datasets are representative of the data collected by clinics and hospitals during the routine of treating patients.

Another type of data that is readily available, although proprietary, is claims data. It is more complicated than the data in the nationally collected databases. In particular, different types of providers use different coding methods to list patient diagnosis information. Hospitals use ICD9 codes; physicians tend to use CPT or HCPCS codes. Inpatients receive bills from the hospital, and from each physician who provides any type of treatment while the patient is in the hospital, even if that treatment is just to examine the patient record. The different claims, providers, and codes need to be combined in some way to define an episode of care so that different episodes can be sequenced, and the different outcomes of care can be considered.

In fact, the number one issue in any definition of a patient severity index is to determine the best way to handle all of the codes that are used to represent patient conditions, and patient treatments. There are thousands of possible codes. There is no good way to include all of them in a statistical model. For this reason, some method of compression must be used; the most common compression method is to limit the number of codes used in the model, either to the codes that are the most frequent, or the ones that are the most crucial. The Charson Index, discussed in Chapter 5, is a good representative of this type of compression.

A second method is to examine each and every diagnosis code and related co-morbidities, and to assign a level of severity to each combination of conditions. This can be very difficult to do. The APRDRG index defined in Chapter 6 utilizes this method. Panels of physicians are used to arrive at a consensus as to the level of a patient's condition based upon co-morbidities to the primary diagnosis. Another method is to use patient outcomes to assign a level of severity as opposed to using the patient diagnoses, under the assumption that a more severe patient will use more treatment resources and have a higher risk of mortality. This approach is used in the disease staging measures discussed in Chapter 7.

It is important that patient severity indices convey accurate information. Unfortunately, there is no "gold standard" that allows us to compare models of patient severity to a standardized outcome. Therefore, any severity index must be considered carefully, and the statistical methodology used to develop the index must be adequate. The results should be validated in some way in the absence of a gold standard. All of these issues will be developed in this text. However, we will discuss in more detail the issue of validating the model in Chapter 11.

In addition, we will examine the ranking of quality providers while adjusting for the severity of a patient's condition. Moreover, we will demonstrate additional uses for the process of defining severity indices. It is important to investigate thoroughly just how well patient severity indices accurately identify a patient's true severity and how accurate the resulting ranking of provider quality actually is. It is particularly important to ensure that the indices are truly meaningful and that the amount of gaming is limited so that those who provide high quality care are identified as providing high quality.

Chapter 1
Introduction to Ranking Models

INTRODUCTION

In this text, we will discuss how patient risk adjustment models are defined, their shortcomings, and their benefits. We will also provide some innovative methods to improve on the currently used risk adjustment methods. Risk adjustment is necessary to examine the differences between healthcare providers. Suppose, for example, that hospital A has a higher mortality rate compared to hospital B. Without looking at whether or not hospital A treats sicker patients at higher risk for mortality compared to hospital B, it is impossible to determine whether hospital A has better or worse outcomes compared to hospital B for treating any one patient. According to the Society of Thoracic Surgeons, risk adjustment is a way of "leveling the playing field" to adjust for differences in risk among specific patients. Risk adjustment makes it possible to compare different healthcare providers in terms of quality.

However, because patients are so different from each other, it is very difficult to define the "typical" patient. How does a patient with severe heart disease compare to a patient with kidney failure? Do they have similar risk, or does the heart patient have a higher risk than the kidney patient? Without finding some way to determine "comparable risk", there are just too many combinations of patient co-morbidities to compare two providers on a nearly identical patient.

DOI: 10.4018/978-1-60566-752-2.ch001

Because there are so many possible patient conditions, the results of risk adjustment are more likely to reflect the definition of the model rather than to reflect actual comparisons of patient severity. No matter what patient conditions are included in the model, there are many more excluded that could be just as crucial when considering patient risk. Moreover, the few that are included will cover only a small percentage of patients.

In addition, risk adjustment models only consider patient condition and not patient compliance with treatment.(Rosen, Reid, Broemeling, & Rakovski, 2003) This paper suggests that health status is dependent upon health behaviors and psychosocial factors as well as the social environment and socioeconomic status of the patients themselves. Therefore, a physician with more lower-income and minority patients will have health outcomes that are not as strong as a physician with mostly affluent patients. However, that brings up another issue. Just how should health behaviors be identified and ranked? In other words, risk is an extremely complex issue that has multiple dimensions, and all dimensions contribute to risk. Without looking at all of these factors and dimensions, risk adjustment models will continue to be questionable.

Moreover, any model that defines risk should be subject to strict scrutiny to determine its validity. Otherwise, it is possible to decide that heart patients are sicker than cancer patients, and both are sicker than dialysis patients. The degree of "sickness" is usually defined in a model by assigning weights to each condition. The greater the weight, the greater the sickness. However, this proposed model of heart, career, and dialysis patients uses three conditions only. Would it be a better model to include pneumonia and asthma? At some point, every model includes some conditions but excludes others. It is possible that excluded conditions can be more severe than included conditions.

In this text, we will discuss some common methods for defining patient severity and compare results using different models. In addition, we will propose a technique that uses all patient diagnoses and procedures to define a patient index. Since there are many different methods of risk adjustment, the different methods can give very different results.(L. Iezzoni, Shwartz, Ash, & Mackieman, 1994) However, if the results can be so different, how can any risk adjustment model be validated? Indeed, can it be validated when the results can be so different?

It is not enough to simply use a statistical measure to claim validation because of a number of problems, including over-fitting by including too many diagnoses. Another problem is caused by using too few diagnoses; unfortunately, both problems commonly occur.(Singh et al., 2003) A previously published edited text on risk adjustment discusses at length several indices with different choices of patient diagnoses. The chapter written by Lisa Iezzoni states that patients with comorbidities have higher risks of death and complications as is logical, usually have higher rates of functional disability, and often require additional diagnostic testing and treatment interventions. (Iezzoni, 2003) However, the text goes on to say that using comprehensive criteria to specify diagnoses is not reasonable, and that it is not possible to identify specific diagnoses usually because of a lack of knowledge or information. The number one issue for any model of patient severity is how to handle all possible combinations of diagnoses.

Using publicly available data and coded information about patient conditions, quality can be defined in many ways. However, it is primarily defined as the difference between predicted and actual mortality, although the ratio of predicted and actual mortality can also be used. (Ash et al., 2003) Other information might be given as well and used to modify the ranking. For example, the Texas Hospital Checkup makes available the following information: (Anonymous-TGBH, 2008; Arca, Fusco, Barone, & Perucci, 2006)

- Actual vs. expected mortality
- Number of procedures done a year
- Average length of stay
- Average total charges
- Average charge per day

Since providers are ranked by the difference between actual and predicted mortality, then, if a provider has zero actual mortality, and zero predicted mortality, then the difference is zero. For this reason, a provider with zero mortality can actually rank lower in quality compared to providers that have high levels of actual mortality. We will demonstrate this seeming contradiction in subsequent chapters.

However, if the magnitude of difference between actual and expected mortality is the measure of quality, it is clear that providers can improve their quality ranking either by decreasing the actual mortality, or by increasing the expected mortality. Increasing the expected mortality is easier, using what is known as "upcoding". (Yuill, 2008) That means that the provider can add diagnosis codes to describe the patient condition that increases the level of identifiable risk. Although considered fraud, upcoding remains widely practiced.(Lorence & Spink, 2004)

Accuracy in identifying risk is more important than ever since these risk adjustment models are used to set health insurance premiums, and Medicare hospital payment rates as well as to measure provider performance. (O'Leary, Keeler, Damberg, & Kerr, 1998). Because of the relationship of quality ranking to reimbursements, there is substantial pressure to upcode patient conditions.

We also need to determine whether to focus on errors, or upon optimal care. We need to decide whether to focus on inputs, meaning adherence to treatment guidelines, or upon outcomes. Because outcomes are often difficult to examine, many measures tend to focus only upon inputs. Did the patient receive necessary tests and medications given the defined diagnosis, or did the provider minimize conditions that result in a spread of infection? However, ultimately, patient outcomes are more important than inputs, and we should concentrate upon outcomes. A focus on inputs assumes that the correct inputs will result in the best outcomes. Not every decision or procedure is subject to guidelines; therefore, outcomes depend on more than just an adherence to known guidelines.

BACKGROUND IN CODED INFORMATION

The datasets used to define patient severity indices rely upon patient conditions as identified through coding systems and these codes must be integrated. There are a number of coding systems that are used in administrative data. The first is the DRG, or diagnosis related group. These codes are used by Medicare and other insurance providers to provide reimbursements. Generally, a value is negotiated between the insurer and the provider for a particular DRG. Generally, DRG grouper software uses "the principal diagnosis, secondary diagnoses (as defined using ICD9 codes), surgical procedures, age, sex and discharge status of the patients treated" to assign inpatient records to a specific DRG. (Anonymous-DRG, 2008b). Examples of DRG codes are listed below:(Anonymous-DRG, 2008a)

424 Operating room procedure with principal diagnoses of mental illness
425 Acute adjustment reaction & psychosocial dysfunction
426 Depressive neuroses

427 Neuroses except depressive

428 Disorders of personality & impulse control

429 Organic disturbances & mental retardation

430 Psychoses

431 Childhood mental disorders

432 Other mental disorder diagnoses

433 Alcohol/drug abuse or dependence, left, against medical advice

434 Alcohol/drug abuse or dependence, detoxification or other symptom treatment with complications, comorbidities

435 Alcohol/drug abuse or dependence, detoxification or other symptom treatment without complications, comorbidities

436 Alcohol/drug dependence with rehabilitation therapy

437 Alcohol/drug dependence combined rehabilitation & detoxification therapy

ICD9 codes are developed by the World Health Organization. They represent a very detailed method of classifying patient conditions and procedures. A complete listing is readily available on the internet. (Anonymous-ICD9, 2008) For patient diagnoses, each ICD9 code has a form of xxx.xx, where the first three digits represent the general patient condition and the last two digits give specifics of that diagnosis. The first digit may be a 'v' or an 'e'. The 'v' represents a pre-existing factor that can influence the current health status; the 'e' represents external causes of injury and poisoning. For procedures, the code is of the form of xx.xx. Some providers and organizations have adopted the ICD10 coding system, although ICD9 remains the standard in the United States. It will shortly be abandoned and the US will adopt ICD10 codes.

For example, the ICD9 codes for different conditions of diabetes are

250 Diabetes mellitus

    1 type I [juvenile type], not stated as uncontrolled

    2 type II or unspecified type, uncontrolled

    3 type I [juvenile type], uncontrolled

250.0 Diabetes mellitus without mention of complication

250.1 Diabetes with ketoacidosis

250.2 Diabetes with hyperosmolarity

250.3 Diabetes with other coma

250.4 Diabetes with renal manifestations

250.5 Diabetes with ophthalmic manifestations

250.6 Diabetes with neurological manifestations

250.7 Diabetes with peripheral circulatory disorders

250.8 Diabetes with other specified manifestations

250.9 Diabetes with unspecified complication

Similarly, the procedure codes for surgery on the joints are

81 Repair and plastic operations on joint structures

    81.0 Spinal fusion

81.1 Arthrodesis and arthroereisis of foot and ankle
81.2 arthrodesis of other joint
81.3 Refusion of spine
81.4 Other repair of joint of lower extremity
81.5 Joint replacement of lower extremity
81.6 Other procedures on spine
81.7 Arthroplasty and repair of hand, fingers, and wrist
81.8 Arthroplasty and repair of shoulder and elbow
81.9 Other operations on joint structures

Each one of the above codes can be further refined by the remaining digit. For example, 81.5 has the following refinements:

81.51 Total hip replacement
81.52 Partial hip replacement
81.53 Revision of hip replacement, not otherwise specified
81.54 Total knee replacement
81.55 Revision of knee replacement,not otherwise specified
81.56 Total ankle replacement
81.57 Replacement of joint of foot and toe
81.59 Revision of joint replacement of lower extremity, not elsewhere classified

CPT codes were developed by the American Medical Association for procedures.(Smith, 2008) These codes are 5 digits and numeric in format. They have considerable detail in the coding system, more so than that available using ICD9 codes. Some examples are given in Table 1.

HCPCS codes include all CPT codes, which are 5 digit numbers. In addition, other HCPCS codes are available to describe more precise procedures. They have an added alphabetic code.

There are many thousands of these codes, and we must organize them in some manner in order to be able to use them for defining a risk adjustment measure. For the most part, the risk adjustment measures choose a group of procedures and/or diagnoses, and base their results on the mortality (or complications) score. For example, healthgrades.com uses the codes shown in Table 2 (Anonymous-healthgrades, 2008).

ICD9 codes (or CPT equivalents) are used to identify the specific diagnoses/procedures on the list. Once identified, they are given weights, with more severe conditions given higher weights.

The ability of a model to predict patient outcomes will depend almost entirely on how well it can handle all of the patient diagnosis and procedure codes. While risk adjustment can be performed for each and every procedure, there are still thousands of possible patient diagnoses and co-morbidities that must be considered. In this text, we will demonstrate a technique that can be used to accommodate all potential diagnoses in a risk adjustment model.

The Department of Health and Human Services (HHS) just announced a timeline to transition from ICD9 codes to ICD10 codes, which will require transitioning the severity index formulas. Implementation is to take place as of October 1, 2011. Another proposal will require the adoption of a standard (X12 standard, Version 5010) for all electronic transactions, including healthcare claims. HHS claims that adoption of ICD10 codes absolutely requires the adoption of this X12 standard. The present ICD9 coding

Table 1.

73218	Magnetic resonance (eg, proton) imaging, upper extremity, other than joint; without contrast material(s)
73219	Magnetic resonance (eg, proton) imaging, upper extremity, other than joint; with contrast material(s)
73220	Magnetic resonance (eg, proton) imaging, upper extremity, other than joint; without contrast material(s), followed by contrast material(s) and further sequences
73221	Magnetic resonance (eg, proton) imaging, any joint of upper extremity; without contrast material(s)
73222	Magnetic resonance (eg, proton) imaging, any joint of upper extremity; with contrast material(s)
73223	Magnetic resonance (eg, proton) imaging, any joint of upper extremity; without contrast material(s), followed by contrast material(s) and further sequences
73225	Magnetic resonance angiography, upper extremity, with or without contrast material(s)

system contains 17,000 codes, and all possible code combinations will be exhausted by early 2009. In contrast, the ICD10 coding system will allow up to 155,000 new code combinations. The United States is virtually the last industrialized country to adopt the ICD10 standard. With the adoption of this new coding system, methods to compress codes into a meaningful index will become even more important. (Anonymous-ICD10, 2008)

REQUIREMENTS OF DATA PREPROCESSING

We want to discuss some of the more recent studies concerning the use of claims data to examine treatment and outcomes for cancer. Claims data are difficult to work with and require considerable prepro-

Table 2.

Appendectomy	Heart failure
Atrial fibrillation	Hip fracture repair
Back and neck surgery (except spinal fusion)	Pancreatitis
Back and neck surgery (spinal fusion)	Peripheral vascular bypass
Bariatric surgery	Pneumonia
Bowell obstruction	Prostatectomy
Carotid surgery	Resection/replacement of abdominal aorta
Cholecystectomy	Respiratory failure
Chronic obstructive pulmonary disease	Sepsis
Coronary bypass surgery	Stroke
Diabetic acidosis and coma	Total hip replacement
Gastrointestinal bleed	Total knee replacement
Gastrointestinal surgeries and procedures	Valve replacement surgery
Heart attack	

cessing before they are ready to use. It is a necessary component of research using administrative data; yet few studies discuss the process in detail. For this reason, the preprocessing methodology cannot be validated. Since the conclusions in the study depend upon the validity of the preprocessing, without some knowledge of the preprocessing performed, the conclusions must always remain in doubt. We consider a paper by Loughlin, et. al. in detail.(Loughlin et al., 2002) In this study, patients with an ICD9 diagnosis code contained within the interval 140 through 208 were extracted for a 210-day period, and then only included patients with a prescription for transdermal fentanyl in the period. However, there were no details provided as to how this extraction was performed. Moreover, the study goes on to define a propensity score by first identifying factors that were statistically significant with respect to transdermal fentanyl use. While stating that patient diagnoses were significant, the paper did not discuss how the number of diagnoses that exist in the patient dataset was reduced to three. Once the sub-population of patients was identified, the extracted factors were used to examine costs. However, without knowing if the sub-population was correctly identified, it is not possible to conclude that the results are correct. Similar problems exist in other studies.(Dobie et al., 2008; Epstein, Knight, Epstein, Bride, & Nichol, 2007; Hoy et al., 2007)

A study by Carsos, Zhu, and Zavras used ICD9 codes to define the study population, and also the treatment outcomes. (Cartsos, Zhu, & Zavras, 2008) It stratified the sample by using the outcomes, identifying a control population as not having these outcomes. Stratifying outcomes virtually guarantees that the model results will be statistically significant. However, the biggest problem with this analysis is that the outcome is a rare occurrence, and there is no indication in the paper that the statistical model was modified to account for the rare occurrence. Unfortunately, ignoring needed modifications to examine rare occurrences is a fairly common practice in retrospective studies. (Gross, Galusha, & Krumholz, 2007; West, Behrens, McDonnell, Tielsch, & Schem, 2005) As a result, the model will inflate the results, and the results will all be statistically significant while of no real practical importance. A study concerning the relationship between patient outcome and hospital volume did not clearly define how volume was computed from the data.(Xirasagar, Lien, Lee, Liu, & TC Tsai, 2008) Moreover, it is very possible that hospitals with higher volume also have higher risk patients, suggesting that results must be modified based upon patient severity.(Gilligan et al., 2007)

Wynn, Chang, and Peipins provided more details about the CPT and ICD9 codes used to extract the patient population. (Wynn, Chang, & Peipins, 2007) It matched a cohort of women with ovarian cancer to a control cohort matched on age, geographic region, Medicare eligibility, and health plan type. It did not match on co-morbidities; instead, it examined the difference between the two cohorts only on the co-morbidities related to women's health. It did examine some other co-morbid conditions such as diabetes, but excluded others such as previous myocardial infarction. Moreover, it used a 3:1 ratio of treatment to control group without explaining why 3:1 is optimal as opposed to say, a 1:1 or a 10:1 match.

Claims data can also be used to examine health disparities and access to services, especially when matched to census data.(Halliday, Taira, Davis, & Chan, 2007) Such studies are particularly relevant to the study of cancer screening, and compliance with that screening. (Mariotto, Etzioni, Krapcho, & Feuer, 2007) These studies can become time-oriented, looking at the time to screening, or the time between screening and treatment. In this case, it is possible to introduce the methodology of survival data mining with multiple time events. We can also have multiple time events when examining the data for the occurrence of adverse events after surgery. (Baxter et al., 2007)

Another part of the decision is to determine both the inputs and outcomes under study. Many studies focus on adherence to guidelines without going to the next step of investigating outcomes with respect to that adherence (or the lack thereof).(Hoy et al., 2007) However, by examining the time between physician visits, or the time between prescription refills, we can get an idea of patient compliance.(Darkow et al., 2007) We can also use the further access of services to determine whether adverse effects have occurred.(Hartung et al., 2007)

Once a claims database has been investigated, it should be validated through the use of an additional data source. This can be self-reports, or it can be the use of a secondary database.(Setoguchi et al., 2007; Wolinsky et al., 2007) If the same database is used, but say for the next year, results will tend to be very similar. This will show that the model is reliable, meaning that results will continue to be similar. This does not, however, demonstrate validity.

There are only a handful of papers that discuss data preprocessing. Gold and Do examine three algorithms to extract patient sub-groups from claims databases. (Gold & Do, 2007) However, the paper does not discuss the algorithms themselves. Therefore, we go to the original papers that were referenced by Gold and Do. Freeman, et. al. developed a logistic regression of diagnosis codes to predict the occurrence of a breast cancer case in the Medicare-SEER database.(Freeman, Zhang, Daniel H Freeman, & Goodwin, 2000) The included codes were 174xx, 2330, v103, 8541-8549, 8521-8523, 403, 8511-8512, 8735-8737, 8873, 8885, 9221-9229, 9985, 9925. Corresponding CPT and HCPCS codes were also used. The study showed that there was a 99.86% specificity rate but a sensitivity of 90%. There were a total of 62 false positives, although it suggests that half of the false positives were in fact for recurrent breast cancer that was previously diagnosed and treated outside of the SEER database. These 62 cases represent just under 2% of the whole, which will not significantly impact the study of patient outcomes. However, while giving the algorithm, the paper does not provide the actual SAS coding used to extract the data.

Nattinger, et. al. developed a different algorithm, using ICD9 codes 174-174.9, 233.0, v10.3, 238.3, 239.3, 198.2, 198.81, 140-173.9, 175-195.8, 197-199.1 excluding 198.2, 198.81, 200-208.91, 230-234.9, excluding 233.0 and 232.5, 235-239.9, excluding 238.3, 239.3, 85.1-85.19, 85.20-85.21, 85.22-85.23, 40.3, 85.33-85.48, and 92.2-92.29. This list is somewhat more expansive than the list of Freeman, et.al. Yet the study reports lower sensitivity and specificity compared to Freeman's study. Again, the actual coding is not provided with the study.(Nattinger, Laud, & Rut Bajorunaite, 2004) Therefore, these studies provide little to serve as a template to extract patient sub-groups from the datasets. Because they were also created to extract breast cancer patients, these algorithms also cannot be generalized to other cancer types. Welch, et. al. provide a flow chart to indicate how the patients were identified, again with no coding.(Welch, Fisher, Gottlieb, & Barry, 2007) Norton, et.al. indicated that all diagnoses that occurred in 0.5% of the population or more were considered.(Garfinkel et al., 1998) However, their objective was to determine whether the diagnoses were complications of a surgical procedure, or not. The purpose was to investigate the proportion of complications by hospital to determine the quality of care.

Because so little information is given concerning data preprocessing, we are generally left to assume that it has been done correctly, and that someone qualified in data preprocessing performed the required operations and wrote the correct program code.(West et al., 2005) We will provide SAS code throughout this text when preprocessing is needed. The code can be used as a basic template that you can adapt to your own data.

PATIENT RISK MEASURES

Because some patients are at higher risk compared to others, differences in patients can mask differences across healthcare providers. In many cases, higher volume is correlated with better outcomes. However, higher volume can also mean a higher proportion of higher risk patients. If this is the case, then comparing just volume to outcome may not end up statistically significant. (Enzinger et al., 2007) Sometimes, the attempt at risk adjustment is fairly simple, defined by just using a count of co-morbid conditions.(Shugarman, Bird, Schuster, & Lynn, 2007) However, it is not usually given just how the co-morbid conditions were decided upon. Other choices for co-morbid conditions will result in different risk adjustment values.(Cerrito, 2006) Still other studies just give a very vague idea of how patient co-morbidities are accounted for in the study without providing specific codes that are used to define them.(Fang et al., 2006) Occasionally, the paper will give a reference to a defined severity index without going into much detail.(Donald H Taylor & Hoenig, 2006; Ellis et al., 1996)

In a study by Schlenker, et. al., a list of 37 different risk factors was defined; most by using a 0-1 indicator function, but others on a scale of 0-5, including urinary incontinence severity and disability in ambulation.(Schlenker, Powell, & Goodrich, 2005) Treatments such as the use of oxygen and the presence of a urinary catheter are also included. This list is derived from the OASIS, or Outcome and Assessment Information Set that is routinely collected by home health agencies. The measures, as defined through a consensus of experts, include the following: (Anonymous-OASIS, 2007)

- Three measures related to improvement in getting around:
  - Percentage of patients who get better at walking or moving around
  - Percentage of patients who get better at getting in and out of bed
  - Percentage of patients who have less pain when moving around
- Four measures related to meeting the patient's activities of daily living:
  - Percentage of patients whose bladder control improves
  - Percentage of patients who get better at bathing
  - Percentage of patients who get better at taking their medicines correctly (by mouth)
  - Percentage of patients who are short of breath less often
- Two measures about how home health care ends:
  - Percentage of patients who stay at home after an episode of home health care ends
  - Percentage of patients whose wounds improved or healed after an operation
- Three measures related to patient medical emergencies:
  - Percentage of patients who had to be admitted to the hospital
  - Percentage of patients who need urgent, unplanned medical care
  - Percentage of patients who need unplanned medical care related to a wound that is new, is worse, or has become infected

Unfortunately, it is difficult to determine the magnitude of "better" without more specifics.

Daley, Iezzoni, & Shwartz (2003) suggests that we can use the following strategies to find potential risk factors to include in a patient severity model:

- Published reports from randomized trials and clinical studies
- Ask clinical experts or panels of practicing clinicians

Both methods are limited because panels may reach consensus without examining the validity of the choices. If one provider has very severe patients with comorbidities that are not included in the list, these patients will appear to have a very low severity level.

In an interesting study concerning the use of high deductible/medical savings plans, Humana used the utilization of healthcare services as identified through claims data to segment its employees into risk clusters to compare the introduction of a new type of insurance. It was found that those who utilized services less often were more likely to switch to the new plan.(Tollen, Ross, & Poor, 2004) Another study used the incidence of a ruptured appendix in children as a marker for the quality of care. However, there was no discussion of how to validate the use of just one diagnosis factor to rank the provider quality. (Gadomski & Jenkins, 2001)

Given patients with similar conditions, we should be able to rank the quality of hospitals and other medical providers by the outcomes of their patients. However, there is considerable variability in patient conditions, so much so that it is rare to have similar patients at different hospitals. Numerous attempts have been made to develop a method to equate patients at specific levels of risk so that outcomes can be compared. In many cases, these measures are used to define those providers of highest quality, and to rank the providers in order of quality. They are also used to compare different providers directly to see if one is better than another.(Reilly, Chin, Berkowitz, Weedon, & Avitable, 2003)

Other measures of patient severity are used to determine those patients at highest risk, and those who will be the most costly to treat, so that reimbursements to hospitals and providers can be adjusted by risk levels. (Macario, Vitez, Dunn, McDonald, & Brown, 1997) However, different measures of patient severity can lead to different rankings of provider quality, making these rankings of questionable validity. We should expect that rankings are invariant of the measure used to define the rankings. In the absence of such consistency, the validity of ranking may be restricted to the top and bottom of the ranking list. (Daley, Ash, & Iezzoni, 2003) In the absence of such consistency, we need to understand the limitations of defining risk-adjusted quality, and to be careful when assigning reimbursements based on the outcomes of these models.

Still other measures were developed to predict patient outcomes, and to develop standard measures for specific patient populations.(Monami et al., 2007) This seems to be reasonable for some procedures, but not for others. Can we define one risk adjustment method that works for heart patients and elderly patients with dementia, but also for labor and delivery patients? Should risk be age, race, and gender specific? This is probably not reasonable, which is why a risk adjustment model is defined for a specific patient procedure.

Some measures are defined as composites of other measures to see if the multiple measures predict better than just using one measure.(Azarisman et al., 2007; Inouye et al., 1998; O'Connell & Lim, 2000) Similarly, different risk adjustment measures are compared directly.(Rochon et al., 1996)

Generally, a set of patient diagnoses is assembled, and a different weight is assigned to each of the diagnoses. Then, a linear combination of weights is defined for each patient, with the combination consisting of only those defined diagnoses that apply to that patient. The question to ask is how the set of diagnoses is defined. Different sets will result in different risk adjustments; often, the different methods will contradict each other. In some cases, a patient defined as having low risk in one measure can be defined as having high risk in another measure.(L. I. Iezzoni et al., 1995) Assigning weights presents another problem. Should diabetes have higher or lower weight compared to kidney disease? If each diagnosis is given the same weight, then the risk adjustment method is essentially a count of the number of diagnoses for each patient; again, the number is based upon a defined set of diagnoses.

Once a method of risk adjustment is defined, a logistic regression is used to see if patient mortality outcomes can be predicted.(Cher & Lenert, 1997) Linear regression is used to predict patient costs, and also length of stay. (Shwartz & Ash, 2003) That is the reason that only a small number of patient diagnoses can be used to define the score; logistic regression cannot use all of the thousands of codes that are assigned to patients. However, while p-values are statistically significant, the correlation coefficient, or r^2 value, tends to be low in a linear regression, suggesting that most of the variability in the outcome is not predicted by the severity of patient condition. (Rochon et al., 1996) Logistic regression will have a high accuracy level, reflecting only the fact that mortality is a rare occurrence. This rare occurrence is almost never taken into consideration when developing the model, when some model adjustments are required.

One of the more public risk adjustment measures is available at healthgrades.com. There, you can find rankings of hospitals all over the United States. For a fee, you can also get a report on any physician. The developers at healthgrades.com discuss their methodology at www.healthgrades.com/media/DMS/pdf/HospitalQualityGuideMethodology20072008.pdf so that we can examine in detail some of the problems as well as the benefits of using this methodology. As discuss in their methodology, they do use a logistic regression, and the document provides the patient diagnoses used to examine patient outcomes. In some cases, healthgrades.com examines specific procedures such as cardiac bypass, and then creates a risk adjustment for the remaining general patient population. For most of their ratings, their measures examine mortality. If the procedure has virtually no mortality, then it ranks based upon the occurrence of complications.

Another consideration in defining provider quality is the proportion of medical errors and complications resulting from an inpatient stay. If a hospital has a high rate of nosocomial infection, then it should probably not rank as high in terms of quality with a hospital with a much lower rate of nosocomial infection. Therefore, in addition to risk adjusted severity models, additional measures should also be computed and compared by provider.

DATASETS USED

Throughout this text, we will be relying on two different databases. The first is the Medical Expenditure Panel Survey (MEPS). The second is the National Inpatient Sample (NIS). The MEPS is available through a download from http://www.meps.ahrq.gov/mepsweb/data_stats/download_data_files.jsp. It is very complete data for a cohort of patients. It is also available for ten years and contains information on inpatient and outpatient treatment as well as physician visits, medications, and detailed patient demographics. The NIS is available for a small fee from http://www.hcup-us.ahrq.gov/nisoverview.jsp. It contains all inpatient visits from a stratified sample of hospitals from a total of 37 different states. In addition, we will discuss some proprietary data as needed. In particular, we will discuss how Claims data can be used to determine patient severity. The two databases that are publicly available represent the different types of information that can be found in claims data, or in the electronic medical record.

MEPS Data

In the case of MEPS data, the datasets are available in SAS format, or in SPSS format. SAS and SPSS coding are provided to translate the datasets into usable files. In addition, data dictionaries are readily available to enable you to understand the data. MEPS currently has two major components for which data are released: the Household Component and the Insurance Component. The Household Component data are based on questionnaires to individual household members and their medical providers; the Insurance Component estimates come from a survey of employers conducted to collect health insurance plan information. These MEPS datasets have detailed cost information concerning all facets of healthcare utilization, including physician visits, inpatient and outpatient care, medications, laboratory usage, eye and dental care, and so on. The data for 2006 are available in December, 2008, with each subsequent year added by December of each year. The data are available from the year 1996. Table 3 gives a list of datasets available for the year 2005.

In the prescribed medicines file, there are a number of variables related to cost (Table 4). The RX in the name relates to prescriptions. For the inpatient costs, 'RX' is replaced by 'OP', and by 'IP' for inpatient costs. The '01' represents the year 2001; '05' is used for the 2005 data.

With such detailed cost information, we can examine the relationship between patient condition and costs. Care must be taken when examining these datafiles, especially when merging cost information from the different datasets.(Cerrito, 2008a)

NIS DATA

NIS data come only in ascii format, and the SAS coding needed to translate the datasets into standard SAS format is available on the NIS web site. There is exactly one observation per patient, with no longitudinal linkage between observations. There are two methods of coding patient conditions in the

Table 3. MEPS datasets for 2005

Dataset Name	Description
HC-097	Full year consolidated file
HC-096	Medical conditions file
HC-095	Person round plan public use file
HC-094I	Appendix to MEPS 2005 event files
HC-094H	Home health file
HC-094G	Office-based medical provider visits file
HC-094F	Outpatient visits file
HC-094E	Emergency room visits file
HC-094D	Hospital inpatient stays file
HC-094C	Other medical expenses
HC-094B	Dental visits
HC-094A	Prescribed medicines file
HC-091	Jobs file
HC-090	Full year population characteristics
HC-084	Population characteristics
HC-036BRR	Replicates for calculating variances
HC-036	MEPS 1996-2005 pooled estimation linkage file

dataset, ICD9 and CCS codes. We will discuss the use of the ICD9 codes with an available translation at http://icd9cm.chrisendres.com or at http://www.icd9coding1.com/flashcode/home.jsp. There are three outcomes available for each patient observation: mortality in the hospital, total charges, and length of stay. There is information concerning patient age, race, and gender. There are fifteen columns to record diagnosis codes and another fifteen columns to record procedure codes. There are thousands of possible diagnoses. One of the problems with defining a risk adjustment model is to work with these codes to define a risk score. They must be compressed in some manner, either by restricting attention to a small subset of the diagnosis codes, or by other methods. One novel method using text analysis will be discussed in Chapter 8.

In particular, NIS data contain patient severity indices defined using the APRDRG, a proprietary code available through a software purchase. It contains other severity indices as well that are also proprietary. Although proprietary, the index values are publicly available in the NIS datasets. Its date information is more complete compared to the MEPS. Some of the variables we will work with in the NIS data include patient demographics:

- Age (in years)
- Female (0=male, 1=female)
- Race(1=White, 2=Black, 3=Hispanic, 4=Asian/Pacific Islander, 5=Native American, 6=Other)
- DRG
- Patient diagnoses in ICD9 codes (DX1-DX15, fifteen columns)
- Patient procedures in ICD9 codes (PR1-PR15, fifteen columns)
- TOTCHG (Total Charges)
- LOS (Length of Stay)

In order to work with these variables, there are some preprocessing issues, especially to work with 15 columns of diagnoses and procedure codes. We will discuss these requirements briefly. For more details we refer you to *The Little SAS Book,* available from SAS Press or to Cerrito (Cerrito, 2008b). The severity measures available in the NIS are listed in Table 5.

Table 4. Cost variable definitions for the year 2001

Variable Name	Variable Definition
RXSF01X	Self-pay
RXMR01X	Medicare
RXMD01X	Medicaid
RXPV01X	Private insurance
RXTR01X	TRICARE
RXOF01X	Other federal sources
RXSL01X	State and local government sources
RXWC01X	Worker's compensation
RXOT01X	Other private source of insurance
RXOU01X	Other public source of insurance
RXXP01X	Sum of payments for each prescribed medication

Table 5. Severity index measures

Data Element	Variable Name	Description
AHRQ Comorbidity	CM_AIDS	Acquired immune deficiency syndrome
AHRQ Comorbidity	CM_ALCOHOL	Alcohol abuse
AHRQ Comorbidity	CM_ANEMDEF	Deficiency anemias
AHRQ Comorbidity	CM_ARTH	Rheumatoid arthritis/collagen vascular diseases
AHRQ Comorbidity	CM_BLDLOSS	Chronic blood loss anemia
AHRQ Comorbidity	CM_CHF	Congestive heart failure
AHRQ Comorbidity	CM_CHRNLUNG	Chronic pulmonary disease
AHRQ Comorbidity	CM_COAG	Coagulopathy
AHRQ Comorbidity	CM_DEPRESS	Depression
AHRQ Comorbidity	CM_DM	Diabetes, uncomplicated
AHRQ Comorbidity	CM_DMCX	Diabetes with chronic complications
AHRQ Comorbidity	CM_DRUG	Drug abuse
AHRQ Comorbidity	CM_HTN_C	Hypertension, uncomplicated and complicated
AHRQ Comorbidity	CM_HYPOTHY	Hypothyroidism
AHRQ Comorbidity	CM_LIVER	Liver Disease
AHRQ Comorbidity	CM_LYMPH	Lymphoma
AHRQ Comorbidity	CM_LYTES	Fluid and electrolyte disorders
AHRQ Comorbidity	CM_METS	Metastatic cancer
AHRQ Comorbidity	CM_NEURO	Other neurological disorders
AHRQ Comorbidity	CM_OBESE	Obesity
AHRQ Comorbidity	CM_PARA	Paralysis
AHRQ Comorbidity	CM_PERIVASC	Peripheral vascular disorders
AHRQ Comorbidity	CM_PSYCH	Psychoses
AHRQ Comorbidity	CM_PULMCIRC	Pulmonary circulation disorders
AHRQ Comorbidity	CM_RENLFAIL	Renal failure
AHRQ Comorbidity	CM_TUMOR	Solid tumor without metastasis
AHRQ Comorbidity	CM_ULCER	Peptic ulcer disease excluding bleeding
AHRQ Comorbidity	CM_VALVE	Valvular disease
AHRQ Comorbidity	CM_WGHTLOSS	Weight loss
All Patient Refined DRG (3M)	APRDRG_Risk_Mortality	Risk of mortality subclass
All Patient Refined DRG (3M)	APRDRG_Severity	Severity of illness subclass
All-Payer Severity-adjusted DRG (Hss, Inc.)	APSDRG_Mortality_Weight	Mortality weight
All-Payer Severity-adjusted DRG (Hss, Inc.)	APSDRG_LOS_Weight	Length of stay weight
All-Payer Severity-adjusted DRG (Hss, Inc.)	APSDRG_Charge_Weight	Charge weight
Disease Staging (Medstat)	DS_DX_Category1	Stage of principal disease category
Disease Staging (Medstat)	DS_LOS_Level	Length of stay level
Disease Staging (Medstat)	DS_LOS_Scale	Length of stay scale
Disease Staging (Medstat)	DS_Mrt_Level	Mortality level

Table 5. continued

Data Element	Variable Name	Description
Disease Staging (Medstat)	DS_Mrt_Scale	Mortality scale
Disease Staging (Medstat)	DS_RD_Level	Resource demand level
Disease Staging (Medstat)	DS_RD_Scale	Resource demand scale
Linkage Variables	HOSPID	Hospital identification number
Linkage Variables	KEY	Patient identification number

We will be discussing these data elements in later chapters.

Claims Data

Claims data is usually messier compared to the MEPS and to the NIS data. Unlike these two datasets provided by the government, claims data are drawn from a variety of sources, including hospitals, physician offices, laboratories, radiology centers, and pharmacies. The different sources use different coding systems, with hospitals relying primarily upon ICD9 codes and physician offices using CPT codes. Pharmacies do not generally provide diagnosis information with their medications.

A severity index using claims data must be able to handle the different coding schemes simultaneously. We will demonstrate how this can be done in Chapter 9. In addition, claims related to just one treatment episode, including follow up visits needs to be isolated within the data in order to investigate patient outcomes. Because claims are for specific services, episodes of treatment are not clear in the data.

DATA MINING AND HEALTHCARE DATABASES

Clinical trials have always represented the gold standard in healthcare. However, there are limitations that include cost, time, question, randomization, and sample size. Clinical trials are expensive to conduct; therefore, not every question concerning medical decisions, new drug treatments, and surgical procedures can be answered with clinical trials. Also because of the expense, clinical trials tend to examine short term effects only, often relying upon surrogate rather than actual endpoints, and then making the assumption that the surrogate is exactly related to the actual patient outcomes. Clinical trials also focus on one treatment at a time, usually excluding subjects who are taking combinations of medications. Also because of the expense, clinical trials do not enroll enough subjects to detect rare occurrences of adverse events. Moreover, clinical trials must rely upon volunteers. If the treatment is for a life-threatening illness that cannot be treated with currently available methods, the majority of patients will undoubtedly volunteer. However, in other treatments, there can still be a self-selection bias in the volunteer sample. Therefore, we cannot always be certain that a randomized, controlled clinical trial is unbiased.

When the gold standard is not available, we must rely upon information that we do have for analysis purposes. Clinical and administrative databases that are collected routinely have considerable value in terms of patient treatments and outcomes. However, these data are observational, and observational data can always introduce the possibility of confounding factors. Potential confounders need to be examined in the analysis, increasing the number of variables to be considered. Such studies can examine adverse events, long term follow up and treatment interactions that are not possible with clinical trials.(Tirkkonen et al., 2008)

Another factor that must be considered is that clinical databases tend to very large. They are so large that the standard measure of a model's effectiveness, the p-value, will become statistically significant with an effect size that is nearly zero. Therefore, other measures need to be used to measure a model's effectiveness. In linear regression or the general linear model, it would not be unusual to have a model that is statistically significant but with an r^2 value of 2% or less, suggesting that most of the variability in the outcome variable remains unaccounted for.(Loebstein, Katzir, Vasterman-Landes, Halkin, & Lomnicky, 2008) It is a sure sign that there are too many patient observations when most of the p-values are equal to '<0.00001'.

Large datasets are also required to examine rare occurrences. There need to be a sufficient number of rare occurrences in the database to be comparable. For example, if a condition occurs 0.1% of the time, there would be approximately 1 such occurrence for every 1000 patients and 10 occurrences for 10,000 patients. It would require a minimum of 100,000 patients in the dataset to find 100 occurrences. However, all 100,000 patients cannot be used in a model to predict the occurrences. The problem of rare occurrences will be discussed in more detail in Chapter 3. The model would be nearly 99% accurate, but would predict nearly every patient as a non-occurrence. In the absence of large samples and long-term follow up, surrogate endpoints are still used.(Sabate, 1999)

Another advantage of using data mining techniques on large datasets is that we can investigate outcomes at the patient level rather than at the group level. Typically in regression, we look to patient type to determine those at high risk. Patients above a certain age represent one type. Patients who smoke represent a type. However, with data mining, we can examine a patient of a specific age who smokes 10 cigarettes a week, who drinks one glass of wine on weekends, and who is physically in good shape to predict specific outcomes.

Another measure we can consider is the fact that physicians vary in how they treat similar patients. That variability itself can be used to examine the relationship between physician treatment decisions and patient outcomes. Once we determine which outcome is "best" from the patient's viewpoint, we can determine which treatment decisions are more likely to lead to that decision. This is particularly true for patients with chronic illness where there is a sequence of treatment decisions followed by multiple patient outcomes. For example, a patient with diabetes can start with medication, progressing to insulin injections as the disease itself progresses. Moreover, patients with diabetes can end up with organ failure: heart, kidney, and so on. We can examine treatments that prolong the time to such organ failure.

Another important problem in healthcare that can be examined using data mining has to do with scheduling of personnel given patient needs. To examine solutions, we can use time series methods. We can also examine physician prescribing habits to determine the impact of new drugs, or new procedures and how they change patient care. Time series methods currently are under-utilized in the data analysis of clinical databases.

Because of the value of these large databases, many professional medical societies are developing registries.(Andaluz & Zuccarello, 2008; Hamilton et al., 2008; Wax, Srivastava, Shubikha, & Joashi, 2008) The SEARCH database discussed in Hamilton, et.al.(Hamilton et al., 2008) is quite popular in the medical literature for outcomes research.(Turley et al., 2008) It is, however, propriety to a research study group. It is not clear in Hamilton, et.al. that the statistical methods used to investigate the databases take the large size into consideration. In many cases, it is difficult to tell if the extracted data are meaningful because none of the preprocessing steps are clearly identified. The programming code necessary for the extraction is also not provided. Consider a recent study on heart failure. The total number of subjects was 278,214. The number was reduced to 70,571 subjects for a logistic regression to test the relationship between length of stay and treatment. With such a large sample size, the independent variables will be statistically significant with an effect size of almost zero. Other studies have similar problems with large sample sizes and all independent variables statistically significant. (Delaney, Chang, Senagore, & Broder, 2008)

In a study of length of stay for the treatment of lung cancer, the sample size was 4979, but the treatment under consideration was performed in 351 patients (7%), indicating a rare occurrence.(Wright et al., 2008) The study did not adjust for the rare occurrence, nor did it report on the difference in the false positive versus the false negative rate. Therefore, it is doubtful if the study has any real predictive capabilities. Any model that predicts 100% as non-occurrences will be 93% accurate, so a good prediction model would have to be more accurate than 93%. Another aspect of predictive modeling is that multiple models are used and compared, defining a holdout sample (or minimizing costs) to find the optimal choice. In traditional statistics, one model is chosen and used without any attempt to validate the model choice, or to compare to other models. (Odueyungbo, Browne, Akhtar-Danesh, & Thabane, 2008)

The Society of Thoracic Surgeons has an excellent database repository; however, the statistical methods used need to include predictive modeling rather than to just rely on logistic regression. In particular, a study of atrial fibrillation from this dataset used dozens of variables. (Gammie et al., 2008) Predictive modeling techniques are available to reduce the number of variables and to avoid the hazard of over-fitting the model. However, these techniques are not commonly employed in medical research studies. One such study started with 708,593 patients but did not define a holdout sample to validate the results, nor did it compensate for the rare occurrence.(Mehta et al., 2008) One of the problems with the analyses is that the database remains proprietary to a select group of investigators, similar to the case with the SEARCH database, so there is no independent examination of the data or of the results. (Boffa et al., 2008)

One of the great advantages of using these large databases is that it is possible to examine long-term consequences of treatment for chronic illnesses. (Raaijmakers et al., 2008) It is also possible to investigate treatment decisions in relationship to patient demographics, and to investigate the possibility in disparities in treatment choices by gender. (Aron, Nguyen, Stein, & Gill, 2008; Cho, Hoogwere, Huang, Brennan, & Hazen, 2008), race or ethnicity, and by socio-economic status. It is also possible to use the entire database and to use variable reduction techniques that are part of the data mining process rather than to continue to use inclusion/exclusion criteria.(Hauptman, Swindle, burroughts, & Schnitzler, 2008) These criteria can overlook important confounding factors that are always important to investigate in observational studies. Dividing a study population on just one factor tends to neglect any examination of confounders.(Good, Holschub, Albertson, & Eldridge, 2008) In this study by Good et.al., the determining factor was grain consumption, completely overlooking the fact that there are many factors involved in nutrition and diet, and they are all highly dependent on each other.(Good et al., 2008)

Occasionally, some studies use some data mining techniques, particularly the technique of separating a holdout sample from the data used to define the model.(Moran, Bristow, Solomon, George, & Hart, 2008) One such study conducted in Australia examined mortality in intensive care (ICU). In addition, by using receiver operating curves (ROC), the study examines the difference between false positives and false negatives. However, this study still does not consider the fact that mortality remains a fairly rare occurrence and the group sizes between mortality and non-mortality are quite different, influencing model choice and results.

SAS PROGRAMMING AND DATA MINING

In order to define the different indices used in this text, the data sources require some preprocessing. Some of the processing code will be given here. More details are provided in workbooks developed for preprocessing the datasets.(Cerrito, 2008a, 2008b) We do assume that the reader either has some experience in working with SAS software, or collaborates with a user of SAS software to preprocess the data. For a general introduction to programming SAS using the point-and-click interface, Enterprise Guide, we refer the reader to Exploratory Data Analysis: An Introduction to Data Analysis Using SAS. (P. Cerrito, 2007)

We will also be using the SAS component, SAS Enterprise Miner for all data mining. This is a data mining add-on to SAS software. It, too, has a point-and-click interface similar to that in SAS Enterprise Guide. We will give a brief introduction to Enterprise Miner as we will be using several of the components in this book. For more information, we refer the interested reader to a text on Enterprise Miner. (P. B. Cerrito, 2007)

In particular, we will make use of a feature in SAS Enterprise Miner called Text Miner. The purpose of this component is to analyze unstructured, non-standardized text. It can also be used to examine patient information that is identified using ICD9 codes. In particular, SAS Text Miner has the ability to cluster patients into groups that can be ranked by order of severity. Once ranked, they can be validated by using patient outcomes to determine if the most severe patients have the greatest proportion of detrimental outcomes.

Figure 1 shows the login screen for Enterprise Miner. For a desktop install, the password is the Windows login user id and password.

Figure 1. Login for Enterprise Miner (created with SAS® software. Copyright 2009, SAS Institute Inc., Cary, NC, USA. All Rights Reserved. Reproduced with permission of SAS Institute Inc., Cary, NC)

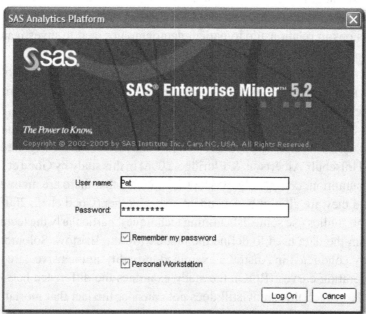

Figure 2 shows the next screen where you have the option of setting up a new project or referencing a previously created project.

If you choose to Open Project, you are next directed to a list of available projects to choose. Figure 3 shows a project window.

Startup code is important because it is executed with every procedure in Enterprise Miner. It is particularly important to define a library name to contain the datasets used in the project. Figure 4 shows this code, defining a library called NIS.

Figure 2. New Project Screen for Enterprise Miner (created with SAS® software. Copyright 2009, SAS Institute Inc., Cary, NC, USA. All Rights Reserved. Reproduced with permission of SAS Institute Inc., Cary, NC)

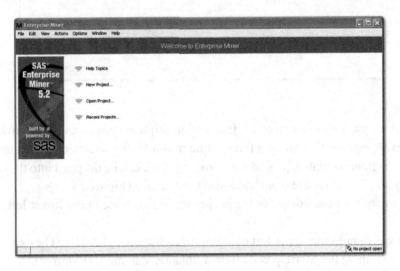

Figure 3. Project Window in Enterprise Miner (created with SAS® software. Copyright 2009, SAS Institute Inc., Cary, NC, USA. All Rights Reserved. Reproduced with permission of SAS Institute Inc., Cary, NC)

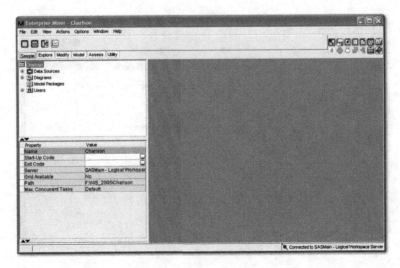

Figure 4. Startup code in Enterprise Miner (created with SAS® software. Copyright 2009, SAS Institute Inc., Cary, NC, USA. All Rights Reserved. Reproduced with permission of SAS Institute Inc., Cary, NC)

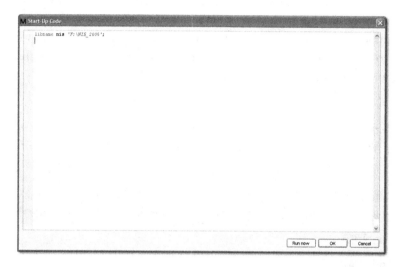

There can be multiple datasets in each project, and multiple diagrams as well. However, Enterprise Miner can only examine one diagram at a time, while multiple datasets can be open and available in a diagram. When a diagram is created, procedure icons, or nodes, can be dropped into the diagram window to define an analysis. The nodes are connected using the mouse (Figure 5).

Highlighting any of the nodes displays the properties of that node in the lower left window (Figure 6).

The Data Sources item in the upper left contains all of the open datasets. They can only be entered from the libraries set up on the StartUp code with a libname statement (Figure 7).

Figure 5. A diagram in Enterprise Miner (created with SAS® software. Copyright 2009, SAS Institute Inc., Cary, NC, USA. All Rights Reserved. Reproduced with permission of SAS Institute Inc., Cary, NC)

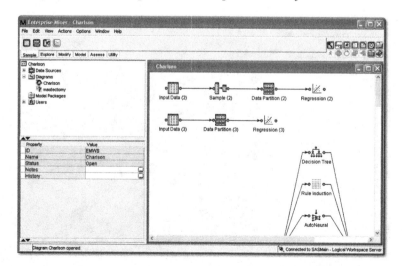

Figure 6. Property Window (created with SAS® software. Copyright 2009, SAS Institute Inc., Cary, NC, USA. All Rights Reserved. Reproduced with permission of SAS Institute Inc., Cary, NC)

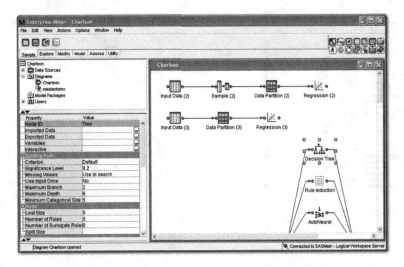

Note that there are items for the variables, the decisions, and the role for the dataset. The default role is "Raw". It can be changed to "Score" when using additional data to predict patient outcomes. The Variables option gives a list of the variables in the dataset as well as the properties of the variables (Figure 8).

In this example, there are a number of variables defined as rejected, meaning that the default is not to use them in an analysis. The outcome, or Target variables is "Died" (mortality). Currently, it is defined as an Interval variable. In order to use it as the dependent variable in a logistic regression, it will need to be

Figure 7. Dataset in Enterprise Miner (created with SAS® software. Copyright 2009, SAS Institute Inc., Cary, NC, USA. All Rights Reserved. Reproduced with permission of SAS Institute Inc., Cary, NC)

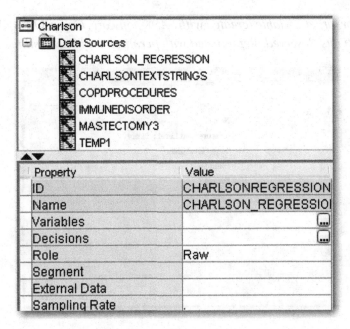

Figure 8. Dataset variables (created with SAS® software. Copyright 2009, SAS Institute Inc., Cary, NC, USA. All Rights Reserved. Reproduced with permission of SAS Institute Inc., Cary, NC)

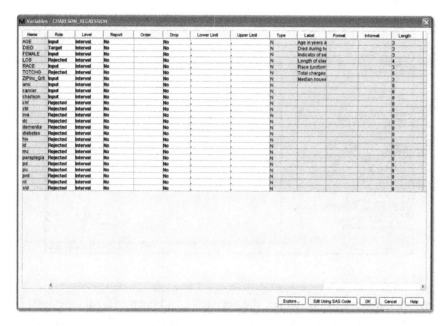

changed to "binary". This is done by right clicking on the level that needs changing. Multiple options will be displayed, with "binary" as one of the choices. Note the "Explore" button in the lower right. You can highlight the variables in the dataset that you want to examine in more detail and then press "Explore".

Once the "Died" variable has been changed to binary, we can investigate the decisions (Figure 9), and the importance of each decision.

Figure 9. Decisions for target variable (created with SAS® software. Copyright 2009, SAS Institute Inc., Cary, NC, USA. All Rights Reserved. Reproduced with permission of SAS Institute Inc., Cary, NC)

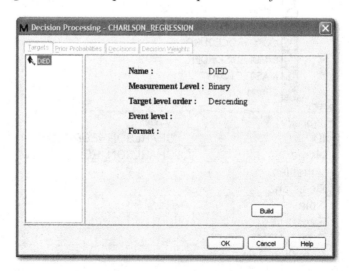

We want to build the decisions, including prior probabilities and weights. The prior probabilities are those that exist in the population (Figure 10). In this example, mortality is a rare occurrence (approximately 2% of all patients in the dataset). A discussion of how to accommodate a rare occurrence with these prior probabilities is given in Chapter 4.

One of the things we need to consider is whether we want to weight a false negative differently from a false positive in terms of cost. While this will be discussed in more detail in Chapter 4, we want to demonstrate how the information is entered (Figure 11).

Decision one is to predict mortality; decision zero predicts non-mortality. Currently, the cost of error

Figure 10. Prior probabilities for target variable (created with SAS® software. Copyright 2009, SAS Institute Inc., Cary, NC, USA. All Rights Reserved. Reproduced with permission of SAS Institute Inc., Cary, NC)

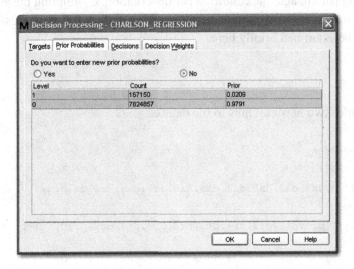

Figure 11. Decision weights (created with SAS® software. Copyright 2009, SAS Institute Inc., Cary, NC, USA. All Rights Reserved. Reproduced with permission of SAS Institute Inc., Cary, NC)

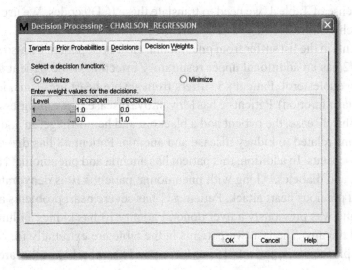

is the same, whether that error is a false positive or a false negative. When the weights are symmetric as they are in Figure 11, the problem defaults to one of misclassification.

If we want to predict those at highest risk for mortality so that interventions can be used to prevent it, it would be better to have more false positives, which will increase the cost of treatment, rather than false negatives, which will result in greater unexpected mortality. In this case, we can change the values to reflect the cost that we want to give. A positive value indicates a profit; a negative value indicates a cost. Therefore, for medical treatment, we want to have a negative value to indicate the cost. Then there is the option of whether to maximize or to minimize. We maximize profit when the weights are positive; we minimize cost when the weights are negative.

The NIS and the MEPS datasets have two different types of listings of diagnosis and procedure codes. The NIS data have 15 columns of both procedures and diagnoses for each patient. They can easily be combined using the CATX function in SAS. The MEPS data include a patient condition file with multiple conditions per patient and one condition per observation. Combining these conditions into one observation per patient requires a bit more coding. While the coding will be discussed in more detail in later chapters, it will be examined briefly here.

NIS Data

The following code adds two new columns to the dataset:

```
Data NIS.combinecodes;
Set nis.datafor2005;
Diagnoses=catx(' ',dx1,dx2,dx3,dx4,dx5,dx6,dx7,dx8,dx9,dx10,dx11,
dx12,dx13,dx14,dx15) ;
    procedures=catx(' 'pr1,pr2,pr3,pr4,pr5,pr6,pr7,pr8,pr9,pr10,pr11,pr12,
pr13,pr14,pr15) ;
    run ;
```

Table 6 shows the results of the above code for the diagnoses. The result is to create a text string consisting of all the codes for an individual patient.

In order to make sense of Table 4, we need to translate these ICD9 codes. We use the online information at http://icd9cm.chrisendres.com. The codes are given in Table 7.

The first four patients in the list suffer from pneumonia. However, patient #1 also suffers from asthma and obesity. Patient #2 has an additional upper respiratory infection while patient #3 also suffers from asthma and from high cholesterol. Patient #5 suffers from severe heart problems, including a previous heart attack (myocardial infarction). Patient #6 has Moyamoya disease, a rare, progressive cerebrovascular disorder. Along with this disease, the patient had a blackout and hemorrhage. In addition to pneumonia, patient #7 has problems related to kidney disease and anemia. Patient #8 has diabetes and cellulitis in the leg due to staphylococcus. In addition, this patient has anemia and pneumonia. Number 9 has severe hypertension, edema, and diabetes. Along with pneumonia, patient #10 is dehydrated with asthma and pleurisy, having had a previous heart attack. Patient #11 has severe heart problems as well as a sexually transmitted disease, and was previously a liver donor. Patient #13 has kidney failure, heart failure, and is in need of physical therapy. The last two patients in the table are extremely ill. Number 14 has both spina bifida and multiple sclerosis; patient #15 has kidney and heart problems that are related to diabetes.

Table 6. Concatenated diagnoses

Patient	Concatenated Diagnoses
1	486 4932 7863 2780 486 493 786 278
2	486 4661 4659 486 466 465
3	486 4932 2720 486 493 272
4	486 486
5	7298 4273 4534 4598 4019 412 729 427
6	7802 2865 4375 7803 40199 412 729
7	486 4031 2852 2720 3860 5198 7805
8	6826 486 4534 4939 0411 2500 7823
9	4010 2500 2780 7823 401 250 278 782
10	486 2765 4939 5110 4019 412 486 276
11	2765 4241 4280 1122 4589 2500 v586
12	3310 2765 2941 2888 5751 4019 4140
13	V571 486 5849 4280 v586 4019 2449
14	7221 7419 340 7373 722 741 340 737
15	4280 5849 4039 2504 v586 4140 2859

MEPS Data

The following SAS code is used to combine the diagnosis codes into one column. In order to perform text analysis on HC-078, Medical Conditions data file from MEPS. The data must first be pre-processed. In this data file, each patient condition is an observational unit, and each patient will have multiple observations in the dataset. In order to put all of the patient conditions into one observation per patient, and then to define a text string of patient conditions, the data must first be transposed. Proc Transpose creates one observation per patient by creating a string of variables. The total number of variables created is equal to the maximum number of patient conditions listed for any one patient.

```
libname meps 'c:\Meps';
proc Transpose data=meps.h78codes
          out=work.tran (drop=_name_ _label_)
               prefix=med_ ;
     var icd9codx ;
     by dupersid;
run;
```

The next step is to concatenate all of the variables created by Proc Transpose. The creation of the chconcat array allows for this combination. The different codes are separated by spaces in the text string.

```
data work.concat(keep= dupersid icd9codx) ;
   length icd9codx $32767 ;
```

Table 7. Translated codes

Patient	Concatenated Diagnoses
1	Pneumonia, organism unspecified, Chronic obstructive asthma, Hemoptysis, Overweight and obesity, Asthma, Symptoms involving respiratory system and other chest symptoms, Overweight, obesity and other hyperalimentation
2	Pneumonia, organism unspecified, Acute bronchiolitis, Acute upper respiratory infections of multiple or unspecified sites
3	Pneumonia, organism unspecified, Chronic obstructive asthma, Pure hypercholesterolemia
4	Pneumonia, organism unspecified
5	Other musculoskeletal symptoms referable to limbs, Atrial fibrillation and flutter, Venous embolism and thrombosis of deep vessels of lower extremity, Other specified disorders of circulatory system, Essential hypertension, Old myocardial infarction
6	Syncope and collapse, Hemorrhagic disorder due to intrinsic circulating anticoagulants, Moyamoya disease, Convulsions, Essential hypertension, Viral exanthem, unspecified, Fever
7	Pneumonia, organism unspecified, Hypertensive kidney disease, benign, Anemia in chronic illness, Pure hypercholesterolemia, Méniére's disease, Other diseases of respiratory system, not elsewhere classified, Sleep disturbances
8	Other cellulitis and abscess, ankle, not foot, Pneumonia, organism unspecified, Venous embolism and thrombosis of deep vessels of lower extremity, Asthma, unspecified, Staphylococcus, Diabetes mellitus without mention of complication, Other hemolytic anemias due to enzyme deficiency
9	Essential hypertension, malignant, Diabetes mellitus without mention of complication, Overweight and obesity, Edema, Essential hypertension, Diabetes mellitus
10	Pneumonia, organism unspecified, Volume depletion, Asthma, unspecified, Pleurisy without mention of effusion or current tuberculosis, Essential hypertension, Old myocardial infarction
11	Volume depletion, Aortic valve disorders, Congestive heart failure, unspecified, Candidiasis, Hypotension, unspecified, Diabetes mellitus without mention of complication, liver donor
12	Alzheimer's disease, Volume depletion, Dementia in conditions classified elsewhere, Diseases of white blood cells, Other cholecystitis, Essential hypertension, Coronary atherosclerosis
13	Other physical therapy, Pneumonia, organism unspecified, Acute renal failure, unspecified, Congestive heart failure, unspecified, Long-term (current) drug use, Essential hypertension, Coronary atherosclerosis
14	Displacement of thoracic or lumbar intervertebral disc without myelopathy, Spina bifida, Multiple sclerosis, Kyphoscoliosis and scoliosis
15	Congestive heart failure, unspecified, Acute renal failure, unspecified, Hypertensive kidney disease, Diabetes with renal manifestations, Long-term (current) drug use, Coronary atherosclerosis, Anemia, unspecified

```
   set work.tran ;
   array chconcat {*} med_: ;
   icd9codx = left(trim(med_1)) ;
   do i = 2 to dim(chconcat) ;
       icd9codx = left(trim(icd9codx)) || ` ` || left(trim(chconcat[i])) ;
   end ;
run ;
```

Because it is unknown just how many variables need to be concatenated, the maximum possible length was used. Proc SQL is used to reduce the length of the text string to its minimum possible.

```
proc sql ;
    select max(length(icd9codx)) into:icd9codx_LEN from work.concat ;
quit ;
%put icd9codx_LEN=&icd9codx_LEN ;
```

```
data meps.icd9codes ;
    length icd9codx $ &icd9codx_LEN ;
    set work.concat ;
run ;
```

Negative numbers in the code columns indicate that there are no ICD9 codes in the designated columns. The final resuls will be quite similar to those given in tables 4 and 5. Each patient will have a defined text string, and that text string contains all diagnoses that have been assigned to that patient.

FUTURE TRENDS

As healthcare providers and physicians implement an electronic medical record, more and larger databases will become available for analysis. As is already done in many other businesses, data mining techniques will be adopted to "know your customer (patient)". Data mining will greatly enhance the use of patient data to improve decision making. It will be extremely important to ensure that the modeling techniques used to analyze the data will return accurate, meaningful results.

In addition, providers will become more accountable for how they treat patients. As patient severity indices improve, they will be used to decide upon provider reimbursements, which will be tied to performance goals and quality rankings.

DISCUSSION

In this chapter, we provided a basic introduction of patient severity indices as well as a brief discussion of data mining and SAS Enterprise Miner, which is used to examine large, complex databases. We will expand upon this information considerably in subsequent chapters.

Information codes are used in billing and administrative data to define patient conditions, and also to define patient treatments. These codes are used to define patient severity indices. Therefore, it is absolutely essential to both understanding the severity indices, and to defining such severity indices to be able to work with these codes. The most difficult data to work with are contained within claims databases where different coding methods are used by different providers; the different codes must be reconciled in some manner.

The standard method to define a patient severity index is to use a number of patient demographics and diagnoses in a linear or logistic regression, comparing patient information to outcomes. Unfortunately, the only way to determine reliability is by using fresh data. There is no good way to validate the model. We will demonstrate several types of patient severity indices to show the current state of the science. While attempts are made to validate the indices by comparing several methods to each other; however different methods can lead to very different outcomes.

In addition, we will propose a novel technique that depends upon predictive modeling and text mining. It makes use of the text strings that were defined, with each text string containing all diagnoses related to that individual. Unlike the standard procedure, text mining does not rely on outcomes to define a patient severity index. Therefore, it is possible to examine the validity of a patient severity index defined using this technique.

REFERENCES

Andaluz, N., & Zuccarello, M. (2008). Recent trends in the treatment of cerebral aneurysms: analysis of a nationwide inpatient database. *Journal of Neurosurgery, 108*(6), 1163–1169.

Anonymous-DRG. (2008a). DRG (Diagnosis Related Group) [Electronic Version]. Retrieved 2008 from http://health.utah.gov/opha/IBIShelp/codes/DRGCode.htm.

Anonymous-DRG. (2008b). *DRG Desk Reference 2008: The Ultimate Resource for Improving the New Ms-drg Assignment Practices* (Vol. 2008). Salt Lake City, UT: Ingenix.

Anonymous-healthgrades. (2008). *Healthgrades.com.* 2008. Retrieved from healthgrades.com

Anonymous-ICD10. (2008). *Transaction and Code Sets Standards.* Retrieved 2008, from http://www.cms.hhs.gov/TransactionCodeSetsStands/02_TransactionsandCodeSetsRegulations.asp#TopOfPage

Anonymous-ICD9. (2008). *ICD9 Codes* [Electronic Version]. Retrieved 2008 from http://icd9cm.chrisendres.com/index.php.

Anonymous-OASIS. (2007). *Home Health compare* [Electronic Version]. Retrieved February, 2008 from http://www.medicare.gov/HHCompare/Home.asp?dest=NAV|Home|About#TabTop.

Anonymous-TGBH. (2008). *The Texas Hospital Checkup* [Electronic Version]. Retrieved June, 2008 from http://tbgh.org/checkup/HowCreated.htm.

Arca, M., Fusco, D., Barone, A., & Perucci, C. (2006). Introduction to risk adjustment methods in comparative evaluation of outcomes. *Epidemiologia e Prevenzione, 30*(4-5), 5–47.

Aron, M., Nguyen, M. M., Stein, R. J., & Gill, I. S. (2008). Impact of gender in renal cell carcinoma: an analysis of the SEER database. *European Urology, 54,* 133–142.

Ash, A. S., Shwartz, M., & Pekoz, E. A. (2003). Comparing Outcomes Across Providers. In L. I. Iezzoni (Ed.), *Risk Adjustment* (3rd Ed., pp. 297-333). Chicago: Health Administration Press.

Azarisman, M. S., Fauzi, M. A., Faizal, M. P. A., Azami, Z., Roslina, A. M., & Roslan, H. (2007). The SAFE (SGRQ score, air-flow, limitation and exercise tolderance) Index: a new composite score for the stratification of severity in chronic obstructive pulmonary disease. *Postgraduate Medical Journal, 83,* 492–497.

Baxter, N. N., Hartman, L. K., Tepper, J. E., Ricciardi, R., Durham, S. B., & Virnig, B. A. (2007). Postoperative irradiation for rectal cancer increases the risk of small bowl obstruction after surgery. *Annals of Surgery, 245,* 553–559.

Boffa, D. J., Allen, M. S., Grab, J. D., Gaissert, H. A., Harpole, D. H., & Wright, C. D. (2008). Data from the society of thoracic surgeons general thoracic surgery database: the surgical management of primary lung tumors. *The Journal of Thoracic and Cardiovascular Surgery, 135*(2), 247–254.

Cartsos, V. M., Zhu, S., & Zavras, A. I. (2008). Bisphosphonate use and the risk of adverse jaw outcomes. *The Journal of the American Dental Association, 139*(1), 23–30.

Cerrito, P. (2006). Text mining coded information. In H. A. D. Prado & E. Ferneda (Eds.), *Emerging Technologies of Text Mining: Techniques and Applications* (pp. 268-296). New York: Idea Group Publishing.

Cerrito, P. (2007). *Exploratory Data Analysis: An Introduction to Data Analysis Using SAS*. Morrisville, NC: Lulu.com.

Cerrito, P. (2008a). *Step by Step Instructions to Extract Coded Information from the Medical Expenditure Panel Survey (MEPS)*. Morrisville, NC: Lulu.com.

Cerrito, P. (2008b). *Step by Step Instructions to Extract Coded Information from the National Inpatient Sample (NIS)*. Morrisville, NC: Lulu.com.

Cerrito, P. B. (2007). *Introduction to Data Mining with Enterprise Miner*. Cary, NC: SAS Press.

Cher, D. J., & Lenert, L. A. (1997). Method of medicare reimbursement and the rate of potentially ineffective care of critically ill patients. *Journal of the American Medical Association, 278*(12), 1001–1007.

Cho, L., Hoogwere, B., Huang, J., Brennan, D. M., & Hazen, S. L. (2008). Gender differences in utilization of effective cardiovascular secondary prevention: a Cleveland Clinic prevention database study. *Journal of Women's Health, 17*(4), 515–521.

Daley, J., Ash, A. S., & Iezzoni, L. I. (2003). Validity and Reliability of Risk Adjusters. In L. I. Iezzoni (Ed.), *Risk Adjustment* (3rd Ed., pp. 207-230). Chicago: Health Administration Press.

Daley, J., Iezzoni, L. I., & Shwartz, M. (2003). Conceptual and Practical Issues in Developing Risk-Adjustment Methods. In L. I. Iezzoni (Ed.), *Risk Adjustment* (3rd ed., pp. 179-205). Chicago: Health Administration Press.

Darkow, T., Henk, H. J., Thomas, S. K., Feng, W., Baladi, J.-F., & Goldberg, G. A. (2007). Treatment interruptions and non-adherence with imatinib and associated healthcare costs: a retrospective analysis among managed care patients with chronic myelogenous leukaemia. *PharmacoEconomics, 25*(6), 481–496.

Delaney, C. P., Chang, E., Senagore, A. J., & Broder, M. (2008). Clinical outcomes and resource utilization associated with laparoscopic and open colectomy using a large national database. *Annals of Surgery, 247*(5), 819–824.

Dobie, S. A., Warren, J. L., Matthews, B., Schwartz, D., Baldwin, L.-M., & Billingsley, K. (2008). Survival benefits and trends in the use of adjuvant therapy among elderly stage II and III rectal cancer patients in the general population. *Cancer, 112*(4), 789–799.

Donald, H., Taylor, J., & Hoenig, H. (2006). Access to health care services for the disabled elderly. *Health Sciences Research, 41*(3, Part 1), 743–758.

Ellis, R., Pope, G., Iezzoni, L., Ayanian, J., Bates, D., & Burstin, H. (1996). Diagnosis-based risk adjustment for medicare capitations payments. *Health Care Financing Review, 17*, 101–128.

Enzinger, P. C., Benedetti, J. K., Meyerhardt, J. A., McCoy, S., Hundahl, S. A., & Macdonald, J. S. (2007). Impact of hospital volume on recurrence and survival after surgery for gastric cancer. *Annals of Surgery, 245*, 426–434.

Epstein, D., Knight, T. K., Epstein, J. B., Bride, M. A., & Nichol, M. B. (2007). Cost of care for early- and late-stage oral and pharyngeal cancer in the California Medicaid population. *Head & Neck, 30*(2), 178–186.

Fang, Y., Chien, L., Ng, Y., Chu, H., Chen, W., & Cheng, C. (2006). Association of hospital and surgeon operation volume with the incidence of postoperative endophthalmitis: Taiwan experience. *Eye (London, England), 20*, 900–907.

Freeman, J. L., Zhang, D., Daniel, H., Freeman, J., & Goodwin, J. S. (2000). An approach to identifying incident breast cancer cases using Medicare claims data. *Journal of Clinical Epidemiology, 53*, 605–614.

Gadomski, A., & Jenkins, P. (2001). Ruptured appendicitis among children as an indicator of access to care. *Health Services Research, 36*(1, Part 1), 129–142.

Gammie, J. S., Haddad, M., Milford-Beland, S., Welke, K. F., Bruce, T., & Ferguson, J. (2008). Atrial fibrillation correction surgery: lessons from the Society of Thoracic Surgeons national cardiac database. *The Annals of Thoracic Surgery, 85*, 909–915.

Gilligan, M. A., Neuner, J., Zhang, X., Sparapani, R., Laud, P. W., & Nattinger, A. B. (2007). Relationship between number of breast cancer operations performed and 5-year survival after treatment for early-stage breast cancer. *American Journal of Public Health, 97*, 539–544.

Gold, H., & Do, H. (2007). Evaluation of three algorithms to identify incident breast cancer in Medicare claims data. *Health Services Research, 42*(5), 2056–2069.

Good, C. K., Holschub, N., Albertson, A. M., & Eldridge, A. L. (2008). Whole grain consumption and body mass index in adult women: an analysis of NHANES 1999-2000 and the USDA Pyramid Servings Database. *Journal of the American College of Nutrition, 27*(1), 80–87.

Gross, C. P., Galusha, D. H., & Krumholz, H. M. (2007). The impact of venous thromboembolism on risk of death or hemorrhage in older cancer patients. *Journal of General Internal Medicine, 22*(3), 321–326.

Halliday, T., Taira, D. A., Davis, J., & Chan, H. (2007). Socioeconomic Disparities in Breast Cancer Screening in Hawaii. *Preventing Chronic Disease: Public health research, practice, and policy, 4*(4), 1-9.

Hamilton, R. J., Aronson, W. J., Terris, M. K., Kane, C. J., Joseph, C., & Presti, J. (2008). Limitations of prostate specific antigen doubling time following biochemical recurrence after radical prostatectomy: results from the SEARCH database. *The Journal of Urology, 179*, 1785–1790.

Hartung, D. M., Middleton, L., Haxby, D. G., Koder, M., Ketchum, K. L., & Chou, R. (2007). Rates of adverse events of long-acting opioids in a state Medicaid program. *The Annals of Pharmacotherapy, 41*(6), 921–928.

Hauptman, P. J., Swindle, J., Burroughts, T. E., & Schnitzler, M. A. (2008). Resource utilization in patients hospitalized with heart failure: insights from a contemporary national hospital database. *American Heart Journal, 155*, 978–985.

Hoy, T., Fisher, M., Barber, B., Borker, R., Stolshek, B., & Goodman, W. (2007). Adherence to K/DOQI practice guidelines for bone metabolism and disease. *The American Journal of Managed Care, 13*(11), 620–625.

Iezzoni, L., Shwartz, M., Ash, A., & Mackieman, Y. (1994). *Risk adjustment methods for examining in-hospital mortality.* Paper presented at the AHSR FHSR Annual Meeting.

Iezzoni, L. I. (2003). Range of Risk Factors. In L. I. Iezzoni (Ed.), *Risk Adjustment* (3rd ed., pp. 33-70). Chicago: Health Administration Press.

Iezzoni, L. I., Ash, A. S., Shwartz, M., Daley, J., Hughes, J. S., & Mackiernan, Y. D. (1995). Predicting who dies depends on how severity is measured: implications for evlauating patient outcomes. *Annals of Internal Medicine, 123*(10), 763–770.

Inouye, S. K., Peduzzi, P. N., Robison, J. T., Hughes, J. S., Horwitz, R. I., & Concato, J. (1998). Importance of functional measures in predicting mortality among older hospitalized patients. *Journal of the American Medical Association, 279*(15), 1187–1193.

Loebstein, R., Katzir, I., Vasterman-Landes, J., Halkin, H., & Lomnicky, Y. (2008). Database assessment of the effectiveness of brand versus generic rosiglitazone in patients with type 2 diabetes mellitus. *Medical Science Monitor, 14*(6), CR323–CR326.

Lorence, D. P., & Spink, A. (2004). Regional Variation in Medical Systems Data: Influences on Upcoding. *Journal of Medical Systems, 26*(3), 369–381.

Loughlin, J. E., Cole, A., Dodd, S. L., Schein, J. R., Thornhill, J. C., & Walker, A. M. (2002). Comparison of resource utilization by patients treated with transdermal fentanyl and long-acting oral opioids for nonmalignant pain. *Pain Medicine, 3*(1), 47–55.

Macario, A., Vitez, T. S., Dunn, B., McDonald, T., & Brown, B. (1997). Hospital costs and severity of illness in three types of elective surgery. *Anesthesiology, 86*(1), 92–100.

Mariotto, A. B., Etzioni, R., Krapcho, M., & Feuer, E. J. (2007). Reconstructing PSA testing patterns between black and white men in the US from Medicare Claims and the National Health Interview Survey. *Cancer, 109*, 1877–1886.

Mehta, R. H., Grab, J. D., O'Brien, S. M., Glower, D. D., Haan, C. K., & Gammie, J. S. (2008). Clinical characteristics and in-hospital outcomes of patients with cardiogenic shock undergoing coronary artery bypass surgery. *Circulation, 117*, 876–885.

Mittnacht, A. J., Wax, D. B., Srivastava, S., Nguyen, K., & Joashi, U. (2008). Development and implementation of a pediatric cardiac anesthesia/intensive care database. *Seminars in Cardiothoracic and Vascular Anesthesia, 12*(1), 12–17.

Monami, M., Lambertucci, L., Lamanna, C., Lotti, E., Marsili, A., & Masotti, G. (2007). Are comorbidity indices useful in predicting all-cause mortality in Type 2 diabetic patients? Comparison between Charlson index and disease count. *Aging Clinical and Experimental Research, 19*(6), 492–496.

Moran, J. L., Bristow, P., Solomon, P. J., George, C., & Hart, G. K. (2008). Mortality and length-of-stay outcomes, 1993-2003, in the binational Australian and New Zealand intensive care adult patient database. *Critical Care Medicine, 36*(1), 46–61.

Nattinger, A. B., Laud, P. W., & Rut Bajorunaite, R. A. S., Jean L Freeman. (2004). An algorithm for the use of Medicare claims data to identify women with incident breast cancer. *Health Services Research, 39*(6 (part 1)), 1733-1749.

Norton, E. C., Garfinkel, S. A., McQuay, L. J., Heck, D. A., Wright, J. G., Dittus, R., & Lubitz, R. M. (1998). The effect of hospital volume on the in-hospital complication rate in knee replacement patients. *Health Services Research, 33*(5), 1191–1210.

O'Connell, R., & Lim, L. (2000). Utility of the Charlson comorbidity index computed from routinely collected hospital discharge diagnosis codes. *Methods of Information in Medicine, 39*(1), 7–11.

O'Leary, J., Keeler, E. B., Damberg, C., & Kerr, E. A. (1998). An Overview of Risk Adjustment. In *Health Information Systems: Design Issues and Analytic Applications* (pp. 1-37). Santa Monica, CA: Rand Corporation.

Odueyungbo, A., Browne, D., Akhtar-Danesh, N., & Thabane, L. (2008). Comparison of generalized estimating equations and quadratic inference functions using data from the Nationalo Longitudinal Survey of Children and Youth (NLSCY) database. *BMC Medical Research Methodology, 8*(28), 1–10.

Raaijmakers, R., Noordam, C., Karagiannis, C., Gregory, G., Hertel, J., & Sipila, N. (2008). Response to growth hormone treatment and final height in Noonan syndrom in a large cohort of patients in the KIGS database. *Journal of Pediatric Endocrinology & Metabolism, 21*(3), 267–273.

Reilly, J. J., Chin, B., Berkowitz, J., Weedon, J., & Avitable, M. (2003). Use of a state-wide administrative database in assessing a regional trauma system: the New York City experience. *Journal of the American College of Surgeons, 198*, 509–518.

Rochon, P., Katz, J., Morrow, L., McGlinchey-Berroth, R., Ahlquist, M., & Sarkarati, M. (1996). Comorbid illness is associated with survival and length of hospital stay in patients with chronic disability. A prospective comparison of three comorbidity indices. *Medical Care, 34*(11), 1093–1100.

Rosen, A. K., Reid, R., Broemeling, A.-M., & Rakovski, C. C. (2003). Applying a Risk-Adjustment Framework to Primary Care: Can We Improve on Existing Measures? *Annals of Family Medicine, 1*, 44–51.

Sabate, J. (1999). Nut consumption, vegetarian diets, ischemic heart disease risk, and all-cause mortality: evidence from epidemiologic studies. *The American Journal of Clinical Nutrition, 70*(Suppl), 500S–503S.

Schlenker, R. E., Powell, M. C., & Goodrich, G. K. (2005). Initial Home Health Outcomes Under Prospective Payment. *Health Services Research, 40*(1), 177–193.

Setoguchi, S., Solomon, D. H., Glynn, R. J., Cook, F. E., Levin, R., & Schneeweiss, S. (2007). Agreement of diagnosis and its date for hematologic malignancies and solid tumors between medicare claims and cancer registry data. *Cancer Causes & Control, 18*(5), 561–569.

Shugarman, L. R., Bird, C. E., Schuster, C. R., & Lynn, J. (2007). Age and gender differences in Medicare Expenditures at the end of life for colorectal cancer decedents. *Journal of Women's Health, 16*(2), 214–227.

Shwartz, M., & Ash, A. S. (2003). Evaluating Risk-Adjustment models Empirically. In L. I. Iezzoni (Ed.), *Risk Adjustment* (3rd ed., pp. 231-273). Chicago: Health Administration Press.

Singh, M., Rihal, C. S., Selzer, F., Kip, K. E., Detre, K., & Holmes, D. R. (2003). Validation of Mayo clinic risk adjustment model for in-hospital complications after percutaneous coronary interventions, using the National Heart, Lung, and Blood Institute dynamic registry. *Journal of the American College of Cardiology, 42*, 1722–1728.

Smith, G. I. (2008). *Basic CPT/HCPCS Coding 2008*. Chicago: American Health Information Management Association.

Tirkkonen, T., Ryynanen, A., Vahlberg, T., Irjala, K., Klaukka, T., & Huupponen, R. (2008). Frequency and clinical relevance of drug interactions with lovastatin and simvastatin; an obervational database study. *Drug Safety, 31*(3), 231–240.

Tollen, L. A., Ross, M. N., & Poor, S. (2004). Evidence about utilization and expenditures. *Health Services Research, 39*(4, Part II), 1167–1187.

Turley, R. S., Hamilton, R. J., Terris, M. K., Kane, C. J., Aronson, W. J., & Joseph, C. (2008). Small transrectal ultrasound volume predicts clinically significant Gleason score upgrading after radical prostatectomy: results from the SEARCH database. *The Journal of Urology, 179*, 523–528.

Welch, H. G., Fisher, E. S., Gottlieb, D. J., & Barry, M. J. (2007). Detection of prostate cancer via biopsy in the Medicare-SEER population during the PSA era. *Journal of the National Cancer Institute, 99*, 1395–1400.

West, E. S., Behrens, A., McDonnell, P. J., Tielsch, J. M., & Schem, O. D. (2005). The incidence of endophthalmitis after cataract surgery among the US Medicare population increased between 1994 and 2001. *Ophthalmology, 112*, 1388–1394.

Wolinsky, F. D., Miller, T. R., An, H., Geweke, J. F., Wallace, R. B., & Wright, K. B. (2007). Hospital episodes and physician visits: the concordance between self-reports and Medicare claims. *Medicare Care, 45*(4), 300–307.

Wright, C. D., Gaissert, H. A., Grab, J. D., O'Brien, S. M., Peterson, E. D., & Allen, M. S. (2008). Predictors of prolonged length of stay after lobectomy for lung cancer: a Society of Thoracic Surgeons general thoracic surgery database risk-adjustment model. *The Annals of Thoracic Surgery, 85*, 1857–1865.

Wynn, M. L., Chang, S., & Peipins, L. A. (2007). Temporal patterns of conditions and symptoms potentially associated with Ovarian cancer. *Journal of Women's Health, 16*(7), 971–986.

Xirasagar, S., Lien, Y., Lee, H., Liu, H., & Tsai, TC, J. (2008). Procedure volume of gastric cancer resections versus 5-year survival. *European Journal of Surgical Oncology, 34*(1), 23–29.

Yuill, M. (2008). *Risk adjustment-what is in it for doctors?* [Electronic Version] from http://www.hccblog.com/?p=20.

Chapter 2
Data Visualization and Data Summary

INTRODUCTION

Data visualization is an important concept in data mining. It enables you to understand the data, and to begin to formulate questions that you need to answer in order to make reasonable decisions. In traditional statistics, models and hypothesis tests provide proof; visualization is used to accompany the model in an attempt to explain it. In the data mining approach, visualization may provide essential information about the patterns in the data.

Patients in a clinic or geographic area are very heterogeneous. Therefore, the distribution of patient factors will not have a normal distribution. Generally, the distribution will have a heavy tail since every patient population will have those extreme patients who need extraordinary care; there will be more patients who need considerable care than those whose treatment can be discontinued early. Thus, unlike the normal distribution assumption, distributions of patient populations will not be symmetric. Therefore, great care must be used when considering a model that assumes normality, or even symmetry. We will look at alternative methods of analysis and visualization that do not depend upon the assumption of normality.

DOI: 10.4018/978-1-60566-752-2.ch002

Figure 1. Length of hospital stay for patients with diabetes

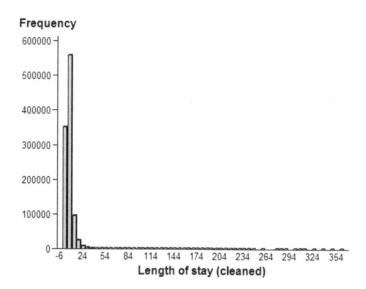

In this chapter, we look at bar graphs of patient length of stay. As will be clearly demonstrated, these distributions are not normally distributed. Therefore, we will need some way to model these patient distributions. We will show a method, called kernel density estimation, that makes no assumption about the shape of the underlying population distribution; instead, it provides a way to define a model that can be used to examine the entire population instead of just its average.

Probability is usually defined in terms of a density function. The most common such density function is the bell-shaped curve. The Probability that a value x is less than some pre-determined value, X (P(x≤X)=C), is equal to the integral between -∞ and the value X of the density function. In the past, tables were provided with the integral value of the standard normal density function. More recently, most statistical or graphing calculators provide the values as more and more mathematical tables are no longer printed. A brief summary of kernel density estimation is available online.(Anonymous-kde, 2008)

Kernel density estimation follows the same principal as integral calculus. The area under a curve can be estimated using a series of rectangles, with the total area assumed to be the sum of the areas of the rectangles. As the width of the rectangles becomes smaller, the sum of the rectangles comes closer and closer to the actual area under the curve. As the width of the rectangles approaches zero, the sum of rectangles approaches the area. There are a number of calculus formulas available that can be used to estimate the area under the curve. The simplest, but still relatively effective method is known as Simpson's Rule.(Anonymous-simpson, 2008)

BACKGROUND

Bar Graphs of Population Distributions

We start with Figure 1, the bar graph of the hospital length of stay for all patients with diabetes. In the National Inpatient Sample, that includes just over 1 million patient stays. Note that the distribution has

Figure 2. Length of stay limited to 50 days maximum

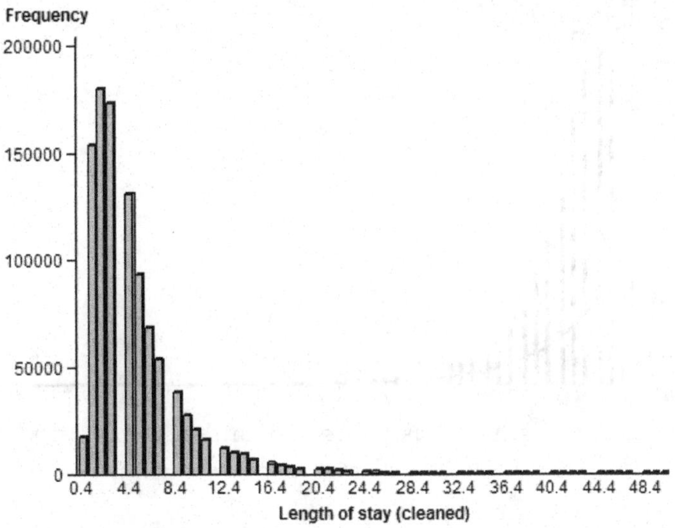

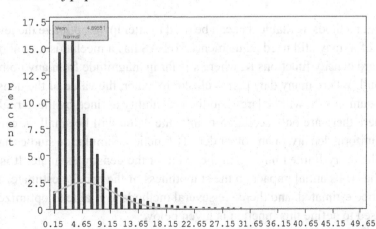

a very heavy tail with the maximum stay of about 354 days. The average length of stay is equal to 5 days with a standard deviation of 5.8 days. Figure 2 reduces the values on the x-axis to a maximum of 50 days so that we can focus on this part of the graph.

In Figure 2, note the gaps that occur because of rounding in the length of stay. It suggests that the information is not completely accurate because of this rounding.

Figure 3 gives the best normal estimate of the population distribution. It significantly under-values the probability at the low end, but also does not adequately estimate the outliers, or extreme patient outcomes.

Figure 4 gives an exponential distribution estimate. It better follows the pattern of the bar graph, but it still under-values the height of the bars.

Figure 3. Normal estimate of population distribution

Figure 4. Exponential estimate of population distribution

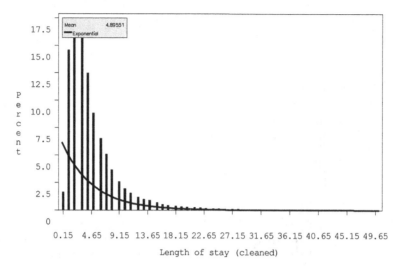

Kernel Density Estimation

When a known distribution does not work to estimate the population, we can just use an estimate of that distribution. (Silverman, 1986) The histograms demonstrated in Figures 1-4 can be smoothed into a probability density function. The formula for computing a kernel density estimate at the point x is equal to

$$f(x) = \frac{1}{na_n} \sum_{j=1}^{n} K\left(\frac{x - X_j}{a_n}\right)$$

where n is the size of the sample and K is a known density function. The value, a_n, is called the bandwidth. It controls the level of smoothing of the estimate curve. As the value of a_n approaches zero, the curve, f(x) becomes very jagged. As the value of a_n approaches infinity, the curve becomes closer to a straight line.

There are different methods available that can be used to attempt to optimize the level of smoothing. However, the value of a_n may still need adjustments, so SAS has a mechanism to allow you to do just that. For most standard density functions K, where x is far in magnitude from any point X_j, the value of f(x) will be very small. Where many data points cluster together, the value of the density function will be high because the sum of x-X_j will be large and the probability defined by the kernel function will be large. However, where there are only scattered points, the value will be small. K can be the standard normal density, the uniform density, or any other density function. Simulation studies have demonstrated that the value of K has very limited impact on the value of the density estimate. It is the value of the bandwidth, a_n, that has substantial impact on the smoothness of the density estimate. The true value of this bandwidth must be estimated, and there are several methods available to optimize this estimate.

The SAS code used to define this function is given below:

```
proc kde data=nis.diabetesless50los;
univar los/gridl=0 gridu=50 method=srot out=nis.kde50 bwm=3;
run;
```

We specify lower (gridl) and upper grid (gridu) values to bound the estimate. The method=srot attempts to optimize the level of smoothness in the estimate. The option, bwm=3, allows you to modify the optimal smoothness. The 'bwm' stands for bandwidth multiplier. With bwm=3, you take the value of a_n computed through the srot method and multiple it by 3 to increase the smoothness of the graph. The resulting estimate is saved in the nis.kde50 dataset so that it can be graphed. The result is given in Figure 5.

The probability is defined as the area under the curve. Most of the probability occurs for a length of stay between 0 and 10 days, with a much smaller probability of a stay between 10 and 20 days. There is a very small but nonzero probability of a length of stay beyond 20 days. This probability continues beyond the value of 50 days. Without the bwm=3 option, the estimate appears more jagged (Figure 6).

Thus, the more jagged curve has the same general appearance compared to the curve in Figure 5. Therefore, adjusting the bandwidth just gives a better representation of the general pattern of the population distribution.

PROC KDE uses only the standard normal density for K, but allows for several different methods to estimate the bandwidth, as discussed below. The default for the univariate smoothing is that of the Sheather-Jones plug in (SJPI):

$$h = C_3 \left\{ \int f''(x)^2 \, dx, \int f'''(x)^2 \, dx \right\} C_4(K) h^{5/7}$$

where C_3 and C_4 are appropriate functionals. The unknown values depending upon the density function f(x) are estimated with bandwidths chosen by reference to a parametric family such as the Gaussian as

Figure 5. Kernel density estimate of length of stay for patients with diabetes

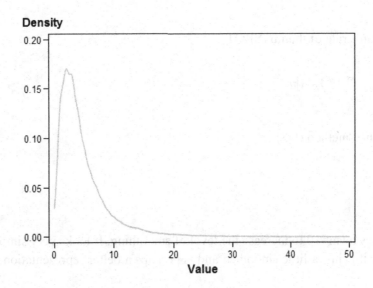

Figure 6. Kernel density estimate of length of stay for patients with diabetes without modifying the level of smoothness

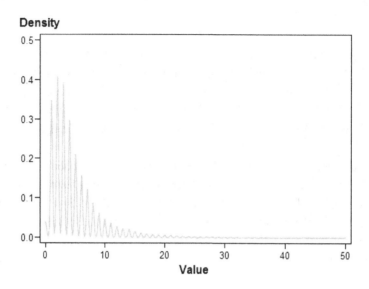

provided in Silverman:

$$\int f''(x)^2\, dx = \sigma^{-5} \int \phi''(x)^2\, dx \approx 0.212\sigma^{-5}$$

However, the procedure can use a different estimator, the simple normal reference (SNR), as the default for the bivariate estimator:

$$h = \hat{\sigma}\left[\frac{4}{(3n)}\right]^{\frac{1}{5}}$$

along with Silverman's rule of thumb (SROT):

$$h = 0.9 \min[\hat{\sigma}, (Q_1 - Q_3)/1.34]n^{-\frac{1}{5}}$$

and the over-smoothed method (OS):

$$h = 3\hat{\sigma}\left[\frac{1}{70\sqrt{\pi n}}\right]^{\frac{1}{5}}.$$

Figure 7 increases bwm=10 to increase the level of smoothing. It looks very similar to the graph in Figure 5. However, it is just a little smoother, and is perhaps a better representation of the population distribution.

Figure 7 appears to have the most optimal level of smoothness. For a bwm<1, the curve becomes more jagged; for bwm>1, it becomes smoother. However, it can be too smooth. Figure 8 has a bwm of 25. If the curve is too smooth, the depiction of the population shows more variability than actually exists in the population. It is optimal to vary the bandwidth and then to choose the best representation of the population.

Although the Central Limit Theorem will allow us to estimate the average length of stay for patients with diabetes, the confidence limits require the assumption of a normal distribution. Without this assumption, we can use numerical methods to estimate the integral. We can use a simple Simpson's Rule

Figure 7. Kernel density estimate of length of stay for patients with diabetes and BWM=10.

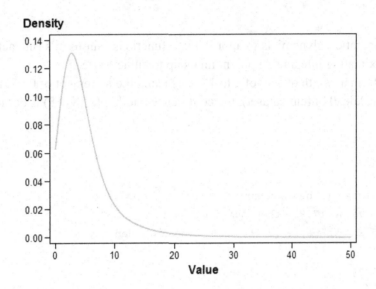

Figure 8. Kernel density estimate of length of stay for patients with diabetes and BWM=25.

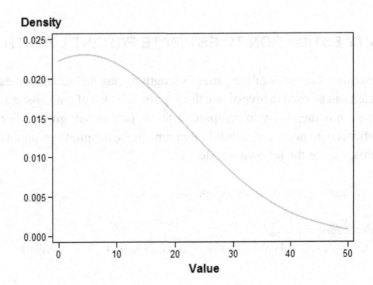

to define the confidence width. Simpson's rule uses quadratic polynomials; that is, it uses parabolic arcs instead of the straight line segments used in the more traditional trapezoidal rule. In particular, let the function f be tabulated at points x_0, x_1, and x_2 equally spaced by distance h, and denote

$$f_n = f(x_n)$$

Then Simpson's rule states that

$$\int_{x_0}^{x_2} f(x)dx = \int_{x_0}^{x_0+2h} f(x)dx \approx \frac{1}{3}h(f_0 + 4f_1 + f_2)$$

Since it uses quadratic polynomials to approximate functions, Simpson's rule actually gives exact results when approximating integrals of polynomials up to cubic degree.

For an integral from a length of stay of 2 to 18 days using the increment of 0.05 (there are 401 data points defined in the kde50 output dataset), the confidence width, p($2 \leq X \leq 18$) is defined by

```
Data work.confidence;
Set nis.kde50;
Sum=0;
If (value<2 or value>18) then sum=sum;
If (value<2.05 or value>17.95) then sum=sum+density;
If (value ge 20.5 and value le 17.95) then sum=sum+4*density);
Data nis.simpson;
Set work.confidence;
Integral=sum*0.05/3;
Run;
```

KERNEL DENSITY ESTIMATION TO ESTIMATE PATIENT LENGTH OF STAY

In this section, we examine estimates of the patient's length of stay and total charges, and demonstrate how visualization itself can be used to investigate the population. One of the biggest advantages in using kernel density estimation is the ability to compare different patient sub-groups. For example, we can examine whether patients with pneumonia spend more time in the hospital compared to patients without pneumonia. To do this, we use the following code:

```
proc sort data=nis.samplepneumonia out=work.pneumonia;
by pneumonia;
proc kde data=work.pneumonia;
univar los/gridl=0 gridu=20 out=nis.kdelospneumonia bwm=3 method=srot;
```

```
univar totchg/gridl=0 gridu=50000 out=nis.kdechgpneumonia method=srot;
by pneumonia;
```

There is considerably more variability in the length of stay for patients with pneumonia compared to patients without pneumonia (Figure 9). A patient with pneumonia, however, has a much higher probability of staying four or more days compared to patients with pneumonia, who are very likely going to stay less than four days. Figure 10 shows the total charges. The peak without pneumonia occurs at $4500; with pneumonia, it occurs at $9125. Patients with pneumonia have a higher probability of $11,000 or more in total charges. However, because of the overlap between the two curves, it is difficult to use just the occurrence or non-occurrence of pneumonia to predict patient outcomes.

We next look at the condition of septicemia. Notice that patients without septicemia have a peak length of stay of 2 days; this increases to a peak of 6.6 days with septicemia (Figure 11). The variability with septicemia is considerable, so that after 5.45 days, the probability is far greater that the patient will have septicemia compared to patients who stay less than 5.45 days. Similarly, the peak at $5500 total charges without septicemia is much less than the peak at $12,500 with septicemia (Figure 12). Moreover, the patient with charges of $20,000 or more has a higher probability of having septicemia.

We want to look at one more diagnosis, that of immune disorder. Figure 13 shows that there is little separation between those with the disorder (peak of 2.9 days) and those without (peak of 2 days). The crossover point occurs at 3.8 days when the probability of having the immune disorder exceeds the probability of not having the disorder. Figure 14 shows the crossover point at $11,500 with the peak of $4625 without the immune disorder, and a peak of $7000 with it. The kernel density shows the added cost when a patient has a diagnosis of immune disorder.

We can also examine two diagnoses simultaneously using kernel density estimation. The following code will divide the patients into 4 groups: those with neither pneumonia nor septicemia, those with one but not the other, and those with both conditions. The following code is used for pneumonia and septicemia.

Figure 9. Probability density of length of stay with and without pneumonia

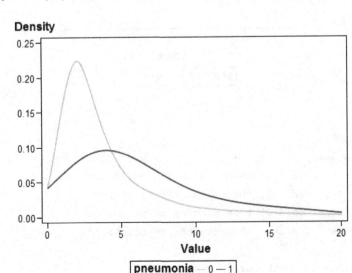

Figure 10. Probability density of total charges with and without pneumonia

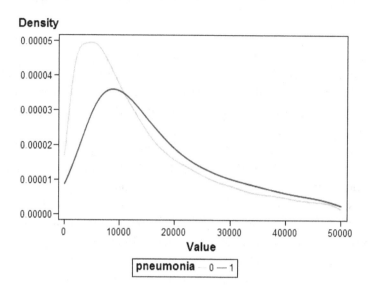

Figure 11. Probability density for length of stay with and without septicemia

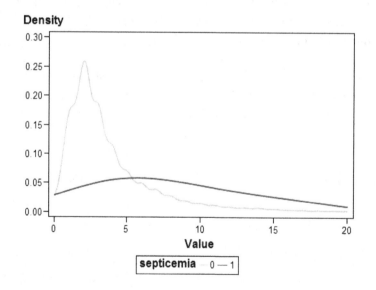

```
data work.septpneucombine;
set nis.samplepneumonia;
if (pneumonia=0 and septicemia=0) then diagnosis='neither';
if (pneumonia=0 and septicemia=1) then diagnosis='septicemia';
if (pneumonia=1 and septicemia=0) then diagnosis='pneumonia';
if (pneumonia=1 and septicemia=1) then diagnosis='both';
run;
proc sort data=work.septpneucombine;
```

Figure 12. Probability density of total charges with and without septecemia

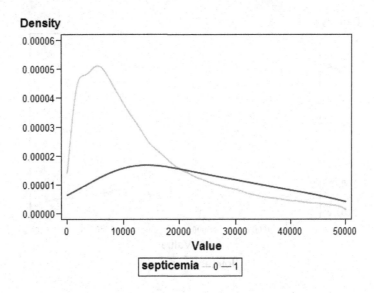

Figure 13. Probability density of length of stay with and without immune disorder

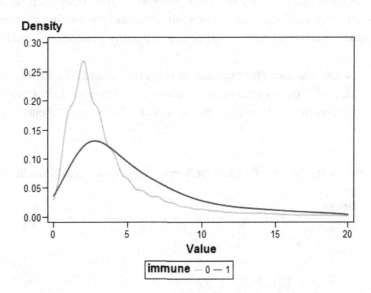

```
by diagnosis;
run;
proc kde data=work.septpneucombine;
univar los/gridl=0 gridu=20 method=srot bwm=1.8 out=nis.kdelosseptpneucombine;
univar totchg/gridl=0 gridu=50000 method=srot bwm=.8 out=nis.kdechgseptneucombine;
by diagnosis;
run;
```

Figure 14. Probability density of total charges with and without immune disorder

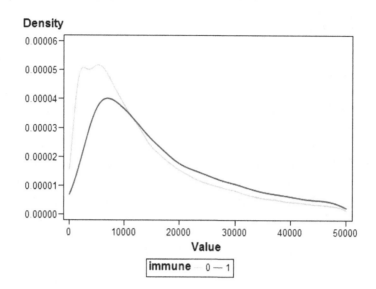

Figure 15 shows the probability density for length of stay; Figure 16 shows it for total charges. Note that the probability curves for septicemia alone, or septicemia and pneumonia are nearly identical. This indicates that septicemia is the more crucial condition, and pneumonia does not add to the required time or cost of treatment.

We next look at immune disorder and pneumonia (Figures 17 and 18). In this case, it is clear that there is a difference. The peak for either the immune disorder or pneumonia is approximately 3.15 days (versus 2 days for neither condition). However, the peak is at 4.9 days for patients with both conditions,

Figure 15. Probability density for length of stay concerning pneumonia and septicemia

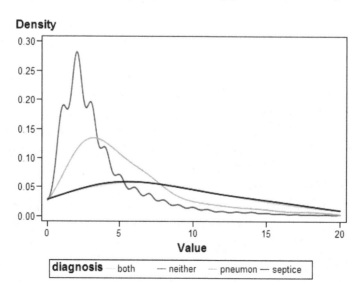

Figure 16. Probability density for total charges concerning pneumonia and septicemia

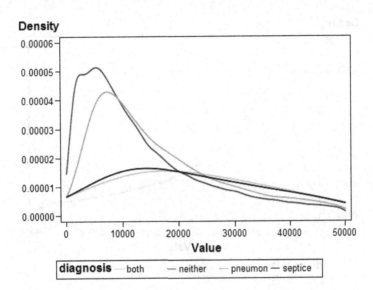

indicating a cumulative effect. For length of stay (Figure 17), the peak total charges for neither condition is $5500, $7000 for immune disorder, and $7125 for pneumonia. However, for both conditions, the peak increases to $9875. Clearly, then, a patient with both conditions utilizes more healthcare services than a patient with just one of the two conditions. The outcomes here contrast significantly to those for septicemia. Combined, these curves indicate the significant cost of septicemia followed by immune disorder.

The next graphs (Figures 19 and 20) consider patients with septicemia or immune disorder or both. Again, it appears that septicemia is the crucial condition; patients with both conditions do not require more healthcare resources than just septicemia by itself. Again, for neither condition, the peak length

Figure 17. Probability density for length of stay concerning pneumonia and immune disorder

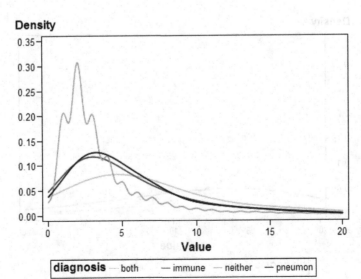

Figure 18. Probability density for total charges concerning pneumonia and immune disorder

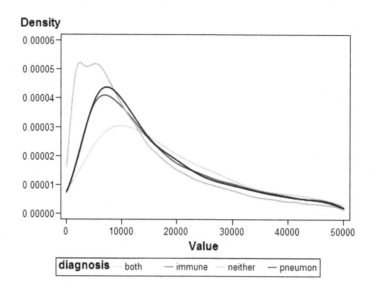

of stay is 2 days; this increases to 2.8 days for an immune disorder, but almost 8 days for septicemia. Similarly, the peak charges for the immune disorder are $6850, and $16,000 for septicemia with or without the added immune disorder.

The next bit of coding allows us to examine all three conditions on the same axes:

```
data work.immseptpnecombine;
set nis.samplepneumonia;
if (septicemia=0 and immune=0 and pneumonia=0) then diagnosis='none';
```

Figure 19. Probability density for length of stay concerning immune disorder and septicemia

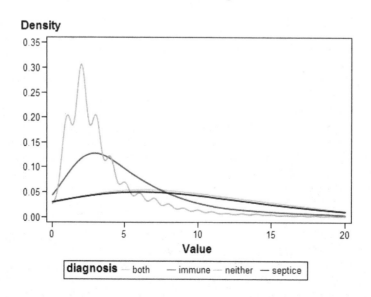

Figure 20. Probability density for total charges concerning immune disorder and septicemia

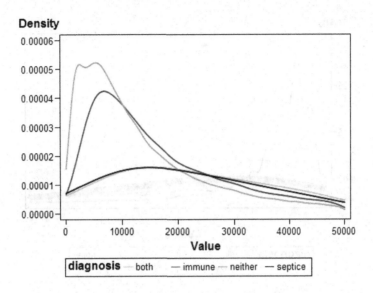

```
if (septicemia=0 and immune=1 and pneumonia=0) then diagnosis='immune';
if (septicemia=1 and immune=0 and pneumonia=0) then diagnosis='septicemia';
if (septicemia=0 and immune=0 and pneumonia=1) then diagnosis='pneumonia';
if (septicemia=1 and immune=1 and pneumonia=0) then diagnosis='sepimm';
if (septicemia=1 and immune=0 and pneumonia=1) then diagnosis='seppne';
if (septicemia=0 and immune=1 and pneumonia=1) then diagnosis='immpne';
if (septicemia=1 and immune=1 and pneumonia=1) then diagnosis='all';
run;
proc sort data=work.immseptpnecombine;
by diagnosis;
run;
proc kde data=work.immseptpnecombine;
univar los/gridl=0 gridu=20 method=srot bwm=2.5 out=nis.kdelosimmseptpne;
univar totchg/gridl=0 gridu=50000 method=srot bwm=.8 out=nis.kdechgimmseptpne;
by diagnosis;
run;
```

The result again shows that the condition of septicemia dominates the other two conditions (Figures 21 and 22). The immune disorder with pneumonia is shown in the two figures to utilize more healthcare resources than either condition alone.

We will use these same three conditions in Chapter 3 to show how statistics, including data summaries and regression models can be used to examine the data; these analyses will be in contrast to the visualization techniques discussed in this chapter.

Figure 21. Probability density for length of stay concerning all three conditions

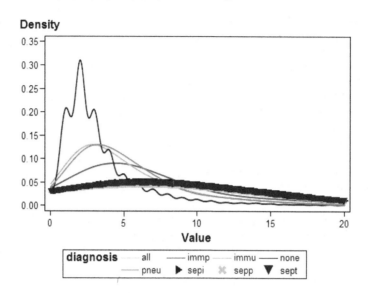

Figure 22. Probability density for total charges concerning all three conditions

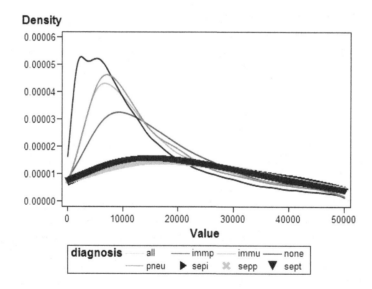

ANALYSIS OF EXAMPLE PROCEDURE OF CARDIOVASCULAR SURGERY

In this example, we restrict our attention to patients undergoing a single procedure, 36.1. This procedure is for heart bypass surgery because of blocked arteries. Patients undergoing this procedure have some very severe problems; the recovery period is considerable even when there are no apparent complications. We use the following code to filter the data down, resulting in approximately 45,000 patients.

```
data work.cardiovascular;
set nis.charlson;
codecabg=0;
if (rxmatch('361',pr1)>0) then codecabg=1;
if (rxmatch('5361',pr1)>0 or rxmatch('8361',pr1)>0 or (rxmatch('9361',pr1)>0) then code-
cabg=0;
run;
data nis.cardiovascular;
set work.cardiovascular;
where codecabg=1;
run;
```

Table 1 gives the resulting frequencies.

There are not enough of 3610 and 3617 to make meaningful comparisons. However, we look at the mortality, average length of stay and charges for each of these procedures. Table 2 gives the mortality in relationship to procedure; Table 3 gives the costs.

Procedure 3619 has the highest probability of mortality; however, the range between procedures is relatively small, ranging from a low of zero to a high of 4%. Note that this 4% translates to just one patient because there are so few patients receiving the procedure. For procedure 3612, 2% translates to 296 deaths.

There is a considerable difference between the average and the maximum values. In particular, at least one patient stayed 150 days or more for procedures 3611, 3612, 3613, and 3614. As suggested here, the distribution is considerably skewed with a few patient outliers having extremely high costs. We use the following code to find the kernel density estimation functions (Figures 23 and 24).

```
proc sort data=nis.cardiovascular out=work.cardiovascular2;
by pr1;
proc kde data=work.cardiovascular2;
univar los/gridl=0 gridu=15 out=nis.kdecardlos;
```

Table 1. Frequency for 36.1 procedure

Procedure	Translation	Frequency	Percent
3610	Aortocoronary bypass for heart revascularization, not otherwise specified	8	0.02
3611	(Aorto)coronary bypass of one coronary artery	5112	11.14
3612	(Aorto)coronary bypass of two coronary arteries	13449	29.30
3613	(Aorto)coronary bypass of three coronary arteries	13176	28.70
3614	(Aorto)coronary bypass of four or more coronary arteries	7208	15.70
3615	Single internal mammary-coronary artery bypass	6419	13.98
3616	Double internal mammary-coronary artery bypass	508	1.11
3617	Abdominal - coronary artery bypass	3	0.01
3619	Other bypass anastomosis for heart revascularization	24	0.05

Table 2. Mortality by Procedure

Table of PR1 by DIED			
Principal procedure	**DIED**		**Total**
Frequency Row Pct Col Pct	**0**	**1**	
3610	8 100.00 0.02	0 0.00 0.00	8
3611	4995 97.85 11.15	110 2.15 11.09	5105
3612	13104 97.79 29.25	296 2.21 29.84	13400
3613	12860 97.82 28.70	287 2.18 28.93	13147
3614	7004 97.37 15.63	189 2.63 19.05	7193
3615	6309 98.42 14.08	101 1.58 10.18	6410
3616	500 98.43 1.12	8 1.57 0.81	508
3617	3 100.00 0.01	0 0.00 0.00	3
3619	23 95.83 0.05	1 4.17 0.10	24
Total	44806	992	45798
Frequency Missing = 109			

```
univar totchg/gridl=20000 gridu=100000 out=nis.kdecardchg bwm=.9;
by pr1;
run;
```

The costs can vary considerably by procedure, and there is also considerable variability within each procedure.

It appears that 3610 has the highest cost followed by 3619 and 3616. However, at the same time, 3610 has a small probability of a stay beyond 9 days while procedures 3615 and 3616 have a much higher probability of a length of stay beyond 12 days.

We want to examine the relationship between procedure and hospital. We want to look at a list of ten hospitals that perform cardiovascular surgery. Therefore, we pick a random list of ten hospitals that are specific to this type of surgery. Table 4 shows the relationship of hospital to procedure. It shows that there

Table 3. Length of stay and total charges by procedure

Principal procedure	N Obs	Variable	Mean	Std Dev	Minimum	Maximum
3610	8	TOTCHG LOS	65496.75 5.8750000	20519.46 1.3562027	39277.00 3.0000000	99584.00 7.0000000
3611	5112	TOTCHG LOS	90656.52 8.9047340	68257.93 7.5870299	84.0000000 0	829195.00 161.0000000
3612	13449	TOTCHG LOS	96585.12 9.3835973	73855.08 7.4754109	534.0000000 0	997836.00 153.0000000
3613	13176	TOTCHG LOS	101269.45 9.5980571	75537.11 7.3233339	2029.00 0	998991.00 188.0000000
3614	7208	TOTCHG LOS	103371.69 9.6594062	74343.53 7.4100765	839.0000000 0	918286.00 155.0000000
3615	6419	TOTCHG LOS	92813.63 8.7963857	66991.61 6.6919820	484.0000000 0	898653.00 114.0000000
3616	508	TOTCHG LOS	89716.19 8.1909449	56349.01 6.1948121	20786.00 1.0000000	461205.00 78.0000000
3617	3	TOTCHG LOS	78057.33 6.3333333	56807.84 2.3094011	43820.00 5.0000000	143632.00 9.0000000
3619	24	TOTCHG LOS	88172.17 8.0833333	56691.47 7.6437907	20741.00 1.0000000	282273.00 32.0000000

Figure 23. Length of stay by procedure

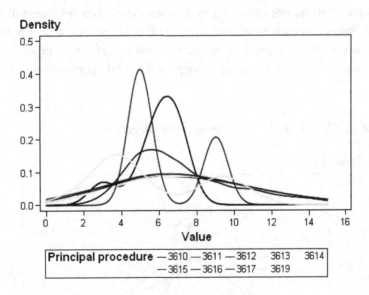

is considerable difference in the procedures performed across the hospitals. For example, #1 has over 50% of procedures identified as 3615, Single internal mammary-coronary artery bypass. The remaining hospitals are more divided in their procedures. Hospital #4 has almost 30% in 3614, (Aorto)coronary bypass of four or more coronary arteries, suggesting that it treats patients with very severe blockage in the coronary vessels. The same hospital has approximately 20% of the procedures in 3611, 3612, and 3613.

Figure 25 shows the length of stay by hospital. As shown, stay differed considerably by procedure

Figure 24. Total charges by procedure

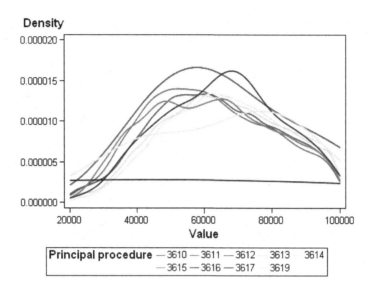

and by hospital. Hospital #6 has the greatest probability of a shorter length of stay compared to the other hospitals. Hospital #2 has the highest probability of a longer length of stay. Hospital #7 tends to be in the middle in probability for both a high and low length of stay, as is hospital #1.

Figure 26 shows the total charges compared by hospital. There is a definite shift in the curves, indicating that some hospitals charge far more compared to other hospitals, especially hospitals #3 and #9. Hospital #1 has the lowest charges, reinforcing the fact that it performs a procedure that is less risky compared to the other procedures. Interestingly, hospital #7, while performing higher risk procedures,

Figure 25. Length of stay by hospital for cardiovascular surgery

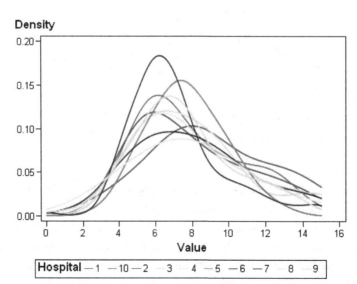

Table 4. Hospital by patient procedure

Table of DSHOSPID by PR1								
HOSPID	**PR1(Principal procedure)**							**Total**
Frequency Row Pct Col Pct	**3611**	**3612**	**3613**	**3614**	**3615**	**3616**	**3619**	
1	16 4.92 14.81	37 11.38 12.85	47 14.46 11.69	24 7.38 9.09	193 59.38 51.47	8 2.46 28.57	0 0.00 0.00	325
2	3 27.27 2.78	4 36.36 1.39	1 9.09 0.25	0 0.00 0.00	2 18.18 0.53	1 9.09 3.57	0 0.00 0.00	11
3	5 4.46 4.63	10 8.93 3.47	19 16.96 4.73	7 6.25 2.65	69 61.61 18.40	2 1.79 7.14	0 0.00 0.00	112
4	22 8.70 20.37	59 23.32 20.49	82 32.41 20.40	75 29.64 28.41	15 5.93 4.00	0 0.00 0.00	0 0.00 0.00	253
5	2 2.27 1.85	14 15.91 4.86	34 38.64 8.46	29 32.95 10.98	9 10.23 2.40	0 0.00 0.00	0 0.00 0.00	88
6	5 2.86 4.63	23 13.14 7.99	51 29.14 12.69	36 20.57 13.64	58 33.14 15.47	2 1.14 7.14	0 0.00 0.00	175
7	21 7.42 19.44	79 27.92 27.43	95 33.57 23.63	60 21.20 22.73	15 5.30 4.00	12 4.24 42.86	1 0.35 100.00	283
8	7 15.56 6.48	11 24.44 3.82	17 37.78 4.23	9 20.00 3.41	1 2.22 0.27	0 0.00 0.00	0 0.00 0.00	45
9	15 19.23 13.89	23 29.49 7.99	23 29.49 5.72	7 8.97 2.65	9 11.54 2.40	1 1.28 3.57	0 0.00 0.00	78
10	12 12.50 11.11	28 29.17 9.72	33 34.38 8.21	17 17.71 6.44	4 4.17 1.07	2 2.08 7.14	0 0.00 0.00	96
Total	108	288	402	264	375	28	1	1466

also tends to charge a lower amount.

Next, we examine the length of stay by procedure for a specific hospital. We contrast hospital #7 to hospital #6. For hospital #6, there is a natural hierarchy that demonstrates the severity of each of the procedures. We restrict our attention to hospital #6 in Figure 27. Procedure 3613 has the highest probability of a long length of stay. Procedures 3611 and 3616 have the highest probability of a short length of stay. Figure 27 shows the length of stay for hospital #7. Figures 28 and 29 show additional hospitals.

First, hospital #6 does only four of the procedures. In contrast to hospital #7, where procedure 3611 has the lowest probability of a low length of stay, procedure 3613 has the highest probability of a low length of stay in hospital #6. The ordering of the procedures is completely different for the two hospitals. We do a final examination in Figure 29 for hospital #1.

In Figure 29, it is clear that procedure 3612 has the highest probability of a long length of stay while

Figure 26. Total charges by hospital for cardiovascular surgery

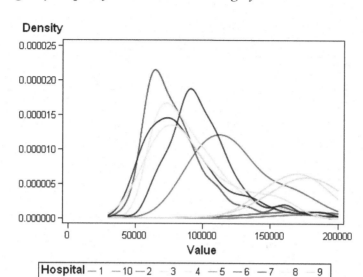

Figure 27. Length of stay for hospital #6 by procedure

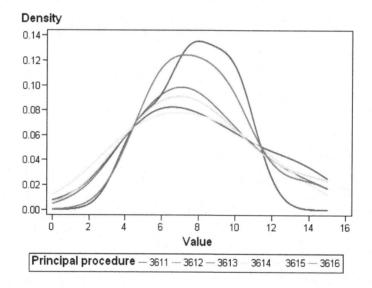

3611 has a high probability of a short length of stay. In other words, we have three different hospitals and they have three very different graphs, indicating that there is almost no relationship between procedure and length of stay when comparing the different hospitals.

Figure 28. Length of stay for hospital #7 by procedure

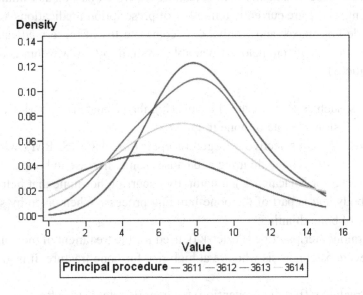

Figure 29. Length of stay for hospital #1 by procedure

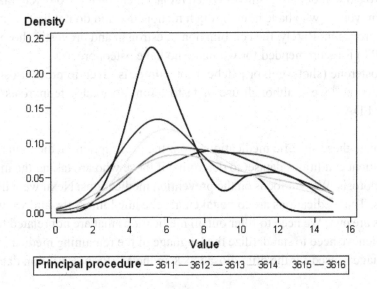

PATIENT COMPLIANCE AND DATA SUMMARIES

Although patient compliance is an important issue in investigating treatment outcomes, it is currently excluded from defining patient severity indices because of the difficulty in computing the level of compliance. We will demonstrate here how data visualization can be used to examine compliance levels. In this section, we use data summaries and data preprocessing to investigate a prescription database. Summaries can be useful when investigating trends in the dataset. For this example, we will use the MEPS data and the prescriptions file. For this analysis, we restrict our attention to the year 2005. We will consider the special case of patients with osteoporosis, which has a small number of medications available for treatment. There are currently a number of prescription medications available to treat the disease. These include Fosamax® and Boniva®. A complete list of these medications used for both treatment and prevention is given below (available from http://www.webmd.com/osteoporosis/tc/osteoporosis-medications):

- Bisphosphonates, such as alendronate (Fosamax®), ibandronate (Boniva®), and zoledronic acid (Reclast®), which slow the rate of bone thinning.
- Raloxifene (Evista®®), a selective estrogen receptor modulator (SERM), which is used only in women. Raloxifene slows bone thinning and causes some increase in bone thickness.
- Calcitonin (Calcimar or Miacalcin®), a naturally occurring hormone that helps regulate calcium levels in your body and is part of the bone-building process. When taken by shot or nasal spray, it slows the rate of bone thinning.
- Parathyroid hormone (teriparatide [Forteo®]), used for the treatment of men and postmenopausal women with severe osteoporosis who are at high risk for bone fracture. It is given by injection.

Medications for treatment (but not prevention) have more potent side effects:

- Estrogen. Estrogen without progestin (estrogen replacement therapy, or ERT) may be used to treat osteoporosis in women who have gone through menopause and do not have a uterus.
- Estrogen and progestin. Rarely, the combination of estrogen and progestin (hormone replacement therapy, or HRT) is recommended for women who have osteoporosis.
- For men, testosterone (shots, gel, or patches) sometimes is given to prevent osteoporosis caused by low testosterone levels, although use of testosterone to treat osteoporosis has not been approved by the FDA.

We will first isolate these specific medications from the prescription medications dataset. Then we will examine the patient conditions dataset to determine if those who are taking the medications have a diagnosis for osteoporosis. We will focus on the prevention medications. Next, we will look at the number of prescriptions. The medications are to be taken at scheduled intervals, and we want to determine whether these goals are met. We need to filter out all medications that are not related to the treatment of osteoporosis, and then we need to standardize the language of the remaining medications. For example, the following language is used for the drug, Fosamax® in the MEPS prescription database:

```
FOSAMAX (UNIT OF USE)
FOSAMAX (UNIT OF USE,BLISTER PCK)
FOSAMAX (UNIT OF USE,BLISTER PK)
```

The above three medications are relabeled simply, "Fosamax®". To preprocess the MEPS dataset HC94a of prescription medications, we use the following SAS code:

```
PROC SQL;
CREATE TABLE SASUSER.Query_for_Query_for_h94a AS SELECT QUERY_FOR_H94A.DUID,
QUERY_FOR_H94A.PID,
```

```
QUERY_FOR_H94A.DUPERSID,
QUERY_FOR_H94A.RXRECIDX,
QUERY_FOR_H94A.LINKIDX,
QUERY_FOR_H94A.PANEL,
QUERY_FOR_H94A.PURCHRD,
QUERY_FOR_H94A.RXBEGDD,
QUERY_FOR_H94A.RXBEGMM,
QUERY_FOR_H94A.RXBEGYRX,
QUERY_FOR_H94A.RXNAME,
QUERY_FOR_H94A.RXNDC,
QUERY_FOR_H94A.RXQUANTY,
QUERY_FOR_H94A.RXFORM,
QUERY_FOR_H94A.RXFRMUNT,
QUERY_FOR_H94A.RXSTRENG,
QUERY_FOR_H94A.RXSTRUNT,
QUERY_FOR_H94A.PHARTP1,
QUERY_FOR_H94A.PHARTP2,
QUERY_FOR_H94A.PHARTP3,
QUERY_FOR_H94A.PHARTP4,
QUERY_FOR_H94A.PHARTP5,
QUERY_FOR_H94A.PHARTP6,
QUERY_FOR_H94A.PHARTP7,
QUERY_FOR_H94A.PHARTP8,
QUERY_FOR_H94A.PHARTP9,
QUERY_FOR_H94A.RXFLG,
QUERY_FOR_H94A.PCIMPFLG,
QUERY_FOR_H94A.CLMOMFLG,
QUERY_FOR_H94A.INPCFLG,
QUERY_FOR_H94A.SAMPLE,
QUERY_FOR_H94A.RXICD1X,
QUERY_FOR_H94A.RXICD2X,
QUERY_FOR_H94A.RXICD3X,
QUERY_FOR_H94A.RXCCC1X,
QUERY_FOR_H94A.RXCCC2X,
QUERY_FOR_H94A.RXCCC3X,
QUERY_FOR_H94A.PREGCAT,
QUERY_FOR_H94A.TC1,
QUERY_FOR_H94A.TC1S1,
QUERY_FOR_H94A.TC1S1_1,
QUERY_FOR_H94A.TC1S1_2,
QUERY_FOR_H94A.TC1S2,
QUERY_FOR_H94A.TC1S2_1,
QUERY_FOR_H94A.TC1S3,
QUERY_FOR_H94A.TC1S3_1,
```

```
    QUERY_FOR_H94A.TC2,
    QUERY_FOR_H94A.TC2S1,
    QUERY_FOR_H94A.TC2S1_1,
    QUERY_FOR_H94A.TC2S1_2,
    QUERY_FOR_H94A.TC2S2,
    QUERY_FOR_H94A.TC3,
    QUERY_FOR_H94A.TC3S1,
    QUERY_FOR_H94A.TC3S1_1,
    QUERY_FOR_H94A.RXSF05X,
    QUERY_FOR_H94A.RXMR05X,
    QUERY_FOR_H94A.RXMD05X,
    QUERY_FOR_H94A.RXPV05X,
    QUERY_FOR_H94A.RXVA05X,
    QUERY_FOR_H94A.RXTR05X,
    QUERY_FOR_H94A.RXOF05X,
    QUERY_FOR_H94A.RXSL05X,
    QUERY_FOR_H94A.RXWC05X,
    QUERY_FOR_H94A.RXOT05X,
    QUERY_FOR_H94A.RXOR05X,
    QUERY_FOR_H94A.RXOU05X,
    QUERY_FOR_H94A.RXXP05X,
    QUERY_FOR_H94A.PERWT05F,
    QUERY_FOR_H94A.VARSTR,
    QUERY_FOR_H94A.VARPSU,
    ((CASE WHEN "ACTONEL" = QUERY_FOR_H94A.RXNAME THEN "Actonel" WHEN "ACTONEL
(DOSEPACK,FILM-COATED)" = QUERY_FOR_H94A.RXNAME THEN "Actonel" WHEN "ACTONEL (FILM-COAT-
ED)" = QUERY_FOR_H94A.RXNAME THEN "Actonel" WHEN "BONIVA" = QUERY_FOR_H94A.RXNAME THEN
"Boniva" WHEN "BONIVA (FILM-COATED)" = QUERY_FOR_H94A.RXNAME THEN "Boniva" WHEN "CALCI-
TONIN SALMON" = QUERY_FOR_H94A.RXNAME THEN "Calcitonin" WHEN "ESTROGEN CON" = QUERY_FOR_
H94A.RXNAME THEN "Estrogen" WHEN "ESTROGEN CONJUGATED" = QUERY_FOR_H94A.RXNAME THEN "Es-
trogen" WHEN "ESTROGENS" = QUERY_FOR_H94A.RXNAME THEN "Estrogen" WHEN "ESTROGENS CONJ"
= QUERY_FOR_H94A.RXNAME THEN "Estrogen" WHEN "ESTROGENS CONJUGATED" = QUERY_FOR_H94A.
RXNAME THEN "Estrogen" WHEN "ESTROGENS, CONJ." = QUERY_FOR_H94A.RXNAME THEN "Estrogen"
WHEN "ESTROGENS, CONJUGATED CR" = QUERY_FOR_H94A.RXNAME THEN "Estrogen" WHEN "EVISTA" =
QUERY_FOR_H94A.RXNAME THEN "Evista" WHEN "EVISTA (UNIT OF USE)" = QUERY_FOR_H94A.RX-
NAME THEN "Evista" WHEN "FORTEO" = QUERY_FOR_H94A.RXNAME THEN "Forteo" WHEN "FOSAMAX" =
QUERY_FOR_H94A.RXNAME THEN "Fosamax" WHEN "FOSAMAX (RASPBERRY)" = QUERY_FOR_H94A.RXNAME
THEN "Fosamax" WHEN "FOSAMAX (UNIT OF USE)" = QUERY_FOR_H94A.RXNAME THEN "Fosamax" WHEN
"FOSAMAX (UNIT OF USE,BLISTER PCK)" = QUERY_FOR_H94A.RXNAME THEN "Fosamax" WHEN "FOSAMAX
(UNIT OF USE,BLISTER PK)" = QUERY_FOR_H94A.RXNAME THEN "Fosamax" WHEN "FOSAMAX PLUS D" =
QUERY_FOR_H94A.RXNAME THEN "Fosamax" ELSE QUERY_FOR_H94A.RXNAME END)) AS RevisedRXName
FROM SASUSER.QUERY_FOR_H94A AS QUERY_FOR_H94A;
QUIT;
```

Fosamax® is generally used once weekly, so there are four tablets prescribed for a month with 12 prescriptions a year if the patient is taking the medication properly. Once the data have been preprocessed, we can examine the relationship of medication to patient prescriptions and to the quantity of doses in the prescription. Table 5 shows the number of pills given for a prescription dose of Actonel®.

Almost 80% of the patients receive a 30-day supply with 9.5% receiving less than a 30-day supply and 4% receiving a 90-day supply. Because of the standard dispensing practices, the 30-day and 90-day prescriptions should be the norm in the dataset. If we limit our analysis to these patients, omitting the remaining as perhaps in error, we can examine whether these patients are complying by looking at the total number of prescriptions in a year. For Boniva®, which is taken once a month, 22 patients receive 1 dose, 14 receive 2 doses, and 2 receive 3 doses in the prescription. Similarly, Table 6 shows the number of doses for the drug, Fosamax®.

The values of 30, 69, and 300 seem excessive. However, while Fosamax® is most commonly taken once a week, there is a daily version of 10 mg, and the patients beyond 12 doses are probably taking that version. Otherwise, the most common prescriptions are for a 30-day supply (4 pills) and a 90-day supply (12 pills). Prescriptions for other medications are much more scattered, making it more difficult to examine patient compliance.

Given the above information, we next want to examine the total number of doses by patient. One of the difficulties in this dataset is that the RXSTRENG variable is character rather than numeric. The reason for this is because liquid doses are given as a ratio of drug to medium, where the medium is usually some type of saline or dextrose solution. Since we are working with a medication that is almost always given by mouth, we want to remove all non-tablet formulations, and convert the column to numeric. Then we can consider the sum of the quantities, where the sum is taken over all of the prescriptions for any one patient. We can also compute the average number of doses per prescription, and the number of prescriptions in the year to examine the level of patient compliance. Another consideration is that Fosamax® is generally taken once a week, but the 10 mg dose is taken daily. Therefore, when we consider patient compliance, we will need to separate Fosamax® by dose. We use the following code to investigate the total medication prescribed over the one year period of 2005:

Table 5. Number of pills per prescription for Actonel®

Number of Pills	Frequency	Percent of Prescriptions
1	26	2.61
2	18	1.81
3	51	5.12
4	794	79.72
5	9	0.90
8	6	0.60
9	5	0.50
12	39	3.92
20	2	0.20
24	1	0.10
30	35	3.51
90	10	1.00

Table 6. Number of pills per prescription for Fosamax®

Number of Pills	Frequency	Percent of Prescriptions
1	263	13.09
2	109	5.43
3	71	3.53
4	1150	57.24
5	12	0.60
6	3	0.15
7	10	0.50
8	32	1.59
9	60	2.99
12	243	12.10
30	47	2.34
69	4	0.20
300	5	0.25

```
Proc sort data=meps.osteoporosis;
By revisedrxname rxstreng dupersid;
PROC MEANS DATA=meps.osteoporosis;
     NOPRINT
     CHARTYPE
     NWAY
     VARDEF=DF
          MEAN
          STD
          MIN
          MAX
          SUM
          N ;
     VAR RXQUANTY;
     CLASS RevisedRXName / ORDER=UNFORMATTED ASCENDING;
     CLASS RXSTRENG / ORDER=UNFORMATTED ASCENDING;
     CLASS DUPERSID / ORDER=UNFORMATTED ASCENDING;
     OUTPUT OUT=SASUSER.MEANSUMMARYSTATSSUMMARYOFHC_0000(LABEL="Summary Statistics for
ECLIB000.SUMMARYOFHC94A")
          MEAN()=
          STD()=
          MIN()=
          MAX()=
          SUM()=
```

Table 7. Summary of yearly prescriptions

RevisedRXName	STRENGTH OF MED DOSE	N Obs	Mean	Std Dev	Minimum	Maximum
Actonel®	30	6	36.0000000	18.2428068	24.0000000	72.0000000
	35	153	24.9738562	17.8129712	1.0000000	96.0000000
	5	8	246.7500000	288.3825584	30.0000000	900.0000000
Boniva®	150	18	3.1111111	2.5870467	1.0000000	11.0000000
Calcitonin	200	1	6.0000000	.	6.0000000	6.0000000
Estrogen	-9	7	78.9285714	51.6368962	42.5000000	170.0000000
	0.3	18	132.0000000	137.6889077	21.0000000	484.0000000
	0.625	9	169.5555556	113.8322352	12.0000000	360.0000000
Evista®	60	105	241.4761905	196.4417165	11.0000000	864.0000000
Forteo®	250	1	12.0000000	.	12.0000000	12.0000000
	750/3	6	14.6666667	9.9732977	1.0000000	25.0000000
Fosamax®	-9	2	20.0000000	22.6274170	4.0000000	36.0000000
	10	8	187.8750000	173.9609459	6.0000000	450.0000000
	35	46	20.6521739	14.5559723	3.0000000	60.0000000
	5	1	210.0000000	.	210.0000000	210.0000000
	70	320	25.2281250	25.4043382	1.0000000	156.0000000
	70/2800	6	10.6666667	6.0221812	4.0000000	20.0000000
	70/75	1	1500.00	.	1500.00	1500.00

```
     N()=
  / AUTONAME AUTOLABEL WAYS INHERIT
   ;
RUN;
```

The results are summarized in Table 7.

The average sum of doses does not appear to be close to full compliance, which should be 52 doses for the once-per-week medications, and 12 for the once-per-month Boniva®. However, the maximum value of the total prescriptions is much larger than would be expected from full compliance, suggesting that physicians are increasing the dose for some patients.

However, to define a compliance level and to examine the prescribed dose, we also use kernel density estimation. For Actonel® weekly, Figure 30 gives the kernel density at two different dose levels.

Note that the trends in the two doses are very different. For the 30 mg dose, the peak is for 30 doses in a year, but is starting to increase to 60 doses in a year. This indicates that there is a small portion of the patient population that is complying with their medication. However, in the 35 mg dose, there is a peak at 15 doses in a year and a second peak at 30 doses in a year; however, after that point, the probability in the number of doses declines. Figure 31 gives a 5 mg dose of Actonel®, to be taken daily. The trend is almost identical to that of the 30 mg dose. However, one dose per day for 365 doses in a year has a significant amount of probability. Patients who have 600 doses are taking 2 doses in a day.

Figure 30. Number of doses in a year for Actonel®

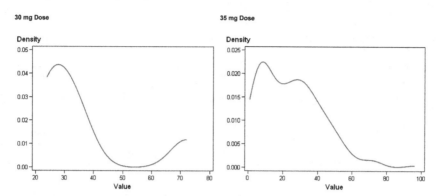

Figure 31. Number of doses in a year for Actonel® daily at 5 mg level

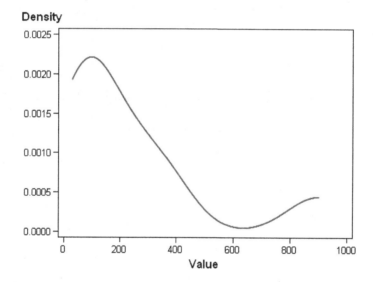

Similarly, we can examine two different doses for Fosamax® at 35 mg and 70 mg. Again, there is a difference in the pattern (Figure 32).

For the 70 mg dose, the peak occurs at 15 doses, and decreases until the probability is virtually zero at 70 doses. In contrast, at the 35 mg dose, there are two peaks; one occurs at 10 doses and a second one occurs at 30 doses, decreasing to 60 doses, which is the maximum number at 30 mg. Figure 33 gives the trend for the 10 mg, daily dose requirement.

This curve, too, has a double peak; the first at 80 doses and the second at 350 doses. The second peak indicates full compliance with the medication. Figure 34 gives the graph for the medication, Boniva®.

There still appears to be an issue with compliance since there should be a total of 12 doses in a year. However, the maximum number of doses is 11. Similarly, Figure 35 gives the distribution for the drug, Evista®.

The pattern is exactly the same as some of the previous patterns in that the major peak occurs at 190

Figure 32. Number of doses in a year for Fosamax®

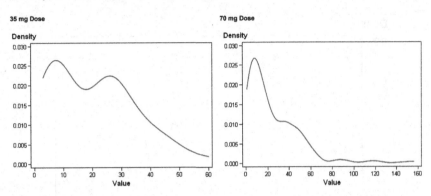

Figure 33. Number of doses in a year for Fosamax® daily at 10 mg level

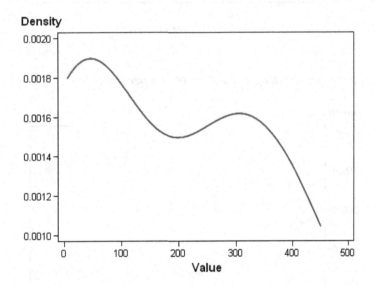

doses with a smaller peak at 380 doses. At once a day, the second peak indicates patient compliance with medication requirements. There is one remaining medication we considered, that of estrogen. Figure 36 gives two different doses.

The dose peaks are very different. For the 0.625 dose, it occurs at 200 doses; for the 0.3 dose, it occurs at 100 doses. There appears to be more compliance at the higher dose.

Once we have these distributions, we can define a level of compliance. We can divide the curve into quantiles, or we can define it in terms of a percentage of full compliance. For example, a patient who is prescribed 20 doses of Fosamax® when 52 are needed can be defined as 20/52=38% compliant.

Whereas estrogen can be prescribed for many different patient complaints, the remaining drugs are prescribed solely for osteoporosis. We need to consider the patient conditions from the MEPS that are listed in the prescription medications datafile. Therefore, we consider the ICD9 codes that are associated with each of the medications. For Actonel®, there are 646 (out of a total of 996) primary codes given as 733, or Other disorders of bone and cartilage. The specific codes for osteoporosis are 733.01 (Senile

Figure 34. Number of doses in a year for Boniva® monthly at 150 mg dose

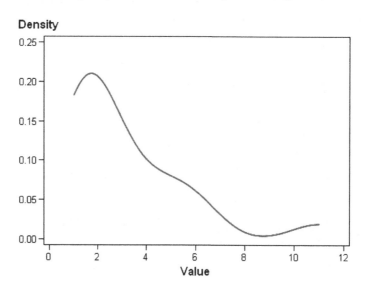

Figure 35. Number of doses for the drug Evista® at 60 mg per dose

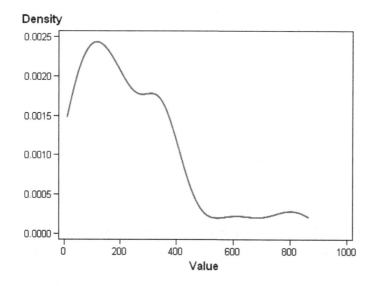

osteoporosis or postmenopausal osteoporosis), V17.81 (Osteoporosis), 733.02 (Idiopathic osteoporosis), 733.03 (Disuse osteoporosis), 733.0 (Osteoporosis), and 733.00 (Osteoporosis, unspecified). However, there are other primary patient conditions listed for Actonel® that include 714 (Rheumatoid arthritis and other inflammatory polyarthropathies), 715 (Osteoarthrosis and allied disorders), 716 (Other and unspecified arthropathies), 718 (Other derangement of joint), and 719 (Other and unspecified disorders of joint). Actonel® is not approved for arthritis and is not considered effective for its treatment. It is possible that arthritis is primary and osteoporosis is secondary. However, 733 is not listed as a secondary

Figure 36. Number of doses for the drug, Estrogen

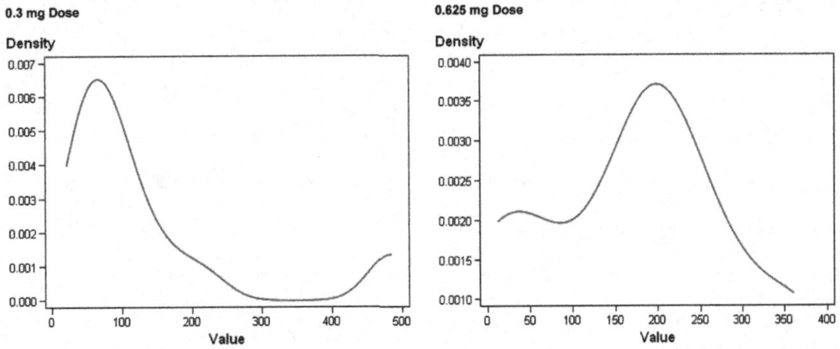

ICD9 code for Actonel®. Either the Actonel® is misprescribed, or the ICD9 code is inappropriately listed.

Evista® similarly has 296 out of 690 primary ICD9 codes listed as 733, but unlike Actonel®, it has 5 secondary codes also listed as 733. While there are also diagnoses listed for arthritis (715-716), there are 88 primary codes for V68 (Encounters for administrative purposes). This code suggests that the purpose of the encounter was to write a new prescription for a recurring medication. For Fosamax®, there are 1531 primary codes out of 2009 for osteoporosis. There are an additional 88 primary codes for arthritis, 46 primary codes for V68, and 61 for V82 (Special screening for other conditions). In contrast, none of the primary codes for estrogen are for osteoporosis or arthritis. The primary code listed is for 627 (Menopausal and postmenopausal disorders). It suggests that the estrogen prescriptions are not for osteoporosis.

Finally, we want to examine the relationship of patient compliance to hospital outcomes. We want to consider whether patients taking these medications have any fractures, particularly hip or ankle fractures, that may have resulted from osteoporosis. Then we can include patient compliance in addition to patient severity to examine these outcomes. We merge the medications dataset to the inpatients dataset. A similar merge to the outpatient dataset is done in the same manner.

```
PROC SQL;
  CREATE TABLE SASUSER.QUERY1_FOR_SUMMARY_STATISTI_0001 AS SELECT MEANSUMMARYSTATSSUMMA-
RYOFHC_00.RevisedRXName,
    MEANSUMMARYSTATSSUMMARYOFHC_00.RXSTRENG,
    MEANSUMMARYSTATSSUMMARYOFHC_00.DUPERSID,
    MEANSUMMARYSTATSSUMMARYOFHC_00._WAY_,
    MEANSUMMARYSTATSSUMMARYOFHC_00._TYPE_,
    MEANSUMMARYSTATSSUMMARYOFHC_00._FREQ_,
    MEANSUMMARYSTATSSUMMARYOFHC_00.RXQUANTY_Mean,
    MEANSUMMARYSTATSSUMMARYOFHC_00.RXQUANTY_StdDev,
    MEANSUMMARYSTATSSUMMARYOFHC_00.RXQUANTY_Min,
    MEANSUMMARYSTATSSUMMARYOFHC_00.RXQUANTY_Max,
    MEANSUMMARYSTATSSUMMARYOFHC_00.RXQUANTY_Sum,
    MEANSUMMARYSTATSSUMMARYOFHC_00.RXQUANTY_N,
    h94f.DUID,
```

```
h94f.PID,
h94f.DUPERSID AS DUPERSID1,
h94f.EVNTIDX,
h94f.EVENTRN,
h94f.FFEEIDX,
h94f.PANEL,
h94f.MPCDATA,
h94f.OPDATEYR,
h94f.OPDATEMM,
h94f.OPDATEDD,
h94f.SEETLKPV,
h94f.SEEDOC,
h94f.DRSPLTY,
h94f.MEDPTYPE,
h94f.VSTCTGRY,
h94f.VSTRELCN,
h94f.PHYSTH,
h94f.OCCUPTH,
h94f.SPEECHTH,
h94f.CHEMOTH,
h94f.RADIATTH,
h94f.KIDNEYD,
h94f.IVTHER,
h94f.DRUGTRT,
h94f.RCVSHOT,
h94f.PSYCHOTH,
h94f.LABTEST,
h94f.SONOGRAM,
h94f.XRAYS,
h94f.MAMMOG,
h94f.MRI,
h94f.EKG,
h94f.EEG,
h94f.RCVVAC,
h94f.ANESTH,
h94f.OTHSVCE,
h94f.SURGPROC,
h94f.MEDPRESC,
h94f.VAPLACE,
h94f.OPICD1X,
h94f.OPICD2X,
h94f.OPICD3X,
h94f.OPICD4X,
h94f.OPPRO1X,
```

```
      h94f:OPPRO2X,
      h94f.OPCCC1X,
      h94f.OPCCC2X,
      h94f.OPCCC3X,
      h94f.OPCCC4X,
      h94f.FFOPTYPE,
      h94f.FFBEF05,
      h94f.FFTOT06,
      h94f.OPXP05X,
      h94f.OPTC05X,
      h94f.OPFSF05X,
      h94f.OPFMR05X,
      h94f.OPFMD05X,
      h94f.OPFPV05X,
      h94f.OPFVA05X,
      h94f.OPFTR05X,
      h94f.OPFOF05X,
      h94f.OPFSL05X,
      h94f.OPFWC05X,
      h94f.OPFOR05X,
      h94f.OPFOU05X,
      h94f.OPFOT05X,
      h94f.OPFXP05X,
      h94f.OPFTC05X,
      h94f.OPDSF05X,
      h94f.OPDMR05X,
      h94f.OPDMD05X,
      h94f.OPDPV05X,
      h94f.OPDVA05X,
      h94f.OPDTR05X,
      h94f.OPDOF05X,
      h94f.OPDSL05X,
      h94f.OPDWC05X,
      h94f.OPDOR05X,
      h94f.OPDOU05X,
      h94f.OPDOT05X,
      h94f.OPDXP05X,
      h94f.OPDTC05X,
      h94f.IMPFLAG,
      h94f.PERWT05F,
      h94f.VARSTR,
      h94f.VARPSU
FROM SASUSER.MEANSUMMARYSTATSSUMMARYOFHC_0000 AS MEANSUMMARYSTATSSUMMARYOFHC_00
   LEFT JOIN EC100008.H94F AS h94f ON (MEANSUMMARYSTATSSUMMARYOFHC_00.DUPERSID = h94f.
```

```
DUPERSID);
WHERE QUERY_FOR_SUMMARY_STATISTIC_00.IPICD1X IN ("808", "812", "820", "821", "822",
"824", "827") OR QUERY_FOR_SUMMARY_STATISTIC_00.IPICD2X IN ("805", "812") OR QUERY_FOR_
SUMMARY_STATISTIC_00.IPICD3X IN ("807", "814");
QUIT;
```

Table 8 lists the inpatients with fractures who are taking medications for osteoporosis.

With the exception of patients #6 and 12, these patients are on the high end of the number of doses. It suggests that patients with osteoporosis, and patients who have broken bones because of it are more diligent in taking their medication compared to patients who are taking it as a preventative medication. We can see if this remains the case for outpatient visits for fractures (Table 9).

There is a red flag on the 156 doses of Fosamax®. These patients are getting far more than is reasonable, and their physicians are ignoring prescription guidelines. And yet, it is very interesting that patients with fractures and problems related to osteoporosis are the ones taking the high doses. It would be of interest to determine whether patients who are taking the medications just as a preventative measure to avoid osteoporosis are the ones with limited compliance compared to patients who already have the disease, and who have complications related to the disease. It is said that "an ounce of prevention is worth a pound of cure". However, if the patients don't accept the prevention, it will do little good.

FUTURE TRENDS

Kernel density remains a rarely used technique in the medical literature to investigate population distributions. One of the reasons for this is that few statistical software packages include it as a technique. When it is used in a Medline article (an article in a medical journal indexed by Medline as provided by

Table 8. Osteoporosis medications by inpatient fractures

Row number	Revised RXName	STRENGTH OF Rx/ PRESCR MED DOSE	QUANTITY OF Rx/ PRESCR MED_Sum	3-DIGIT ICD-9-CM CODE	3-DIGIT ICD-9-CM CODE	3-DIGIT ICD-9-CM CODE
1	Actonel®	35	12	821	-1	-1
2	Actonel®	35	12	821	-1	-1
3	Fosamax®	70	90	822	-1	-1
4	Evista®	60	150	724	733	807
5	Actonel®	35	24	827	-1	-1
6	Fosamax®	70	4	808	922	-1
7	Fosamax®	70	28	820	707	-1
8	Fosamax®	70	12	041	805	787
9	Fosamax®	70	8	824	-1	-1
10	Fosamax®	35	24	824	-1	-1
11	Actonel®	35	12	812	-1	-1
12	Fosamax®	70	4	820	812	814

the National Library of Medicine), it is usually in a technical, non-clinical journal to show improvements in the methodology (Hong, Chen, & Harris, 2008; Pfeiffer, 1985), or in DNA studies. (Fu, Borneman, Ye, & Chrobak, 2005)

Nevertheless, medicine must and will focus more on the study of outlier patients; that is, to investigate patients with extreme conditions instead of focusing just on the average or typical patient. Outlier patient costs can often overwhelm the system even when they form just a small percentage of the total number of patients. However, a keyword search of the term "outlier" in Medline returned just 188 articles total. Most of the returned papers had to do with outlier lab results and quality control (Ahrens, 1999; Novis, Walsh, Dale, & Howanitz, 2004) rather than with patients with extreme treatment needs. Just a handful of papers discussed outlier physician performance. (Harley, Mohammed, Hussain, Yates, & Almasri, 2005)

Exactly one paper considered length of stay and the term, 'outlier'. It examined the length of stay of patients in the intensive care unit; all of the patients in ICU can be considered extreme or outlier.(Weissman, 1997) This paper clearly demonstrated the problem of assuming a normal distribution and estimating averages when the data were clearly skewed. The paper also showed that any current method used to define outliers tended to under-estimate the number of outliers, and the extremes in the added costs of outliers. This result was confirmed in a dissertation on costs and outliers.(Battioui, 2007) Therefore, future trends can only go in the direction of more concern for the impact of the outlier, or most severe patients.

Table 9. Osteoporosis medications by outpatient fractures

Row number	RevisedRXName	STRENGTH OF Rx/PRESCR MED DOSE)	QUANTITY OF Rx/PRESCR MED _Sum	3-DIGIT ICD-9-CM CODE	3-DIGIT ICD-9-CM CODE	3-DIGIT ICD-9-CM CODE
1	Fosamax®	35	4	805	-1	-1
2	Fosamax®	70	12	825	-1	-1
3	Fosamax®	70	156	824	-1	-1
4	Fosamax®	70	156	824	-1	-1
5	Fosamax®	70	156	824	-1	-1
6	Fosamax®	70	156	824	-1	-1
7	Fosamax®	70	156	824	-1	-1
8	Fosamax®	70	156	824	-1	-1
9	Fosamax®	70	156	824	-1	-1
10	Fosamax®	70	156	824	-1	-1
11	Fosamax®	70	156	824	-1	-1
12	Fosamax®	70	156	824	-1	-1
13	Fosamax®	70	156	824	-1	-1
14	Fosamax®	70	156	824	-1	-1
15	Actonel®	30	32	823	-1	-1
16	Actonel®	30	32	823	-1	-1
17	Actonel®	30	32	823	-1	-1
18	Fosamax®	70	4	820	812	814
19	Fosamax®	70	4	820	812	814

DISCUSSION

Kernel density estimation to investigate the entire population distribution is important in a healthcare setting where the distribution is usually not normally distributed. It can be used to examine segments of the population rather than to focus on averages as most traditional statistical methods do currently. We need to examine the costs and demands that are related to the most extreme patients.

Kernel density estimation also allows use to compare subgroups within the population because we can overlay the curves on the same set of axis. As such, it is superior to the use of bar graphs, which depend upon side-by-side comparisons. It is extremely flexible as a technique and can be used to examine a variety of outcome measures, including length of stay, cost, and patient compliance.

REFERENCES

Ahrens, T. (1999). Outlier management. Influencing the highest resource-consuming areas in acute and critical care. *Critical Care Nursing Clinics of North America, 11*(1), 107–116.

Anonymous-kde. (2008). *Kernel Density Estimators* [Electronic Version]. Retrieved from http://homepages.inf.ed.ac.uk/rbf/CVonline/LOCAL_COPIES/AV0405/MISHRA/kde.html.

Anonymous-simpson. (2008). *Simpson's Rule* [Electronic Version]. Retrieved 2008 from http://mathworld.wolfram.com/SimpsonsRule.html.

Battioui, C. (2007). *Cost Models with Prominent Outliers.* University of Louisville, Louisville, USA.

Fu, Q., Borneman, J., Ye, J., & Chrobak, M. (2005). *Improved probe selection for DNA arrays using nonparametric kernel density estimation.* Paper presented at the Annual International Conference of the IEEE Engineering in Medicine & Biology Society, Shanghai, China.

Harley, M., Mohammed, M. A., Hussain, S., Yates, J., & Almasri, A. (2005). Was Rodney Ledward a statistical outlier? Retrospective analysis using routine hospital data to identify gynaecologists' performance. *BMJ (Clinical Research Ed.), 330*(7497), 929.

Hong, X., Chen, S., & Harris, C. J. (2008). A forward-constrained regression algorithm for sparse kernel density estimation. *IEEE Transactions on Neural Networks, 19*(1), 193–198.

Novis, D., Walsh, M. K., Dale, J. C., & Howanitz, P. J. (2004). Continuous monitoring of stat and routine outlier turnaround times: two College of American Pathologists Q-Tracks monitors in 291 hospitals. *Archives of Pathology & Laboratory Medicine, 128*(6), 621–626.

Pfeiffer, K. (1985). Stepwise variable selection and maximum likelihood estimation of smoothing factors of kernel functions for nonparametric discriminant functions evaluated by different criteria. *Computers and Biomedical Research, an International Journal, 18*(1), 46–61.

Silverman, B. W. (1986). *Density Estimation for Statistics and Data Analysis (Monographs on Statistics and Applied Probability.* Boca Raton, FL: Chapman & Hall/CRC.

Weissman, C. (1997). Analyzing intensive care unit length of stay data: problems and possible solutions. *Critical Care Medicine, 25*(9), 1594–1600.

Chapter 3
Statistical Methods

INTRODUCTION

Ultimately, a patient severity index is used to compare patient outcomes across healthcare providers. If the outcome is mortality, logistic regression is used. If the outcome is cost, length of stay, or some other resource utilization, then linear regression is used. A provider is ranked based upon the differential between predicted outcome and actual outcome. The greater this differential, the higher the quality ranking. There are two ways to increase this differential. The first is to improve care to decrease actual mortality or length of stay. The second is to improve coding to increase the predicted mortality or length of stay. Ultimately, it is cheaper to increase the predicted values than it is to decrease the actual values. Many providers take this approach.

However, there are some issues with regression itself when modeling healthcare outcomes. In particular, they require some general assumptions that are rarely satisfied; in many cases, these assumptions are known to be false. All start with an assumption of a random sample. In using billing data, just what are the variables and how can billing information have an assumption of randomness? Patient demographic information is entered into the billing data as are codes related to the patient's diagnoses, and also the procedures performed. What is considered to be random is the patient. Under general model assump-

DOI: 10.4018/978-1-60566-752-2.ch003

tions, any patient is equally likely to enter any hospital to be treated. In reality, a patient usually enters a hospital where their physician has privileges, so the randomization is not complete.

Moreover, we must make the very necessary assumption that any patient's information is entered into the billing record in exactly the same way regardless of the hospital chosen. Yet this assumption is never put to the test by taking a group of patient records to multiple hospitals to see if the billing information extracted is the same. In all likelihood, if such a test were performed, the different billing records would vary considerably. In fact, it is widely known that different providers code differently.

Generally, regression models are used to define severity indices. However, a major problem with traditional statistical methods is that they assume relatively small datasets. They generally do not reach the level of 100,000 or 1 million observations that are typically in the large databases used for outcomes research. When the datasets are so large, the p-value has little meaning and cannot be used to measure the effectiveness of a statistical model; other measurements must be used instead. In this chapter, we will discuss some of the statistical methods and some of the issues with large samples. In addition, we will discuss the issue of model assumptions, and model validity.

Here, we will discuss some of the required assumptions that are involved when using both linear and logistic regression. Regression requires an assumption of normality. The definition of confidence intervals, too, requires normality. However, most healthcare data are exponential or gamma. A gamma distribution is non-symmetric with a very heavy tail. Most patients can be treated within general time guidelines; however, there will always be a few patients who need extraordinary care, which is why health outcomes have skewed, heavy tails in the data distribution. In fact, these extreme patients can overwhelm the available healthcare dollars.

BACKGROUND

Use of the Central Limit Theorem assumes that patients can be treated within 2 standard deviations of the average. However, with a heavy tail, there can be a considerable differential between these two standard deviations and 5-10 percent of the extreme patients.(Battioui, 2007a) One of the reasons for making the assumption of normal distributions is that most of our available statistical models require this assumption. What happens if the assumption of normality is not valid? What happens if the Central Limit Theorem lacks practical meaning? We must be able to work with data in the absence of these assumptions.

According to the Central Limit theorem, the sample mean can be assumed normal if the sample is sufficiently large. If the distribution is exponential, just how large is large enough? We need to examine the requirements of the Central Limit Theorem to explore the concept of large. Also, we want to examine patient-level data rather than group-level data. That will mean that we will want to include information about patient condition in any regression model. A modification of the standard regression, called the generalized linear model can assume population distributions that are not normal. This model can be used to examine gamma and exponential distributions that are often found in medical data.

Additional assumptions for regression are that the mean of the error term is equal to zero, and that the error term has equal variance for different levels of the input or independent variables. While the assumption of zero mean is almost always satisfied, the assumption of equal variance is not. Often, as the independent variables increase in value, the variance increases as well. Therefore, modifications are made to the variables, usually in the form of transformations, substituting the log of an independent variable for the variable itself in an attempt to have equal variances. Transformations require considerable experience to use properly.

Another assumption is that the independent variables are independent of each other. While the model can tolerate some correlation between these variables, too much correlation will result in a poor model that cannot be used effectively on fresh data. It will show statistical significance when such significance does not exist. A similar problem occurs if the independent variables have different range scales. If most of the variables are 0-1 indicator functions with patient's age on a scale of 0-100, the value of age will completely dominate the regression equation. The variable scales should be standardized before the model is developed, or the model will be biased.

Probably the most worrisome requirement is the assumption that the error terms are identically distributed. In order for this assumption to be valid, we must assume the uniformity of data entry. That means that all providers must use the ICD9 codes in exactly the same way. Unfortunately, such an assumption cannot possibly be valid. Consider, for example, the condition of "uncontrolled diabetes". The term, "uncontrolled" is not defined. Therefore, the designation remains at the discretion of the provider to define the term. For this reason, different providers will define it differently, and will try to define it to benefit themselves. For example, one study defined "uncontrolled" to mean that a glycated haemoglobin (A1C) was greater than 7.5%, but less than or equal to 11%, and their fasting plasma glucose (FPG) was less than or equal to 15 mmol/l.(Rosenstock et al., 2006) A second study defined it as plasma glucose over 33 mmol/l and/or venous bicarbonate less than 14 mmol/l.(Gale, Dornan, & Tattersall, 1981) More recently, the definition of uncontrolled diabetes shifted to an HbA(lc) of more than 7%. (Barnett et al., 2007)

However, in a web page designed to optimize coding rather than treatment, it states that optimizing reimbursement requires a focus on the documentation of diabetes as controlled or uncontrolled, identification of previously unrecognized diabetes, and accuracy in the specification of diabetes complications. It suggests still another definition of uncontrolled: blood glucose above 180(–200) mg/dL at admission or two or more measurements while admitted above 180(–200) mg/dL OR lesser persistent hyperglycemia outside guidelines for hospital management. For example, a fasting blood glucose above110 mg/dL and other blood glucose levels above 180 mg/dL of patients in non-critical care units, could also be considered consistent with uncontrolled diabetes.(Anonymous-uncontrolled, 2008) Note that a blood glucose above 110 will increase the proportion of patients identified as uncontrolled when a patient is not considered to have diabetes at all unless a fasting glucose exceeds 126 mg/dL, according to the American Diabetes Association. In other words, the standard for uncontrolled diabetes is now lower than the actual definition of diabetes. In fact, this provides an example of "upcoding" by taking advantage of the vagueness of the terminology to increase the number of patients identified as having a specific coded condition.

This same document also gives suggestions for assigning a diagnosis of diabetes while the patient is in the hospital. The first suggestion is a blood glucose above 200 mg/dL, but the source also suggests that the value of 126 mg/dL can be used if the attending physician so documents. It also states that such a diagnosis must be confirmed once the patient has been discharged. This same report discusses the increased revenue to the hospital if uncontrolled diabetes is better documented. For this reason of financial benefit, uniformity of data entry just cannot be assumed.

Any statistical test has four parameters: Type I error, Type II error (or power), sample size, and effect size. Specifying three of the parameters fixes the fourth. In clinical trials, a power analysis computes the sample size after first fixing Type I error, power, and effect size. The effect size is half the width of the confidence limit surrounding the hypothesized population measure. For a simple test of the mean,

Figure 1. Difference in two curves

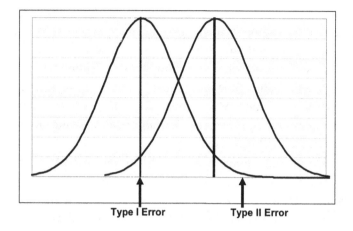

H$_0$: $\mu = \mu_0$, the effect size is equal to $\dfrac{2s}{\sqrt{n-1}}$, where s is the sample standard deviation and n is the sample size. Note that as n increases, the value of $\dfrac{2s}{\sqrt{n-1}}$ decreases so that the effect size begins to converge to zero.

Consider a simple example. The heartbeat of unborn girls tends to be higher than for unborn boys. Then Figure 1 demonstrates the situation of testing the hypotheses:

```
H₀: infant is a girl
H₁: infant is a boy
```

Each infant is a sample of size 1. The curve to the left represents the possible heartbeats for the boys; the curve to the right is for girls. We can reject the null hypothesis if the heartbeat is lower than the leftmost line in the Figure. The amount of the right curve that is to the left of that line represents the Type I error, the probability that the infant is a girl. Similarly, the amount of the left curve that is to the right of the rightmost line is the Type II error. The effect size is the distance between the two curves. It represents the portion of the curve where no decision about H$_0$ and H$_1$ can be made. In this example, since there is only one observation, the observation is equal to the sample mean. Increasing the sample size while holding the Type I and II errors fixed will decrease the effect size. However, it must be remembered that the effect size will only decrease when considering the average; any individual subject can vary considerably more than the mean.

Suppose, for example, that we want to determine whether patients with diabetes have a longer length of hospital stay and higher total charges compared to patients without diabetes. We can use different sample sizes from the National Inpatient Sample to examine this hypothesis H$_0$: $\mu_1 = \mu_2$ where group 1=patients with diabetes and group 2=patients without diabetes. With a sample of size 50 for an unpaired t-test, we get the result that the difference is not statistically significant. The confidence interval for the difference in the length of stay is (-1.819, 2.2194) and for total charges is equal to (-16,438, 6299.50). These are quite large and include the value of zero, the null hypothesis.

To compute a sample that is stratified proportionally to the occurrence of diabetes, we use the following SAS code:

```
PROC SURVEYSELECT DATA=nis.nis_with_diabetescode;
    OUT=NIS.DIABETESSAMPLE50
    METHOD=SRS
    N=50
    NOPRINT
    ;
    STRATA diabetes;
    ID LOS TOTCHG diabetes; RUN;
```

We can modify the above SAS code for different sample sizes. We use this code to generate a sample of size 200. The t-test remains not significant, but the confidence interval is considerably smaller at (-1.298, 0.5078) and (-9344, 2581). At n=1000, the confidence width shrinks even more to (-0.618,0.018) and (-3542,55.64). When n increases to 10,000, the p-values now become highly statistically significant with intervals (-0.579, -0.400) and (-4402, -3453). In other words, the effect size for length of stay is less than 0.15 of a day; the effect size for cost is approximately \$500. If the sample size is increased any more, the effect size will be smaller still. It is already so small, that while it has statistical significance, it has no real practical importance. In fact, if we used the complete data sample, the confidence intervals shrink to (-0.443, -0.429) and (-3783, -3702) for a statistically significant difference of \$80.

THE CENTRAL LIMIT THEOREM AND THE ASSUMPTION OF NORMALITY

Regression requires the assumption that the residuals are normally distributed. However, most healthcare data are exponential or gamma because of the presence of extreme outliers. The mean of a distribution is highly susceptible to the existence of outliers. Usually, it is better to truncate outliers, to use nonparametric tests based upon the median, or to use a model that accepts a skewed distribution. However, nonparametric tests still require symmetry in the distribution and also have difficulty with skewed populations.

Linear regression requires moderately large samples to be effective. Power analysis tends to assume that the population distribution is sufficiently homogeneous to be normally distributed. As healthcare outcomes tend to be exponential or gamma distributions because the populations in outcomes research are heterogeneous, we must consider just how large n has to be before the Central Limit Theorem is realistic.(Battioui, 2007b) To examine the issue, we take samples of different sizes to compute the distribution of the sample mean. The following code will compute 100 mean values from sample sizes starting with 5 and increasing to 10,000.

```
PROC SURVEYSELECT DATA=nis.nis_205 OUT=work.samples METHOD=SRS N=5 rep=100 noprint;
RUN;
proc means data=work.samples noprint;
    by replicate;
    var los;
    output out=out mean=mean;
run;
```

Figure 2. Sample mean with sample=5

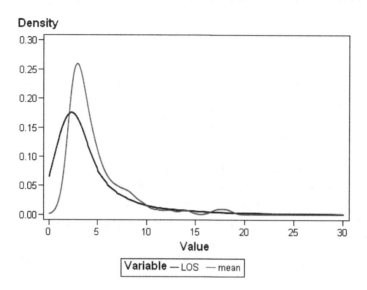

Once we have computed the means, we can graph them using kernel density estimation (a smoothed histogram). We show the difference between the distribution of the population, and the distribution of the sample mean for the differing sample sizes. Figures 2-5 show the distribution of the sample mean compared to the distribution of the population for differing sample sizes. To compute the distribution of the sample mean, we collect 100 different samples using the above code. We compute the mean for the patient length of stay using the National Inpatient Sample.

In Figure 2, the sample mean peaks slightly to the right of the peak of the population distribution; this peak is much more exaggerated in Figure 3. The reason for this shift in the peak is because the sample

Figure 3. Sample mean with sample=30

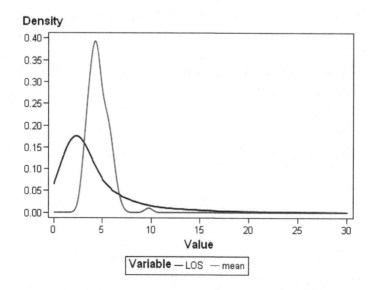

Figure 4. Sample mean with sample=100

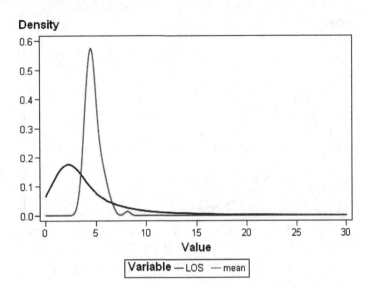

mean is susceptible to the influence of outliers, and the population is very skewed. Because it is so skewed, the distribution of the sample mean is not entirely normal. As the sample increases to 100 and then to 1000, this shift from the population peak to the sample peak becomes much more exaggerated. We use the same sample sizes for 1000 replicates (Figures 6-9).

It is again noticeable that the sample mean is shifted away from the peak value of the population distribution because of the skewed distribution. However, the distribution of the mean is not normally distributed. In other words, the sample converges on a value that is much greater than the actual population peak.

Figure 5. Sample mean with sample=1000

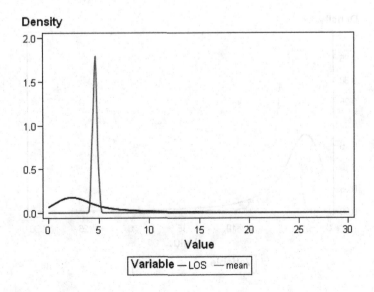

Figure 6. Sample mean for sample size=5 and 1000 replicates

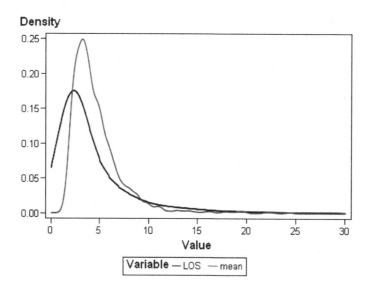

LINEAR REGRESSION

Suppose there are twenty five ICD9 conditions that are included in the linear regession to determine the relationship of patient severity to variables such as length of stay or charges (or cost). Then weights are assigned to the indicator functions. The contribution of these conditions to the linear regression is the sum of the weights of the conditions that are identified with a patient,

$$\alpha_1 X_2 + \alpha_2 X_2 + ... + \alpha_{25} X_{25}$$

Figure 7. Sample mean for sample size=30 and 1000 replicates

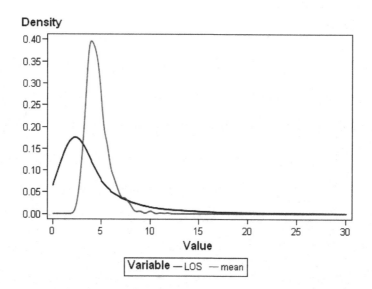

Figure 8. Sample mean for sample size=100 and 1000 replicates

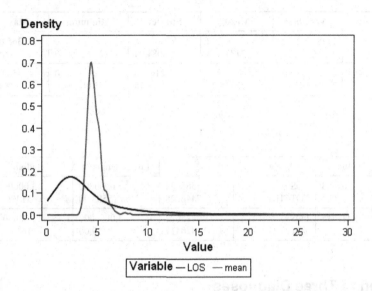

where each X is either 0 or 1 depending upon the presence or absence of an identified condition. This value will clearly increase if more values of X are one, and will increase if more of the values with the highest weights α are one. Therefore, the expected length of stay (or other outcome variable) will be predicted larger if a provider can increase the number of nonzero X's. Since a provider can receive more favorable outcomes, and increased reimbursements, the incentive to upcode is considerable.

Figure 9. Sample mean for sample size=1000 and 1000 replicates

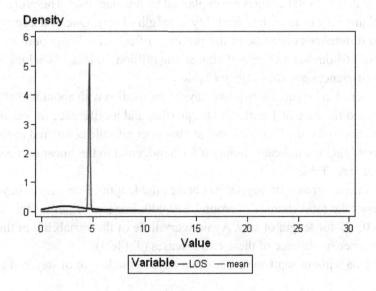

Table 1. Summary statistics for pneumonia

pneumonia	N Obs	Variable	Mean	Std Dev	Minimum	Maximum	N
0	7566548	LOS	4.4941732	6.7191416	0	365.0000000	7566151
		TOTCHG	21779.98	38084.94	25.0000000	999926.00	7443500
1	425459	LOS	7.1067977	8.6216278	0	356.0000000	425421
		TOTCHG	32528.21	53918.78	35.0000000	998514.00	420161

Table 2. Quartile values for pneumonia

pneumonia	N Obs	Variable	N	Lower Quartile	Median	Upper Quartile
0	7569333	LOS	7568934	2.0000000	3.0000000	5.0000000
		TOTCHG	7446228	5583.00	11406.00	23807.00
1	425715	LOS	425677	3.0000000	5.0000000	8.0000000
		TOTCHG	420417	8689.00	16437.00	33982.00

Example Limited to Three Diagnoses

We consider an example where the number of diagnoses is limited to 3 and where the weights, α, are equal to one. We will examine the ability of the model to predict patient outcomes.

When using very large samples, all of the p-values will be statistically significant, but of little importance. For example, we want to consider whether pneumonia will increase the length of stay and the total charges for patients. We also want to know if the linear model will have the outcome that is represented in the kernel density graphs discussed in the previous chapter. Therefore, we look at Table 1, with the summary statistics for length of stay and charges for patients with and without pneumonia.

Note that it appears as if pneumonia adds about two and a half days to a hospital stay at a cost of over $10,000 more compared to patients without pneumonia. However, in a linear regression for length of stay, the correlation coefficient, or r^2 value is equal to 0.007 while pneumonia is statistically significant. For total charges, r^2 is equal to 0.003. This means that 0.7% of the variability in length of stay is explained by the patient diagnoses; 0.3% of total charges are explained by the diagnoses. Therefore, while pneumonia is significant, it explains very little of the variability in length of stay. One of the reasons that the linear model shows such a difference is because of the presence of outliers. These outliers are considerable, with an upper limit of 365 days at a charge of almost one million dollars. If we look at the median and quartile values, the differences are not so great (Table 2).

Note that the difference in length of stay is two days at the median with about $5000 difference in cost. The length of stay is a difference of 1 at the lower quartile, and a difference of 3 at the upper quartile. Therefore, the difference to the median is greater at the upper quartile compared to the lower quartile.

We now consider adding the indicator function for Septicemia to the linear regression for both total charges and length of stay (Table 3).

Unquestionably, the occurrence of Septicemia brings the length of stay to 12 days with or without pneumonia, and brings the total charges to around $70,000. For total charges, this increases the r^2 to 0.038; it is equal to 0.037 for length of stay. Again, very little of the variability in the outcome can be explained by the presence or absence of these two diseases (Table 4).

Note that pneumonia without septicemia adds two days to the length of stay and about $4000 if we

Table 3. Summary statistics for septicemia and pneumonia

pneumonia	septicemia	N Obs	Variable	Mean	Std Dev	Minimum	Maximum	N
0	0	7411485	LOS	4.3245137	6.2727093	0	365.0000000	7411108
			TOTCHG	20759.23	34663.43	25.0000000	999926.00	7291776
	1	155063	LOS	12.6039550	15.9763921	0	361.0000000	155043
			TOTCHG	70837.14	104672.44	29.0000000	998554.00	151724
1	0	390336	LOS	6.6659886	7.7732323	0	356.0000000	390301
			TOTCHG	29305.00	47163.21	35.0000000	997627.00	385543
	1	35123	LOS	12.0056663	14.2393374	0	308.0000000	35120
			TOTCHG	68425.38	95437.36	35.0000000	998514.00	34618

Table 4. Quartiles for pneumonia and septicemia

pneumonia	septicemia	N Obs	Variable	N	Lower Quartile	Median	Upper Quartile
0	0	7411485	LOS	7411108	2.0000000	3.0000000	5.0000000
			TOTCHG	7291776	5501.00	11198.00	23168.00
	1	155063	LOS	155043	4.0000000	8.0000000	15.0000000
			TOTCHG	151724	15748.00	34162.00	79140.00
1	0	390336	LOS	390301	3.0000000	5.0000000	8.0000000
			TOTCHG	385543	8379.00	15545.00	31209.00
	1	35123	LOS	35120	4.0000000	8.0000000	15.0000000
			TOTCHG	34618	16441.00	35630.50	79799.00

use median rather than mean. Septicemia with or without pneumonia has a median stay of 8 days and approximately $23,000 more in cost. We then add Immune Disorder (Table 5).

Again, the greatest costs and length of stay occur for the condition of septicemia with or without the presence of the other two conditions. The linear model for length of stay increases the r^2 value to 0.049; it is 0.045 for total charges. Table 6 gives the corresponding quartiles. Again, it appears that septicemia by itself is extremely costly with 15 days and more than $75,000 in total charges. The median value for septicemia is eight days compared to a mean of 17 days.

Example Restricting Patients to One Diagnosis 2

We next want to consider the procedures that are most closely related to a diagnosis of COPD, and then we want to see if a linear regression with these procedures as explanatory variables can be used to predict length of stay and total charges. We use some SAS code to combine the 15 procedure columns and then find those procedures that occur most frequently with a patient diagnosis of COPD:

```
data work.charlsoncopd;
set nis.charlson;
if (rxmatch('486',diagnoses3digits)>0) then code=1;
else code=0;
data nis.charlsoncopd;
set work.charlsoncopd;
```

Table 5. Summary statistics adding immune disorder

pneumonia	septicemia	immune	N Obs	Variable	Mean	Std Dev	Minimum	Maximum	N
0	0	0	6400742	LOS TOTCHG	4.0293250 19461.52	5.9122481 31835.92	0 25.0000000	365.0000000 999720.00	6400405 6291710
		1	1010743	LOS TOTCHG	6.1938334 28923.46	7.9444937 48033.74	0 27.0000000	365.0000000 999926.00	1010703 1000066
	1	0	85205	LOS TOTCHG	13.0241695 73585.23	17.1073333 111203.96	0 29.0000000	361.0000000 998554.00	85190 83164
		1	69858	LOS TOTCHG	12.0914778 67503.69	14.4616686 96051.33	0 29.0000000	335.0000000 998088.00	69853 68560
1	0	0	271396	LOS TOTCHG	6.2290945 27271.54	7.3532692 44554.49	0 35.0000000	352.0000000 997627.00	271364 267795
		1	118940	LOS TOTCHG	7.6627963 33929.71	8.5725414 52323.63	0 35.0000000	356.0000000 995009.00	118937 117748
	1	0	18583	LOS TOTCHG	12.3906889 71857.44	15.0415450 102026.49	0 35.0000000	297.0000000 998514.00	18580 18270
		1	16540	LOS TOTCHG	11.5731560 64589.81	13.2676578 87331.98	0 75.0000000	308.0000000 993576.00	16540 16348

```
where code=1;
data nis.p1 ;
set nis.charlsoncopd;
pr=pr1;
run;
data nis.p2;
set nis.charlsoncopd;
pr=pr2;
run;
data nis.p3;
set nis.charlsoncopd;
pr=pr3;
run;
data nis.p4;
set nis.charlsoncopd;
pr=pr4;
run;
data nis.p5;
set nis.charlsoncopd;
pr=pr5;
run;
data nis.p6;
set nis.charlsoncopd;
pr=pr6;
run;
```

Table 6. Quartiles when adding immune disorder

pneumonia	septicemia	immune	Variable	Lower Quartile	Median	Upper Quartile
0	0	0	LOS	2.0000000	3.0000000	4.0000000
			TOTCHG	5190.00	10662.00	22040.00
		1	LOS	2.0000000	4.0000000	7.0000000
			TOTCHG	7812.00	15010.00	30922.00
	1	0	LOS	4.0000000	8.0000000	15.0000000
			TOTCHG	15139.50	33496.50	80960.00
		1	LOS	4.0000000	8.0000000	15.0000000
			TOTCHG	16480.50	34870.00	77030.50
1	0	0	LOS	3.0000000	4.0000000	7.0000000
			TOTCHG	7943.00	14552.00	28863.00
		1	LOS	3.0000000	5.0000000	9.0000000
			TOTCHG	9570.00	18134.00	36925.00
	1	0	LOS	4.0000000	8.0000000	15.0000000
			TOTCHG	16335.00	36271.00	84101.00
		1	LOS	4.0000000	8.0000000	14.0000000
			TOTCHG	16528.00	34882.50	75239.00

```
data nis.p7;
set nis.charlsoncopd;
pr=pr7;
run;
data nis.p8;
set nis.charlsoncopd;
pr=pr8;
run;
data nis.p9;
set nis.charlsoncopd;
pr=pr9;
run;
data nis.p10;
set nis.charlsoncopd;
pr=pr10;
run;
data nis.p11;
set nis.charlsoncopd;
pr=pr11;
run;
data nis.p12;
set nis.charlsoncopd;
pr=pr12;
run;
data nis.p13;
```

```
set nis.charlsoncopd;
pr=pr13;
run;
data nis.p14;
set nis.charlsoncopd;
pr=pr14;
run;
data nis.p15;
set nis.charlsoncopd;
pr=pr15;
run;
data nis.procedureforcopd;
set nis.p1 nis.p2 nis.p3 nis.p4 nis.p5 nis.p6 nis.p7 nis.p8 nis.p9
nis.p10 nis.p11 nis.p12 nis.p13 nis.p14 nis.p15;
run;
```

Most (but not all) of the procedures in Table 7 are related to COPD. However, the most frequently occurring procedure is still only performed for just under 8% of the patients.

All of the procedures are rare occurrences since they occur in 8% of the COPD population or less. Table 8 shows the most frequent procedures for a primary diagnosis of COPD. We find the procedure codes by modifying the previous code slightly:

```
data work.charlsoncopd2;
set nis.charlson;
if (rxmatch('486',dx1)>0) then code=1;
else code=0;
data nis.charlsoncopd2;
set work.charlsoncopd2;
where code=1;
```

Usually, once the codes are identified, indicator functions are defined as 1=the diagnosis is present for the patient and 0=the diagnosis is not present. Then the indicator functions are used in a regression equation. Whether the number of codes is 20 or 50, not all potential diagnosis codes can be used; we must limit them in some way.

However, the use of indicator functions requires two additional assumptions when used in regression. First, it must be assumed that all providers code these conditions uniformly the same way. That is, for $X_i=(X_{i1},X_{i2},\ldots,X_{in})$ where X_i represents patient i and $X_{i1},\ldots,X_{in}$ represent the values of the indicator functions; X_i and X_j must be independent and identically distributed. Without the uniformity of data entry, these values are not identically distributed. Another problem occurs if the indicator functions are not independent; that is, if co-morbid conditions are related since the multicollinearity will inflate the variance of the model. If collinearity exists, very likely, the variance, standard error, and parameter estimates are all inflated. In other words, the high variance is not a result of good independent predictors, but a mis-specified model that carries mutually dependent and thus redundant predictors. However, it is well known that many patient factors are co-morbid and related. Consider Tables 9 and 10 showing

Table 7. Most frequent procedures for patients with COPD

pr	Procedure Translation	Frequency	Percent
3893	Venous catheterization, not elsewhere classified	40021	7.54
9904	Transfusion of packed cells	38359	7.22
9604	Insertion of endotracheal tube	27304	5.14
9671	Continuous mechanical ventilation for less than 96 consecutive hours	17065	3.21
9672	Continuous mechanical ventilation for 96 consecutive hours or more	16300	3.07
3995	Hemodialysis	14729	2.77
3324	Closed [endoscopic] biopsy of bronchus	13952	2.63
3491	Thoracentesis	13152	2.48
8872	Diagnostic ultrasound of heart	10356	1.95
9921	Injection of antibiotic	9238	1.74
9394	Respiratory medication administered by nebulizer	8674	1.63
9390	Continuous positive airway pressure	7868	1.48
8856	Coronary arteriography using two catheters	7622	1.44
4516	Esophagogastroduodenoscopy [EGD] with closed biopsy	7516	1.42
966	Enteral infusion of concentrated nutritional substances	7203	1.36
3722	Left heart cardiac catheterization	6652	1.25
8853	Angiocardiography of left heart structures	6350	1.20
4513	Other endoscopy of small intestine	6343	1.19
3404	Insertion of intercostal catheter for drainage	5693	1.07
8741	Computerized axial tomography of thorax	5538	1.04
9915	Parenteral infusion of concentrated nutritional substances	5169	0.97
9907	Transfusion of other serum	4962	0.93
9396	Other oxygen enrichment	4937	0.93
4311	Percutaneous [endoscopic] gastrostomy	4831	0.91
3895	Venous catheterization for renal dialysis	4726	0.89
0331	Spinal tap	4362	0.82
3891	Arterial catheterization	3867	0.73
3327	Closed endoscopic biopsy of lung	3776	0.71
9339	Other physical therapy	3492	0.66
311	Temporary tracheostomy	3406	0.64
4523	Colonoscopy	3404	0.64

the correlation of some of the procedures listed in Table 8.

Unfortunately, many studies simply ignore both the issue of non-uniform data entry and the issue of multicollinearity in the explanatory variables. However, there are techniques available that can utilize all of the procedure and/or diagnosis codes without making either assumption; they will be discussed in Chapter 4. (Cerrito, 2007) In this chapter, we will restrict our attention to regression. To find the relationship of these codes, we combine them using the following SAS code:

Table 8. Most frequent procedures for COPD as primary diagnosis

pr	Procedure Translation	Frequency	Percent
9904	Transfusion of packed cells	17756	7.05
3893	Venous catheterization, not elsewhere classified	16142	6.41
9671	Continuous mechanical ventilation for less than 96 consecutive hours	10528	4.18
3324	Closed [endoscopic] biopsy of bronchus	8315	3.30
9672	Continuous mechanical ventilation for 96 consecutive hours or more	8243	3.27
3491	Thoracentesis	8118	3.22
3995	Hemodialysis	8083	3.21
9604	Insertion of endotracheal tube	7579	3.01
9921	Injection of antibiotic	6786	2.69
9394	Respiratory medication administered by nebulizer	6309	2.50
8872	Diagnostic ultrasound of heart	5419	2.15
4516	Esophagogastroduodenoscopy [EGD] with closed biopsy	4894	1.94
9390	Continuous positive airway pressure	4667	1.85
3327	Closed endoscopic biopsy of lung	3446	1.37
8741	Computerized axial tomography of thorax	3417	1.36
4513	Other endoscopy of small intestine	3277	1.30
3722	Left heart cardiac catheterization	2965	1.18
9396	Other oxygen enrichment	2832	1.12
0331	Spinal tap	2764	1.10
966	Enteral infusion of concentrated nutritional substances	2454	0.97
9339	Other physical therapy	2296	0.91
3404	Insertion of intercostal catheter for drainage	2179	0.87
311	Temporary tracheostomy	2124	0.84
4311	Percutaneous [endoscopic] gastrostomy	1989	0.79
9929	Injection or infusion of other therapeutic or prophylactic substance	1859	0.74
9929	Injection or infusion of other therapeutic or prophylactic substance	1859	0.74
4523	Colonoscopy	1656	0.66
3898	Other puncture of artery	1650	0.66
8703	Computerized axial tomography of head	1644	0.65
8965	Measurement of systemic arterial blood gases	1598	0.63
8622	Excisional debridement of wound, infection, or burn	1580	0.63
387	Interruption of the vena cava	1526	0.61

```
data nis.copdprocedures;
set nis.charlsoncopd2;
prcomb=catx(' ',pr1,pr2,pr3,pr4,pr5,pr6,pr7,pr8,pr9,pr10,pr11,
pr12,pr13,pr14,pr15);
transf=0; vcath=0; ven196=0; biopbronc=0; thorac=0; hemod=0; ventm96=0;
endotrach=0; antibiotic=0; respmed=0; ultrasound=0;
```

Table 9. Correlation of antibiotic and hemodialysis

Table of hemod by antibiotic			
hemod	antibiotic		Total
Frequency Row Pct Col Pct	0	1	
0	220171 97.55 97.99	5535 2.45 98.19	225706
1	4513 97.79 2.01	102 2.21 1.81	4615
Total	224684	5637	230321

Table 10. Correlation of transfusion and venus catheterization

Table of vcath by transf			
vcath	transf		Total
Frequency Row Pct Col Pct	0	1	
0	213265 96.10 96.90	8649 3.90 84.53	221914
1	6824 81.17 3.10	1583 18.83 15.47	8407
Total	220089	10232	230321

```
if (rxmatch('9904',prcomb)>0) then transf=1;
if (rxmatch('3893',prcomb)>0) then vcath=1;
if (rxmatch('9671',prcomb)>0) then ventl96=1;
if (rxmatch('3324',prcomb)>0) then biopbronc=1;
if (rxmatch('9672',prcomb)>0) then ventm96=1;
if (rxmatch('3491',prcomb)>0) then thorac=1;
if (rxmatch('3995',prcomb)>0) then hemod=1;
if (rxmatch('9604',prcomb)>0) then endotrach=1;
if (rxmatch('9921',prcomb)>0) then antibiotic=1;
if (rxmatch('9394',prcomb)>0) then respmed=1;
if (rxmatch('8872',prcomb)>0) then ultrasound=1;
run;
```

Note that for the first table analysis in Table 9, 2% of patients with COPD receiving hemodialysis also receive an antibiotic. Similarly, for Table 10, 18% of patients with COPD receiving a venous catheter also receive a transfusion. The issue of multicollinearity is considerable and cannot just be ignored when defining these indicator functions.

We also want to look at a simple linear regression of total charges versus length of stay. Then Y (total charges)=α+βX+ε, where ε represents the error term. In order for the regression model to be valid, there are some assumptions that need to be considered. The residuals need to be independent and identically distributed such that the mean is zero and the variance is equal to the population variance divided by n. We estimate the population variance by the sample variance.

The best way to examine the assumptions is to look at the residuals. Figure 10 shows the actual versus predicted values; Figure 11 shows the residuals by the total charges. Figure 11 should have no discern-

Figure 10. Actual versus predicted values for total charges

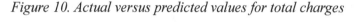

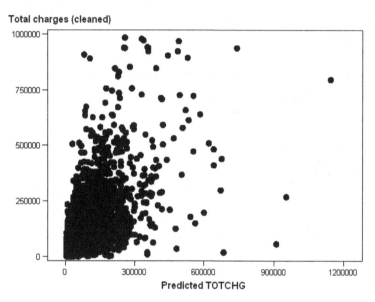

Figure 11. Residuals versus total charges

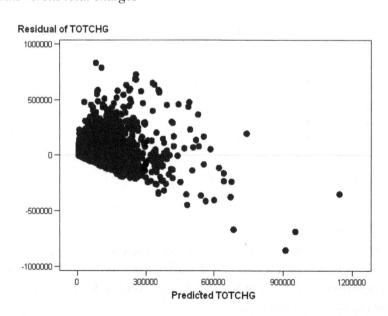

able pattern if the assumptions on the residuals are satisfied. In addition, we examine the r^2 value, which explains the proportion of the variability of Y that can be explained by the variability in X. In this regression, the r^2 value is 47%, indicating that over half of the variability in total charges remains unexplained.

It is quite clear that the assumptions on the residuals are not satisfied since there is a fan-shaped pattern in Figure 11. When that occurs, it is possible to perform a transformation on the variables to see if the transformation will cause the assumptions to be satisfied. When the residuals have this fan shape, one possible transformation is a log function. We can consider the log of total charges, or the log of length of stay. The top of Figure 12 gives the residuals for a log of the length of stay, with an r^2 of 44%; the bottom gives the residuals for a log of total charges, with an r^2 of 26%.

The assumption of randomness is still not satisfied, indicating that the transformation actually makes

Figure 12. Residuals for log of length of stay (top); residuals for log of total charges (bottom)

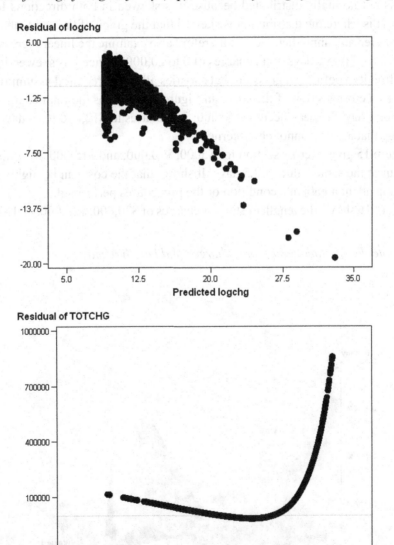

the situation worse as shown by Figure 12.

We investigate the nature of these residuals for the patients with COPD. Recall that the residuals need to be independent and identically distributed normal variables with mean zero and constant variance. If we regress the total charges on the length of stay, the r^2 value is approximately 47%. We want to use bivariate kernel density estimation to examine the basic assumptions. Figure 13 gives the density of total charges and length of stay. To find this bivariate density, we use the following code:

```
proc kde data=sasuser.charlsonsmallersample;
bivar los (gridl=0 gridu=30) totchg (gridl=0 gridu=50000)/ bwm=10 out=sasuser.kdebivar4
plots=all;
run;
```

This density is not normally distributed because it is skewed in both directions for length of stay and total charges. It is where the distribution is skewed that the graph of the residuals in Figures 10, 11 becomes very scattered and unpredictable. We therefore also examine the linear regression for truncated values (length of stay of 0 to 5 days; total charges of 0 to 20,000). Since it is skewed in both directions, it will be very difficult to define a regression that satisfies all of the required assumptions.

Figure 14 gives a cross section of the curve in Figure 13. It gives the total charges for a stay of 1, 5, and 10 days. For 1 day, the peak occurs at $5000; it increases to $12,000 for 5 days. At 10 days, the variable is so large that a peak cannot be discerned.

Similarly, Figure 15 gives a cross section for $5000, $10,000, and $15,000. In contrast to Figure 16, the peaks all occur at the same value of 2.5 days. It shows that the cost can be highly variable without knowing something about a patient's condition or the procedures performed.

Similarly, Figure 16 shows the length of stay for charges of $20,000, $25,000, and $30,000. The peak

Figure 13. Bivariate density function of total charges and length of stay

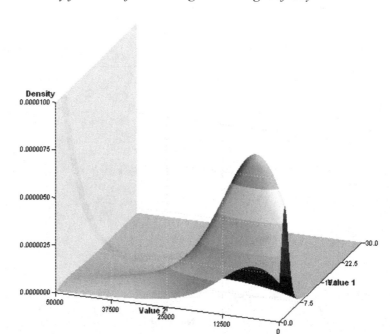

Figure 14. Cross sectional kernel density for 1,5, and 10 days

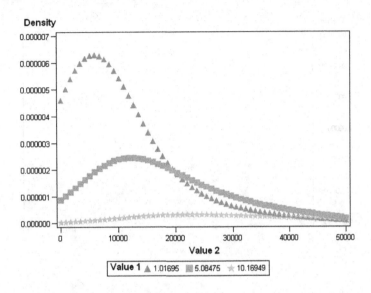

Figure 15. Length of stay for total costs of $5000, $10,000, and $15,000

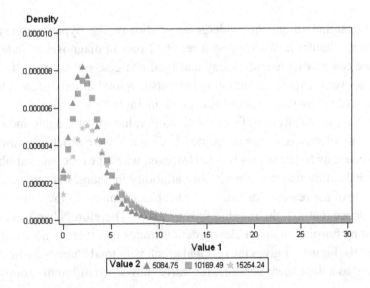

remains at 2.5 days. Because the charges are so variable for a length of stay of 2.5 days, a regression of length of stay to charges will continue to have a low r^2 value. The only way to increase it is to include more variables in the model.

We add more variables when examining mortality in relationship to the example of cardiovascular surgery. This model is 88% accurate even though less than 2% of the patients die in the hospital. However, almost all of the deaths are classified as non-mortality while the false positive rate is somewhat high. We will discuss this example in more detail in Chapter 4.

Figure 16. Length of stay for charges of $20,000, $25,000, and $30,000

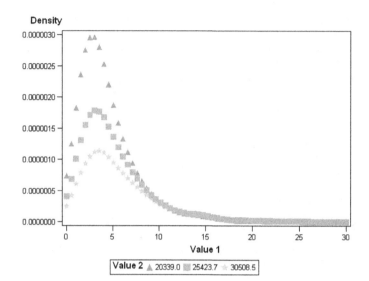

Example Using One Procedure of Cardiovascular Surgery 2

In this example, we examine all patients undergoing cardiovascular bypass surgery; this dataset was previously discussed in Chapter 2. We also use a set of 17 patient diagnoses as independent variables. We want to see if we can predict length of stay and total charges, and we want to see if the hospital makes a difference, so we restrict our attention to patients in a total of ten different hospitals, a total of 1400 patients. The list of independent variables is given in Table 11.

The model is highly statistically significant, with an r^2 value of 0.13, again indicating that most of the variabililty in length of stay is still unaccounted for, even if we restrict the patient procedures and conditions, and limit the data to just ten hospitals. However, when the outcome variable is total charges, the r^2 value is 0.51, indicating that the majority of variability in charges is accounted for by the independent variables. One of the reasons for that is that hospitals tend to set their own charges. If we omit hospital from the independent list, the r^2 value falls to 0.074. Therefore, charges is not determined by patient condition but by hospital. It again clearly demonstrates that there is no uniformity in assessing charges across hospitals. Figure 17 gives the residual graph with total charges as the dependent variable and including hospital as a dependent variable. It clearly shows two different groups in the data.

Outliers in Regression 2

An assumption of normality is required for regression. If we assume normality when the distribution is exponential or gamma, the outliers will be under-counted. Consider the dataset here that is not normally distributed. We use a random sample of 1000 observations. The mean and standard deviation (assuming a normal distribution) are equal to 4.235 and 5.0479 respectively. Then, three standard deviations beyond the mean is equal to 19.3787 days. Two standard deviations beyond the mean is equal to 14.3308. In the random sample, the proportion of patients with length of stay in days beyond two standard deviations is equal to 35% when the normal probability indicates that only 25% should be that large. The proportion

Table 11. Independent variables

Age	Race
Sex	Acute myocardial infarction
Congestive heart failure	Peripheral vascular disease
Cerebral vascular accident	Dementia
Pulmonary disease	Connective tissue disorder
Peptic ulcer	Liver disease
Diabetes	Diabetes with complications
Paraplegia	Renal disease
Cancer	Metastatic cancer
Severe liver disease	HIV
Hospital	

Figure 17. Residuals for linear regression

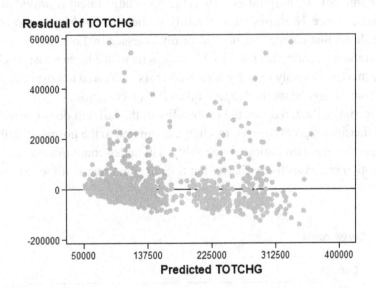

Residual of TOTCHG

beyond three standard deviations is equal to 20%; the probability assuming normality indicates that only 10% should be beyond that point.

This difference in outliers can be extremely important. For example, the Centers for Medicare and Medicaid provide information on how hospitals are reimbursed based upon patient procedures: (Anonymous-PPS, 2008)

The base payment rate is comprised of a standardized amount, which is divided into a labor-related and nonlabor share. The labor-related share is adjusted by the wage index applicable to the area where the hospital is located and if the hospital is located in Alaska or Hawaii, the nonlabor share is adjusted by a cost of living adjustment factor. This base payment rate is multiplied by the DRG relative weight.

Current 2008 weights have been published.(Weights, 2008) Patients designated as "outliers" can have higher reimbursement rates:

To qualify for outlier payments, a case must have costs above a fixed-loss cost threshold amount (a dollar amount by which the costs of a case must exceed payments in order to qualify for outliers).

An example of the computations is given in the Federal Register. (Example, 2003) The computations are linear, making assumptions concerning the normality of the data. They are highly dependent upon a hospital's cost-to-charge ratio, defined by hospital and adjusted on a yearly basis. (Anonymous-KY, 2008) This ratio is defined by CMS and reflects the relationship between actual costs (as determined by an annual audit) and the charges that are billed by the hospital. Therefore, the formula to determine outlier costs includes the value of charges times the cost-to-charge ratio. In addition, a yearly threshold value is set by CMS ($33,560 in 2003) The outlier reimbursement is a linear function of this threshold value and the cost-to-charges ratio.

Therefore, we can look at the outlier charges and the cost-to-charge ratio as determined by the hospital. The cost-to-charge ratio by hospital as well as the wage adjustment is provided with the National Inpatient Sample data. Figure 18 shows the variability in the cost-to-charge ratio across the different hospitals. It clearly shows that charges are not uniformly assessed by hospitals.

Note the considerable variability from 0.1 to 0.8. Hospitals with a higher cost-to-charge ratio tend to bill charges that are more reasonably in line with actual costs compared to hospitals with a rate of 10%. Figure 19 shows a comparison between charges and charges x cost ratio.

The cost-to-charge ratio, then, reduces the probability in the tail, but does not reduce its size. If we compare the kernel density graph of the cost-to-charge compared to the normal distribution assumption (Figure 20), it is clear that the assumption of normality will under-count the outliers.

A normal assumption increases the variance, but fails to count many of the extreme outliers.

Figure 18. Cost-to-charge ratio

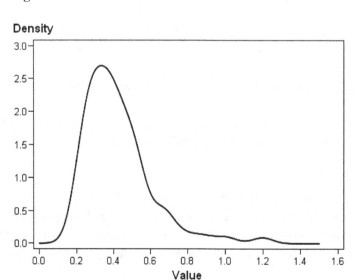

Figure 19. Comparison of charges to estimated costs

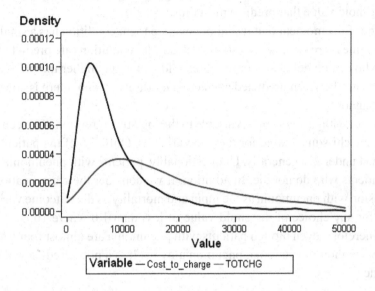

Figure 20. Comparison of kernel estimate to normality assumption

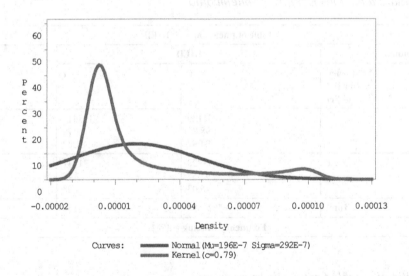

LOGISTIC REGRESSION

We want to see if we can predict mortality in patients using a logistic regression model. The same issue occurs with upcoding. The value,

$$\alpha_1 X_2 + \alpha_2 X_2 + \ldots + \alpha_{25} X_{25}$$

increases as the number of nonzero X's increases. The greater this value, the greater the likelihood that it will cross the threshold value that predicts mortality.

However, consider for a moment that just about every patient condition has a small risk of mortality. Once the threshold value is crossed, every patient with similar conditions are predicted to die. Therefore, the more patients who can be defined over the threshold value, the higher the predicted mortality rate, decreasing the difference between predicted and actual mortality. Again, there is considerable incentive to upcode patient diagnoses.

To simplify, we start with just one input variable to the logistic regression, the occurrence of pneumonia. Table 12 gives the chi-square table for the two variables. Only 7% of the patients with pneumonia died compared to just under 2% generally. Unquestionably, patients with pneumonia are more likely to die compared to patients who do not die. In addition, if we consider the classification table (Table 13) for a logistic regression with pneumonia as the input and mortality as the outcome variable, the accuracy rate is above 90% for any choice of threshold value of less than 1.0 where 100% of the values are to predict mortality. Therefore, even though patients with pneumonia are almost four times as likely to die compared to patients without pneumonia, pneumonia by itself is a poor predictor of mortality because of the rare occurrence.

Table 12. Chi-square table for mortality by pneumonia

Table of pneumonia by DIED				
pneumonia	DIED			Total
Frequency Row Pct Col Pct	0	1		
0	7431129 98.21 94.97	135419 1.79 81.02		7566548
1	393728 92.54 5.03	31731 7.46 18.98		425459
Total	7824857	167150		7992007
Frequency Missing = 3041				

Table 13. Classification table for logistic regression

Classification Table									
Prob Level	Correct		Incorrect		Percentages				
	Event	Non- Event	Event	Non- Event	Correct	Sensi- tivity	Speci- ficity	False POS	False NEG
0.920	782E4	0	167E3	0	97.9	100.0	0.0	2.1	.
0.940	743E4	31731	135E3	394E3	93.4	95.0	19.0	1.8	92.5
0.960	743E4	31731	135E3	394E3	93.4	95.0	19.0	1.8	92.5
0.980	743E4	31731	135E3	394E3	93.4	95.0	19.0	1.8	92.5
1.000	0	167E3	0	782E4	2.1	0.0	100.0	.	97.9

We now add a second patient diagnosis to the regression. Table 14 gives the chi-square table for pneumonia and septicemia.

Of the patients with septicemia only (pneumonia=0), 20% died, increasing to 28% with both septicemia and pneumonia. For patients without septicemia but with pneumonia, 5% died. The classification table for the logistic regression is given in Table 15.

Again, for any threshold value below 98%, the logistic regression model will be over 90% accurate by identifying most of the observations as non-occurrences so that the false negative rate is over 70%. In other words, adding a second input variable did not change the problems with the regression, which are caused by attempting to predict a rare occurrence. We add Immune Disorder to the model (Table 16).

The problem still persists, and will continue to persist regardless of the number of input variables. We need to change the sample size so that the group sizes are close to equal.

The Generalized Linear Model 2

The linear model is one of the most important tools in the statistical analysis of data, but there are types of problems for which the linear model is not appropriate. The main problem occurs when the data are not normally distributed and the variance is not constant. The generalized linear model extends the general linear model and the regression model by solving these issues, and is therefore applicable to a wider range of data analysis problems. The generalized linear model enlarges the class of linear models when the distribution of Y for a fixed x is assumed to be from the exponential family of distributions, which includes important distributions such as the binomial, Poisson, exponential, and gamma distributions in addition to the normal distribution. The exponential family has a probability density function of the form

$$f(y_i) = \exp\left(\frac{y_i \theta_i - b(\theta_i)}{a_i(\phi)} + c(y_i, \phi)\right)$$

where θ_i and φ are parameters and $a_i(\phi)$, $b(\theta_i)$ and $c(y_i, \phi)$ are known functions. A link function can be used to relate the expected value of the outcome to the linear predictor since the effect of the predictors on the dependent variable may not be linear. The equation of the model is given by

Table 14. Chi-square table for pneumonia and septicemia

	Controlling for septicemia=0			Controlling for septicemia=1		
pneumonia	**Died**		**Total**	**DIED**		**Total**
Frequency Row Pct Col Pct	**0**	**1**		**0**	**1**	
0	7307726 98.60 95.20	103759 1.40 82.65	7411485	123403 79.58 83.06	31660 20.42 76.09	155063
1	368553 94.42 4.80	21783 5.58 17.35	390336	25175 71.68 16.94	9948 28.32 23.91	35123
Total	7676279	125542	7801821	148578	41608	190186

Table 15. Classification table for logistic regression with pneumonia and septicemia

Classification Table										
Prob Level	**Correct**		**Incorrect**		**Percentages**					
	Event	**Non-Event**	**Event**	**Non-Event**	**Correct**	**Sensi-tivity**	**Speci-ficity**	**False POS**	**False NEG**	
0.580	782E4	0	167E3	0	97.9	100.0	0.0	2.1	.	
0.600	78E5	9948	157E3	25175	97.7	99.7	6.0	2.0	71.7	
0.620	78E5	9948	157E3	25175	97.7	99.7	6.0	2.0	71.7	
0.640	78E5	9948	157E3	25175	97.7	99.7	6.0	2.0	71.7	
0.660	78E5	9948	157E3	25175	97.7	99.7	6.0	2.0	71.7	
0.680	78E5	9948	157E3	25175	97.7	99.7	6.0	2.0	71.7	
0.700	78E5	9948	157E3	25175	97.7	99.7	6.0	2.0	71.7	
0.720	78E5	9948	157E3	25175	97.7	99.7	6.0	2.0	71.7	
0.740	78E5	9948	157E3	25175	97.7	99.7	6.0	2.0	71.7	
0.760	78E5	9948	157E3	25175	97.7	99.7	6.0	2.0	71.7	
0.780	78E5	9948	157E3	25175	97.7	99.7	6.0	2.0	71.7	
0.800	78E5	9948	157E3	25175	97.7	99.7	6.0	2.0	71.7	
0.820	78E5	9948	157E3	25175	97.7	99.7	6.0	2.0	71.7	
0.840	768E4	41608	126E3	149E3	96.6	98.1	24.9	1.6	78.1	
0.860	768E4	41608	126E3	149E3	96.6	98.1	24.9	1.6	78.1	
0.880	768E4	41608	126E3	149E3	96.6	98.1	24.9	1.6	78.1	
0.900	768E4	41608	126E3	149E3	96.6	98.1	24.9	1.6	78.1	
0.920	768E4	41608	126E3	149E3	96.6	98.1	24.9	1.6	78.1	
0.940	768E4	41608	126E3	149E3	96.6	98.1	24.9	1.6	78.1	
0.960	731E4	63391	104E3	517E3	92.2	93.4	37.9	1.4	89.1	
0.980	731E4	63391	104E3	517E3	92.2	93.4	37.9	1.4	89.1	
1.000	0	167E3	0	782E4	2.1	0.0	100.0	.	97.9	

$$g(\hat{Y}) = X\beta$$

where g() is a non-linear link function. When the response variable follows a normal distribution, the link function is the identity. This identity link explains how this model generalizes the linear model. Examples of link functions for a variety of probability distributions are given in Table 17.

The generalized linear mixed model extends the generalized model when there is a random effect in the data. It also generalizes the linear mixed model when the dependent variable is not normally distributed. However, the random effects must be normal. The generalized linear mixed model has the following form

$$g(E(Y \mid u)) = X\beta + Zu$$

Table 16. Classification table adding immune disorder

Prob Level	Correct		Incorrect		Percentages				
	Event	Non-Event	Event	Non-Event	Correct	Sensi-tivity	Speci-ficity	False POS	False NEG
0.480	782E4	0	167E3	0	97.9	100.0	0.0	2.1	.
0.500	781E4	4907	162E3	11633	97.8	99.9	2.9	2.0	70.3
0.520	781E4	4907	162E3	11633	97.8	99.9	2.9	2.0	70.3
0.540	781E4	4907	162E3	11633	97.8	99.9	2.9	2.0	70.3
0.560	781E4	4907	162E3	11633	97.8	99.9	2.9	2.0	70.3
0.580	781E4	4907	162E3	11633	97.8	99.9	2.9	2.0	70.3
0.600	781E4	4907	162E3	11633	97.8	99.9	2.9	2.0	70.3
0.620	781E4	4907	162E3	11633	97.8	99.9	2.9	2.0	70.3
0.640	781E4	4907	162E3	11633	97.8	99.9	2.9	2.0	70.3
0.660	781E4	4907	162E3	11633	97.8	99.9	2.9	2.0	70.3
0.680	781E4	4907	162E3	11633	97.8	99.9	2.9	2.0	70.3
0.700	781E4	4907	162E3	11633	97.8	99.9	2.9	2.0	70.3
0.720	781E4	4907	162E3	11633	97.8	99.9	2.9	2.0	70.3
0.740	776E4	21322	146E3	65076	97.4	99.2	12.8	1.8	75.3
0.760	775E4	26363	141E3	78618	97.3	99.0	15.8	1.8	74.9
0.780	775E4	26363	141E3	78618	97.3	99.0	15.8	1.8	74.9
0.800	775E4	26363	141E3	78618	97.3	99.0	15.8	1.8	74.9
0.820	775E4	26363	141E3	78618	97.3	99.0	15.8	1.8	74.9
0.840	775E4	26363	141E3	78618	97.3	99.0	15.8	1.8	74.9
0.860	775E4	26363	141E3	78618	97.3	99.0	15.8	1.8	74.9
0.880	775E4	26363	141E3	78618	97.3	99.0	15.8	1.8	74.9
0.900	768E4	41608	126E3	149E3	96.6	98.1	24.9	1.6	78.1
0.920	757E4	51297	116E3	258E3	95.3	96.7	30.7	1.5	83.4
0.940	757E4	51297	116E3	258E3	95.3	96.7	30.7	1.5	83.4
0.960	757E4	51297	116E3	258E3	95.3	96.7	30.7	1.5	83.4
0.980	634E4	103E3	64219	149E4	80.6	81.0	61.6	1.0	93.5
1.000	0	167E3	0	782E4	2.1	0.0	100.0	.	97.9

where again, $u \sim N(0, G)$ is the random effect similar to the linear mixed model and g() is a link function, as in the case of a generalized linear model. However, instead of specifying a distribution for Y, we now specify a distribution for the conditional response, Y / u. An example of the generalized linear mixed model is when randomly sampled patients are measured repeatedly over time; we can model the patient effects by including random intercepts in the model. These intercepts are called G-side components because they contribute to the linear predictor. For a given patient, the correlations over time can be modeled with an autoregressive structure. Combining these elements, the model can be represented as follows:

Table 17. Examples of distributions and their link functions

Outcome	Distribution	Link function
Continuous	Normal	Identity
Binary	Binomial	Logit
Ordinal	Multinomial	Cumulative Logit
Binary	Poisson	Log
Continuous	Gamma	Reciprocal

$$E(Y \, / \, u) = g^{-1}(X\beta + Zu)$$
$$Var(u) = G$$
$$Var(Y \, / \, u) = A^{1/2} R A^{1/2}$$

where $g^{-1}()$ is the inverse link function and A is a diagonal matrix containing the variance functions.

Logistic regression is a special case of the generalized linear model. The link function specified is the logit function. Besides the logit function, we use three different link functions: normal (which is equal to the linear regression), negative binomial, and gamma. The density function for the negative binomial is equal to

$$f(k; r, p) = \binom{k + r - 1}{k} p^r (1 - p^k) \text{ for k=0,1,2....}$$

where

$$\binom{k + r - 1}{k} = \frac{\Gamma(k + r)}{k! \, \Gamma(r)} = (-1)^k \binom{-r}{k} \text{ and } \Gamma(r) = (r-1)!$$

Figure 21 shows the shape of the distribution for different values of r; the distribution for r=1 and r=2 is the closest to that of Figure 2 in Chapter 2.

Similarly, the density of the gamma function is defined by

$$f(x; k, \theta) = x^{k-1} \frac{e^{-x/\theta}}{\theta^k \Gamma(k)}.$$

The distribution is shown in Figure 22.

In the case of the gamma function as well, the density function can take many different shapes depending upon the parameters. We demonstrate using our example of pneumonia, septicemia, and immune disorder. Table 18 shows the estimates of the coefficients for the three link functions.

The gamma link function indicates that having an infection such as septicemia results in a lower length

Figure 21. Negative binomial (http://en.wikipedia.org/wiki/Negative_binomial_distribution)

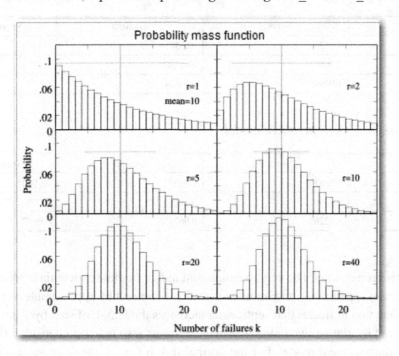

Figure 22. Gamma function (http://en.wikipedia.org/wiki/Image:Gamma_distribution_pdf.png)

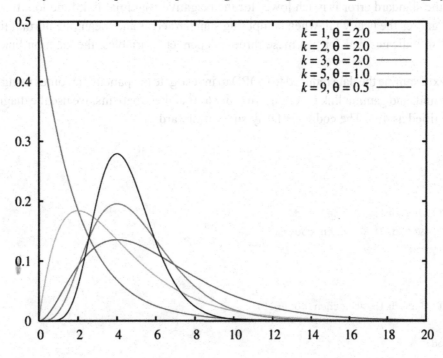

Table 18. Coefficients of independent variables using 3 link functions to estimate length of stay

Coefficient	Normal	Gamma	Negative Binomial
Pneumonia	1.7635	-0.0397	0.3387
Septicemia	7.1664	-0.1036	0.9108
Immune Disorder	1.9484	-0.0624	0.3836

Table 19. Standard error for generalized models

Coefficient	Normal	Gamma	Negative Binomial
Pneumonia	0.0555	0.0397	0.0042
Septicemia	0.0490	0.1036	0.0059
Immune Disorder	0.02209	0.0624	0.0027

of stay; clearly this is erroneous. The negative binomial indicates that septicemia increases the length of stay by almost one day; pneumonia and immune disorder increase it by approximately one third of a day. The normal link function indicates that septicemia increases the length of stay by 7 days; the other two infections increase it by almost two days. However, we must also take into consideration the intercept value of the generalized linear model. For the normal link function, the intercept is equal to -4.0656. For the Negative Binomial, it is 0.2358; for the Gamma, it is 1.4017. The intercept increases the value of the model to a high of 6.8 days for a patient with pneumonia, septicemia, and immune disorder with the normal link function. For the Negative Binomial, it is equal to 4.7 days. The other thing we have to consider is the standard error (Table 19).

Note that the standard error is much lower for the Negative Binomial link function. It suggests that this function ignores the heavy tail when computing standard error and mean; the normal link function does not. It also indicates that for just these three independent variables, the Gamma link function is inadequate.

We will next examine the data reduced to COPD to investigate the patient outcomes using the normal, negative binomial, and gamma link functions. In order to find these patients, we use the diagnosis codes. COPD is identified as 496. The coding is fairly straightforward:

```
Data work.copd;
Set nis.nis;
Code=0;
If (rxmatch('496',dx1)>0) then code=1;
If (rxmatch('496',dx2)>0) then code=2;
.
.
.
If (rxmatch('496',dx15)>0) then code=15;
Run;
Data nis.copd;
Set work.copd;
```

Table 20. Coefficients of independent variables

Coefficient	Normal	Gamma	Negative Binomial
Age	0.0326	-0.0078	-0.0078
Female	0.1746	0.0074	0.0074
Hemodialysis	1.6820	0.4333	0.4333
Continuous Ventilation > 96 Hours	10.6845	1.3606	1.3606
Insertion of endotracheal tube	0.5237	0.0669	0.0669
Injection of antibiotic	0.5237	-0.0149	-0.0149
Respiratory medication administered by nebulizer	0.7881	-0.0076	-0.0076
Diagnostic ultrasound of heart	1.5878	0.4477	0.4477
Esophagogastroduodenoscopy with closed biopsy	2.9541	0.5803	0.5803
Continuous positive airway pressure	2.3769	0.6475	0.6475
Closed endoscopic biopsy of lung	1.1786	0.3529	0.3529
Computerized axial tomography of head	0.9279	0.3149	0.3149
Transfusion of packed cells	2.9279	0.4823	0.4823
Venous catheterization	4.3954	0.7121	0.7121
Continuous Ventilation < 96 Hours	0.7652	0.6255	0.6255
Closed biopsy of bronchus	3.8546	0.6023	0.6023
Thoracentesis	3.8546	0.6195	0.6195

```
Where code>0;
Run;
```

This code not only finds all of the patients with COPD; it identifies the column where COPD is listed. The diagnosis codes are supposed to be entered in their order of importance, which is not always the same for all providers.

Given the sample size, every independent variable is statistically significant. Using the procedures listed in Table 9, we examine the contribution of each procedure to the patient demographic factors. These are listed in Table 20.

For the normal link function, all procedures indicate that the patient will stay longer compared to patients who do not have these procedures. However, the gamma and negative binomial link functions indicate the patients receiving an antibiotic, or medication by a nebulizer will not stay as long compared to patients who do not receive them. Race and income quartile are also statistically significant (Table 21).

Note that the negative binomial and gamma link functions generate the same coefficient estimates. For the three link functions, Caucasian reduces the length of stay; Hispanic patients will stay longer. The normal result indicates that Asians stay less; the gamma and negative binomial indicate that they stay longer.

There is also a considerable difference for each of the standard errors. The normal link function has a much larger error for each coefficient (Table 22).

The standard error for the gamma and negative binomial are smaller because these distributions better fit the shape of the true distribution. The normal distribution assumes a symmetry that does not exist,

Table 21. Coefficients for race and income quartile

Coefficient	Normal	Gamma	Negative Binomial
Quartile 1	-0.0710	-0.2836	-0.2836
Quartile 2	-0.2026	-0.2560	-0.2560
Quartile 3	-0.2506	-0.1382	-0.1382
Caucasian	-0.2337	-0.1095	-0.1095
African American	-0.0298	0.0585	0.0585
Hispanic	0.0485	0.2563	0.2563
Asian	-0.1652	0.2103	0.2103
Native American	-0.5059	-0.1585	-0.1585

and the heavy tail of the distribution inflates the value of the standard error.

We also consider the example for cardiovascular surgery. For a rare occurrence, a Poisson approximation is better than a normal approximation. If we modify the model and assume a Poisson link function, the result is a probability, and we need to find an optimal threshold value. The SAS code for this model is

```
PROC GENMOD DATA=nis.nischarlson
;
    CLASS FEMALE ami chf pvd cva pd ctd pu ld diabetes dc paraplegia rd cancer mc sld
hiv
    ;
    MODEL DIED= AGE FEMALE ami chf pvd cva pd ctd pu ld diabetes dc paraplegia rd cancer
mc sld hiv
        /
        DIST=POISSON
    ;
    OUTPUT OUT=SASUSER.predicted
        PREDICTED=_predicted1
        RESDEV=_resdev1
        RESCHI=_reschi1
        UPPER=_upper1
        LOWER=_lower1
        HESSWGT=_hesswgt1
        XBETA=_xbeta1;
RUN; QUIT;
```

We need to use the predicted value to compute the threshold value. We use kernel density estimation to model the predictions (Figure 23).

If we let 0.05 be the threshold value for prediction, we can compare mortality to predicted mortality. This threshold successfully predicts 50% of the deaths but with 132 (9%) false positives. If we let 0.03 be the threshold value, it predicts 57% of deaths with 213 or 15% false positives. For a threshold value of 0.08, the model successfully predicts 25% of the deaths, but reduces the false positive rate to 5%.

Table 22. Standard error for coefficients for normal compared to gamma (negative binomial)

Coefficient	Normal	Gamma
Age	0.0005	0.0001
Female	0.0232	0.0038
Hemodialysis	0.0815	0.0133
Continuous Ventilation > 96 Hours	0.1570	0.0245
Insertion of endotracheal tube	0.1533	0.0238
Injection of antibiotic	0.0725	0.0117
Respiratory medication administered by nebulizer	0.0795	0.0128
Diagnostic ultrasound of heart	0.0908	0.0148
Esophagogastroduodenoscopy with closed biopsy	0.1119	0.0180
Continuous positive airway pressure	0.1158	0.0188
Closed endoscopic biopsy of lung	0.1377	0.0216
Computerized axial tomography of head	0.1028	0.0166
Transfusion of packed cells	0.0558	0.0090
Venous catheterization	0.0638	0.0100
Continuous Ventilation < 96 Hours	0.1619	0.0255
Closed biopsy of bronchus	0.0802	0.0125
Thoracentesis	0.0868	0.0140
Quartile 1	0.0335	0.0055
Quartile 2	0.0340	0.0055
Quartile 3	0.0346	0.0056
Caucasian	0.0778	0.0126
African American	0.0847	0.0137
Hispanic	0.0852	0.0138
Asian	0.1136	0.0186
Native American	0.1883	0.0304

FUTURE TRENDS

As more complex models come into more common usage in healthcare, they will be adapted to the development of patient severity indices. In particular, the generalized linear model has features that are particularly relevant to healthcare data, namely non-normal distributions. We cannot continue to force the data to fit the model; we must find models that fit the data because the data assumptions are valid. In the past, models have been used regardless of their applicability in terms of assumptions. The results of such studies are highly questionable. There are, in fact, many models that have been developed fairly recently that can be useful in health outcomes research. In chapter 4, we will show some additional models that are relevant to the analysis of healthcare data.

Figure 23. Kernel density estimation for prediction of mortality

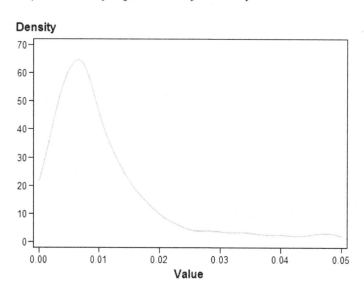

DISCUSSION

Given large datasets, and the presence of outliers, the traditional statistical methods are not always applicable or meaningful. Assumptions can be crucial to the applicability of the model, and assumptions are not always carefully considered. In particular, great care must be taken when performing logistic regression for a rare occurrence. Ideally, the data should be resampled so that the proportion of occurrences and non-occurrences is the same. We will discuss this in more detail in future chapters. However, if we consider the model assumptions carefully, we can usually find a reasonable model that will fit the data.

The data may not give high levels of correlation, and regression may not always be the best way to measure associations. It must also be remembered that associations in the data as identified in regression models do not demonstrate cause and effect. In observational studies for outcomes research, potential confounders should always be considered. It will require considerable domain knowledge to be able to develop a list of potential confounders that should be considered in the study. With the large datasets that are typically used for this type of research, we can include many potential confounders in the analysis. Many of these confounders can be examined through examination of diagnosis and procedure codes. Up to this point, we have just examined a small list of both; in subsequent chapters, we will demonstrate how all of these codes can be used in an outcomes analysis.

REFERENCES

Anonymous-KY. (2008). *Hospital Cost-to-Charge Ratio*. Retrieved June, 2008, 2008, from http://www. labor.ky.gov/workersclaims/medicalservices/hospitalcost/

Anonymous-PPS. (2008). *Acute Inpatient PPS* [Electronic Version]. Retrieved June, 2008 from http://www.cms.hhs.gov/AcuteInpatientPPS/01_overview.asp.

Anonymous-uncontrolled. (2008). *Glycemic Control Resource Room* [Electronic Version]. Retrieved June, 2008 from http://www.hospitalmedicine.org/ResourceRoomRedesign/html/06Track_Perf/08_Business_Case.cfm.

Barnett, A. H., Burger, J., Johns, D., Brodows, R., Kendall, D. M., & Roberts, A. (2007). Tolerability and efficacy of exenatide and titrated insulin glargine in adult patients with type 2 diabetes previously uncontrolled with metformin or a sulfonylurea: a multinational, randomized, open-label, two-period, crossover noninferiority trial. *Clinical Therapeutics, 29*(11), 2333–2348.

Battioui, C. (2007a). *Cost Models with Prominent Outliers.* University of Louisville, Louisville.

Battioui, C. (2007b). *Cost Models with Prominent Outliers: Digital Dissertations.*

Cerrito, P. (2007). Text Mining Coded Information. In H. A. D. Prado & E. Ferneda (Eds.), *Emerging Technologies of Text Mining: Techniques and Applications.* New York: IGI Global.

Example, A.-C. (2003). *Medicare Program; Proposed change in methodology for determinine payment for extraordinarily high-cost cases (cost outliers) under acute care hospital inpatient prospective payment system.* Retrieved 2008, from http://www.cms.hhs.gov/QuarterlyProviderUpdates/downloads/cms1243p.pdf

Gale, E., Dornan, T., & Tattersall, R. (1981). Severely uncontrolled diabetes in the over-fifties. *Diabetologia, 21*(1), 25–28.

Rosenstock, J., Rood, J., Cobitz, A., Biswas, N., Chou, H., & Garber, A. (2006). Initial treatment with rosiglitazone/metformin fixed-dose combination therapy compared with monotherapy with either rosiglitazone or metformin in patients with uncontrolled type 2 diabetes. *Diabetes, Obesity & Metabolism, 8*(6), 650–660.

Weights, A.-D. (2008). *Acute General Inpatient Hospital Reimbursement* [Electronic Version]. Retrieved June, 2008 from http://www.okhca.org/providers.aspx?id=618&menu=74&parts=7675_7677_7679.

Chapter 4
Predictive Modeling Versus Regression

INTRODUCTION

Predictive modeling includes regression, both logistic and linear, depending upon the type of outcome variable. It can also include the generalized linear model. However, there are other types of models also available, including decision trees and artificial neural networks under the general term of predictive modeling. Predictive modeling includes nearest neighbor discriminant analysis, also known as memory based reasoning. These other models are nonparametric and do not require that you know the probability distribution of the underlying patient population. Therefore, they are much more flexible when used to examine patient outcomes. Because predictive modeling uses regression in addition to these other models, the end results will improve upon those found using just regression by itself.

Some, but not all, of the predictive models require that all of the x-variables are independent. Therefore, we can allow some dependency in the indicator functions for diagnosis codes. However, predictive models must still also generally assume the uniformity of data entry. Because of the flexibility in the use of variables to define confounding factors, we can consider the presence or absence of uniformity in the model itself. We can define a variable to model provider, and to see how the provider impacts the severity index.

DOI: 10.4018/978-1-60566-752-2.ch004

Since the datasets used to define severity indices are generally too large for a p-value to have meaning, predictive modeling uses other measures of model fit. Generally, too, there are enough observations so that the data can be partitioned into two or more datasets. The first subset is used to define (or train) the model. The second subset can be used in an iterative process to improve the model. The third subset is used to test the model for accuracy. It is also known as a holdout sample.

The definition of "best" model needs to be considered in this context as well. Just what do we mean by "best"? In a regression model, the "best" model is one that satisfies the criterion of uniform minimum variance unbiased estimator. In other words, it is only "best" in the class of unbiased estimators. As soon as the class of estimators is expanded, "best" no longer exists, and we must define the criteria that we will use to determine a "best" fit. There are several criteria to consider. For a binary outcome variable, we can use the misclassification rate. However, especially in medicine, misclassification can have different costs. For example, a false positive error is not as costly as a false negative error if the outcome involves the diagnosis of a terminal disease.

Another difference when using predictive modeling is that many different models can be used, and compared to find the one that is the best. We can use the traditional regression, but also decision trees and neural network analysis. We can combine different models to define a new model. Generally, use of multiple models has been frowned upon because it is possible to "shop" for one that is effective. Indeed, the nearest neighbor discriminant analysis can always find a model that predicts correctly 100% of the time when defining the model, but predicts 0% of the time for any subsequent data. When using multiple models, it is essential to define a holdout sample that can be used to test the results.

BACKGROUND

Predictive modeling routinely makes use of a holdout sample to test the accuracy of the results. Figure 1 demonstrates predictive modeling. In SAS, there are two different regression models, three different neural network models, and two decision tree models. There is also a memory based reasoning model, otherwise known as nearest neighbor discriminant analysis. These models are discussed in detail in Cerrito (2007). It is not our intent here to provide an introductory text on neural networks; instead, we will demonstrate how they can be used effectively to investigate the outcome data.

Figure 1 shows that many different models can be used. Once defined, the models are compared and the optimal model chosen based upon pre-selected criteria. The node labeled Model Comparison is used for this purpose. It compares all of the models and then chooses the optimal one based upon the pre-selected criterion. Model comparison can use several different statistics for comparison. The default is the misclassification rate on the holdout sample. However, if a false negative that results in an ill patient not getting treatment is more costly to the patient compared to a false positive where a healthy patient gets unnecessary treatment (or conversely), the model can be optimized based upon a minimization of costs. It is up to you to choose which measure you want to use to compare models.

Then, additional data can be scored (using the score node as shown in Figure 1) so that new patients who are admitted subsequently can have a severity level assigned to them. This figture also includes a data partition so that a holdout sample can be extracted in order to test the model results. It is important to be able to use the model to score subsequent data. When a patient severity model is defined, it should be tested on new data to demonstrate reliability.

Figure 1. Predictive modeling of patient outcomes

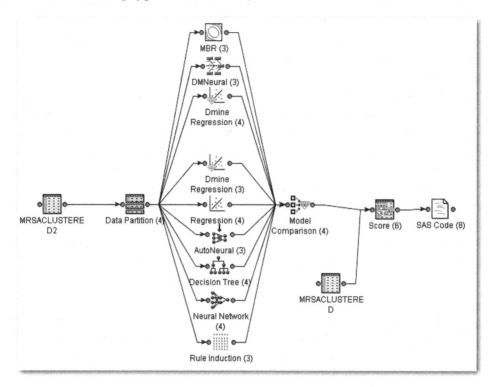

There is still limited use of predictive modeling, with the exception of regression models, in medical studies. Most of the use of predictive modeling is fairly recent. (Sylvia et al., 2006) While most predictive models are used for examining costs (Powers, Meyer, Roebuck, & Vaziri, 2005), they can be invaluable in improving the quality of care. (Hodgman, 2008; Tewari et al., 2001; Weber & Neeser, 2006; Whitlock & Johnston, 2006) One recent study does indicate that predictive modeling can be used to target the most high risk patients for more intensive case management. (Weber & Neeser, 2006) It has also been used to examine workflow in the healthcare environment. (Tropsha & Golbraikh, 2007) Some studies focus on particular types of models such as neural networks. (Gamito & Crawford, 2004) In many cases, administrative (billing) data are used to identify patients who can benefit from interventions, and to identify patients who can benefit the most. Most of the use of predictive modeling is fairly recent.

This chapter is not intended to be a complete discussion of predictive modeling; it provides a basic introduction to its use in defining severity indices and risk models. For a more complete discussion, the reader is referred to Cerrito (2007, 2008). However, we will briefly examine two commonly used predictive models: neural networks and decision trees.

Neural networks act like black boxes. There is no definite model or equation, and the model is not presented in the concise format available for regression. Its accuracy is examined similar to the diagnostics of the regression curve, including the misclassification rate, the AIC (Akaike's Information Criterion), and the average error. The simplest neural network contains a single input (an independent variable) and a single target (a dependent variable) with a single output. Its complexity increases with the addition of hidden layers and additional input variables (Figure 2).

Figure 2. Diagram of a neural network

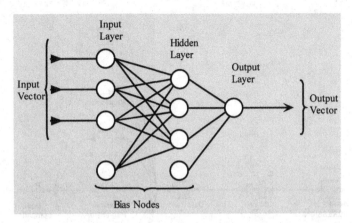

With no hidden layers, the results of a neural network analysis resemble those of regression. Each input variable is connected to each variable in the hidden layer, and each hidden variable is connected to each outcome variable. The hidden layers combine inputs and apply a function to predict outputs. Hidden layers are often nonlinear.

The architecture of the neural network is used to define the model. There are two major types of neural network used, the MLP and the GLIM. MLP, the multi-layer perceptron, is the default model. A perceptron is a classifier that maps an input x to an output, f(x). The GLIM represents the more standard generalized linear model discussed in detail in Chapter 3. You should compare these two models to see the impact on the results. You can also define your own model, although this method is not recommended for beginners.

Decision trees provide a completely different approach to classification. A decision tree develops a series of if-then rules. Each rule assigns an observation to one segment of the tree, at which point another if-then rule is applied. The initial segment, containing the entire data set, is the root node for the decision tree. The final nodes are called leaves. Intermediate nodes (a node plus all its successors) form a branch of the tree. The final leaf containing an observation is its predictive value.

Unlike neural networks and regression, decision trees do not always work with interval data. Decision trees work better with nominal outcomes that have more than two possible results and with ordinal outcome variables. Missing values can be used in creating if-then rules. Therefore, imputation is not required for decision trees, although you can use it when working with decision trees.

PREDICTIVE MODELING IN SAS ENTERPRISE MINER

For predicting a rare occurrence, one more node is added to the model in Figure 1, the sampling node (Figure 3). This node uses all of the observations with the rare occurrence, and then takes a random sample of the remaining data. While the sampling node can use any proportional split, we recommend a 50:50 split. Figure 4 shows how the defaults are modified in the sampling node of SAS Enterprise Miner to make predictions. Starting a project in SAS Enterprise Miner was discussed in Chapter 1.

Rule induction is a special case of a decision tree model. Figure 3 also shows three different neural network models and two regression models. The second regression model automatically categorizes all

Figure 3. Addition of sampling node

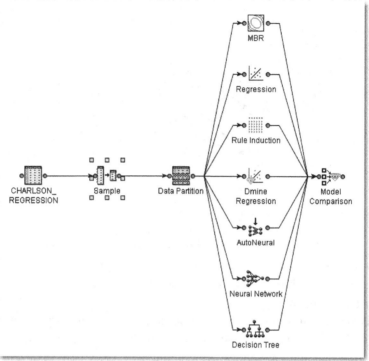

interval independent variables. There is one remaining model in Figure 3; the MBR or memory-based reasoning model. It represents nearest neighbor discriminant analysis. We first discuss the use of the sampling node in the process of predictive modeling. We start with the defaults for sampling node as modified in Figure 4.

The first arrow indicates that the sampling is stratified, and the criterion is level based. The rarest level (in this case, mortality) is sampled so that it will consist of half (50% sample proportion) of the sample to be used in the predictive model.

We consider the same problem of predicting mortality that was discussed in the previous chapter. We use just the three patient diagnoses of pneumonia, septicemia, and immune disorder that we used in Chapter 3. However, unlike the analysis in Chapter 3, we use the sampling node to get a 50/50 split in the data.

We use all of the models depicted in Figure 1. According to the model comparison, the rule induction provides the best fit, using the misclassification criterion as the measure of "best". We first look at the regression model, comparing the results to those in the previous chapter when a 50/50 split was not performed. The overall misclassification rate is 28%, with the divisions as shown in Table 1.

The misclassification becomes more balanced between false positives and false negatives with a 50/50 split in the data. The model gives heavier weight to false positives than it does to false negatives. We will clearly demonstrate the benefits of a 50/50 split in Chapter 5, as we discuss some of the severity indices currently available.

We will first consider the example used in Chapter 3 with just three diagnoses of pneumonia, septicemia, and immune disorder. We will contrast the predictive modeling approach here to the regression

Figure 4. Change to defaults in sampling node

Property	Value
Node ID	Smpl
Imported Data	
Exported Data	
Variables	
Sample Method	Stratify
Random Seed	12345
Size	
Type	Percentage
Observations	
Percentage	10.0
Alpha	0.01
PValue	0.01
Cluster Method	Random
Stratified	
Criterion	Level Based
Ignore Small Strata	No
Minimum Strata Size	5
Level Based Options	
Level Selection	Rarest Level
Level Proportion	100.0
Sample Proportion	50.0
Oversampling	
Adjust Frequency	No
Based on Count	No
Exclude Missing Levels	No

models from Chapter 3. We first want to examine the decision tree model. While it is not the most accurate model, it is one that clearly describes the rationale behind the predictions. This tree is given in Figure 5. The tree shows that the first split occurs on the variable, Septicemia. Patients with Septicemia are more likely to suffer mortality compared to patients without Septicemia. As shown in the previous chapter, the Immune Disorder has the next highest level of mortality, followed by Pneumonia.

Since rule induction is identified as the best model, we examine that one next. The misclassification rate is only slightly smaller compared to the regression model. Table 2 gives the classification table.

The results look virtually identical to those in Table 1. For this reason, the regression model, although not defined as the best, can be used to predict outcomes when only these three variables are used. The similarities in the models can also be visualized in the ROC (received-operating curve) that graphs the

Table 1. Misclassification in regression model

Target	Outcome	Target Percentage	Outcome Percentage	Count	Total Percentage
Training Data					
0	0	67.8	80.1	54008	40.4
1	0	32.2	38.3	25622	19.2
0	1	23.8	19.2	12852	9.6
1	1	76.3	61.7	41237	30.8
Validation Data					
0	0	67.7	80.8	40498	40.4
1	0	32.3	38.5	19315	19.2
0	1	23.8	19.2	9646	9.6
1	1	76.2	61.5	30830	30.7

Figure 5. Decision tree results

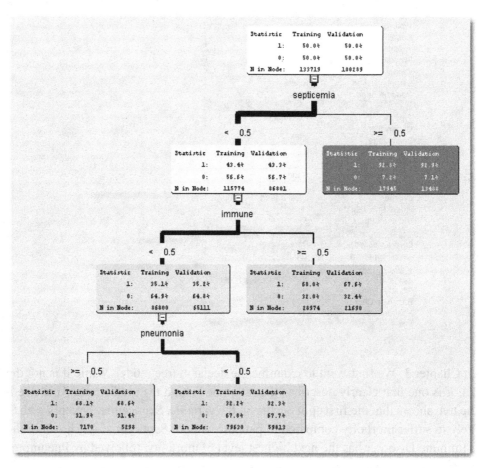

sensitivity versus one minus the specificity (Figure 6). The curves for rule induction and regression are virtually the same.

Table 2. Misclassification in rule induction model

Target	Outcome	Target Percentage	Outcome Percentage	Count	Total Percentage
Training Data					
0	0	67.8	80.8	54008	40.4
1	0	32.2	38.3	25622	19.2
0	1	23.8	19.2	12852	9.6
1	1	76.3	61.7	41237	30.8
Validation Data					
0	0	67.7	80.8	40498	40.4
1	0	32.3	38.5	19315	19.2
0	1	23.8	19.2	9646	9.6
1	1	76.2	61.5	30830	30.7

Figure 6. Comparison of ROC curves

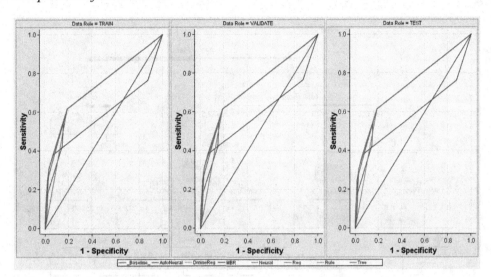

MANY VARIABLES IN LARGE SAMPLES

There can be hundreds if not thousands of variables collected for each patient. There can be far too many to include in any predictive model. We want to include all those variables that are crucial to the analysis, including potential confounders, but the use of too many variables can cause the model to over-fit the results, inflating the outcomes. Therefore, there needs to be some type of variable reduction method. In the past, factor analysis has been used to reduce the set of variables prior to modeling the data. However, there is now a more novel method available (Figure 7).

In our example, there are many additional variables that can be considered in this analysis. Therefore, we use the variable selection technique to choose the most relevant. We first use the decision tree followed by regression, and then regression followed by the decision tree.

Using the decision tree to define the variables, Figure 8 shows the ones that remain for the modeling. Note that age, charges, and length of stay are at the beginning of the tree.

Figure 7. Variable selection

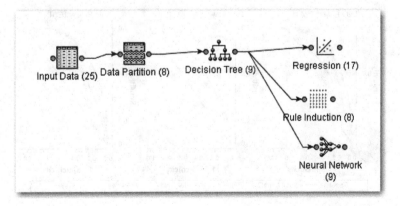

Figure 8. Decision tree variables

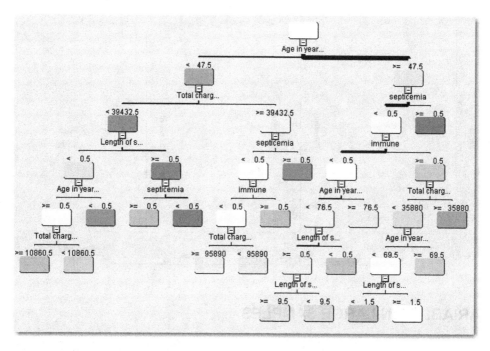

This tree shows that age, length of stay, having septicemia, immune disorder, length of stay and total charges are related to mortality. The remaining variables have been rejected from the model. The rule induction is the best model, and the misclassification rate decreases to 22% with the added variables. The ROC curve looks considerably improved (Figure 9).

The ROC curve is much higher compared to that in Figure 6. If we use regression to perform the variable selection, the results remain the same. In addition, a decision tree is virtually the same when it follows the regression compared to when it precedes regression (Figure 10).

The above example only used three possible diagnosis codes. We want to expand upon the number of diagnosis codes, and also to use a number of procedure codes. In this example, we restrict our atten-

Figure 9. ROC curves for models following decision tree

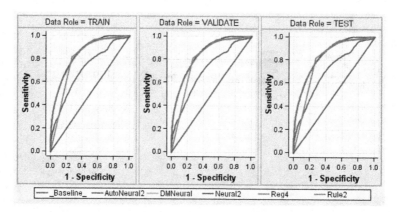

Figure 10. Decision tree following regression

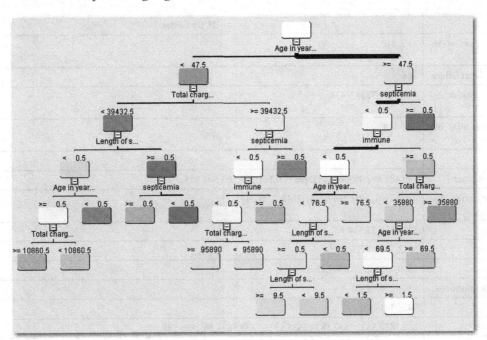

tion to patients with a primary diagnosis of COPD. This is approximately 245,000 patients in the NIS dataset. Table 3 gives the list of diagnosis codes used. The choice of these codes will be discussed in more detail in Chapter 5. Table 4 gives the list of procedure codes taken from Chapter 3. This example was discussed briefly in Chapter 3 for the interval outcomes of length of stay and total charges. Here, we first examine a prediction of mortality.

If we perform standard logistic regression without stratified sampling, the false positive rate remains small (approximately 3-4%), but with a high false negative rate (minimized at 38%). Given the large dataset, almost all of the input variables are statistically significant. The percent agreement is 84% and the ROC curve looks fairly good (Figure 11).

If we perform predictive modeling and stratify the sample to the rarest level, the accuracy rate drops to 75%, but the false negative rate is considerably improved. Figure 12 gives the ROC curve from predictive modeling. It shows that the model predicts considerably better than chance in the testing set.

We will examine the stratified sampling in more detail in the next section.

CHANGE IN SPLIT IN THE DATA

The analyses in the previous section assumed a 50/50 split between mortality and non-mortality. We want to look at the results if mortality composes only 25% of the data, and 10% of the data. Table 5 gives the regression classification breakdown for a 25% sample; Table 6 gives the breakdown for a 10% sample.

Note that the ability to classify mortality accurately is decreasing with the decrease of the split; almost all of the observations are classified as non-mortality, but also at a cost of a high level of false positives.

Table 3. Diagnosis codes used to predict mortality

Condition	ICD9 Codes
Acute myocardial infarction	410, 412
Congestive heart failure	428
Peripheral vascular disease	441,4439,7854,V434
Cerebral vascular accident	430-438
Dementia	290
Pulmonary disease	490,491,492,493,494,495,496,500,501,502,503,504,505
Connective tissue disorder	7100,7101,7104,7140,7141,7142,7148,5171,725
Peptic ulcer	531,532,533,534
Liver disease	5712,5714,5715,5716
Diabetes	2500,2501,2502,2503,2507
Diabetes complications	2504,2505,2506
Paraplegia	342,3441
Renal disease	582,5830,5831,5832,5833,5835,5836,5837,5834,585,586,588
Cancer	14,15,16,17,18,170,171,172,174,175,176,179,190,191,193, 194,1950,1951,1952,1953,1954,1955,1958,200,201,202,203, 204,205,206,207,208
Metastatic cancer	196,197,198,1990,1991
Severe liver disease	5722,5723,5724,5728
HIV	042,043,044

The decision tree for a 25% sample (Figure 13) is considerably different from that in Figure 10 with a 50/50 split. Now, the procedure of Esophagogastroduodenoscopy gives the first leaf of the tree; in Figure 10, the first split was on age followed by charges and length of stay.Thus, a change in the sampling can in and of itself be responsible for the outcomes predicted by the model.

Note that the trend shown in the 25% sample is even more exaggerated in the 10% sample. Figure 14 shows that the decision tree has changed yet again. It now includes the procedure of continuous positive airway pressure and the diagnosis of congestive heart failure.

ADDITION OF WEIGHTS FOR DECISION MAKING

In most medical studies, a false negative is more costly to the patient compared to a false positive. This occurs because a false positive generally leads to more invasive tests; however, a false negative means that a potentially life-threatening illness will go undiagnosed, and hence, untreated. Therefore, we can weight a false negative at higher cost, and then change the definition of a "best" model to one that minimizes costs. The problem is to determine which costs to use.

The best thing to do is to experiment with magnitudes of difference in cost between the false positive and false negative to see what happens. At a 1:1 ratio, the best model is still based upon the misclas-

Table 4. Procedure codes used to predict mortality

pr	Procedure Translation	Frequency	Percent
9904	Transfusion of packed cells	17756	7.05
3893	Venous catheterization, not elsewhere classified	16142	6.41
9671	Continuous mechanical ventilation for less than 96 consecutive hours	10528	4.18
3324	Closed [endoscopic] biopsy of bronchus	8315	3.30
9672	Continuous mechanical ventilation for 96 consecutive hours or more	8243	3.27
3491	Thoracentesis	8118	3.22
3995	Hemodialysis	8083	3.21
9604	Insertion of endotracheal tube	7579	3.01
9921	Injection of antibiotic	6786	2.69
9394	Respiratory medication administered by nebulizer	6309	2.50
9390	Continuous positive airway pressure	7868	1.48
8856	Coronary arteriography using two catheters	7622	1.44
4516	Esophagogastroduodenoscopy [EGD] with closed biopsy	7516	1.42
966	Enteral infusion of concentrated nutritional substances	7203	1.36
3722	Left heart cardiac catheterization	6652	1.25
8853	Angiocardiography of left heart structures	6350	1.20
4513	Other endoscopy of small intestine	6343	1.19
3404	Insertion of intercostal catheter for drainage	5693	1.07
8741	Computerized axial tomography of thorax	5538	1.04
9915	Parenteral infusion of concentrated nutritional substances	5169	0.97
9907	Transfusion of other serum	4962	0.93
9396	Other oxygen enrichment	4937	0.93
4311	Percutaneous [endoscopic] gastrostomy	4831	0.91
3895	Venous catheterization for renal dialysis	4726	0.89
0331	Spinal tap	4362	0.82
3891	Arterial catheterization	3867	0.73
3327	Closed endoscopic biopsy of lung	3776	0.71
9339	Other physical therapy	3492	0.66
311	Temporary tracheostomy	3406	0.64
4523	Colonoscopy	3404	0.64

sification rate. Change to a 5:1 ratio indicates that a false negative is five times as costly compared to a false positive. A 10:1 ratio makes it ten times as costly. We need to determine if changes to this ratio result in changes to the optimal model. We will discuss weights in more detail with additional examples in subsequent sections of this chapter.

Figure 11. ROC curve for traditional logistic regression

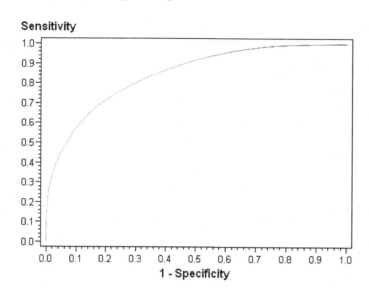

Figure 12. ROC from predictive modeling

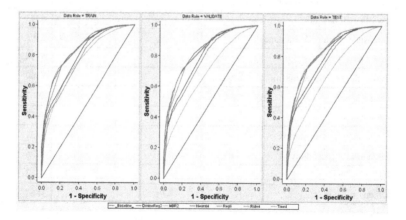

INTRODUCTION TO LIFT

Lift allows us to find the patients at highest risk for occurrence, and with the greatest probability of accurate prediction. This is especially important since these are the patients we would want to take the greatest care for, and who will incur the highest costs and longest length of stay.

Using lift, true positive patients with highest confidence come first, followed by positive patients with lower confidence. True negative cases with lowest confidence come next, followed by negative cases with highest confidence. Based on that ordering, the observations are partitioned into deciles, and the following statistics are calculated:

- The *Target density* of a decile is the number of actually positive instances in that decile divided by the total number of instances in the decile.

Table 5. Misclassification rate for a 25% sample

Target	Outcome	Target Percentage	Outcome Percentage	Count	Total Percentage
Training Data					
0	0	80.4	96.6	10070	72.5
1	0	19.6	70.9	2462	17.7
0	1	25.6	3.3	348	2.5
1	1	74.4	29.1	1010	7.3
Validation Data					
0	0	80.2	97.1	7584	72.8
1	0	19.8	71.7	1870	17.9
0	1	23.7	2.9	229	2.2
1	1	76.2	28.2	735	7.0

- The *Cumulative target density* is the target density computed over the first n deciles.
- The *lift* for a given decile is the ratio of the target density for the decile to the target density over all the test data.
- The *Cumulative lift* for a given decile is the ratio of the cumulative target density to the target density over all the test data.

Given a lift function, we can decide on a decile cutpoint so that we can predict the high risk patients above the cutpoint, and predict the low risk patients below a second cutpoint, while failing to make a definite prediction for those in the center. In that way, we can dismiss those who have no risk, and aggressively treat those at highest risk. Lift allows us to distinguish between patients without assuming a uniformity of risk. Figure 15 shows the lift for the testing set when we use just the three input variables of pneumonia, septicemia, and immune disorder.

Random chance is indicated by the lift value of 1.0; values that are higher than 1.0 indicate that the observations are more predictable compared to random chance. In this example, 40% of the patient

Table 6. Misclassification rate for a 10% sample

Target	Outcome	Target Percentage	Outcome Percentage	Count	Total Percentage
Training Data					
0	0	91.5	99.3	31030	89.4
1	0	8.5	83.5	2899	8.3
0	1	27.3	0.7	216	0.6
1	1	72.6	16.5	574	1.6
Validation Data					
0	0	91.5	99.2	23265	89.3
1	0	8.4	82.4	2148	8.2
0	1	27.8	0.7	176	0.7
1	1	72.2	17.5	457	1.7

Figure 13. Decision tree for 25/75 split in the data

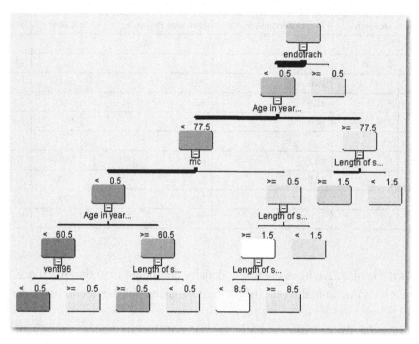

Figure 14. Decision tree for 10% sample

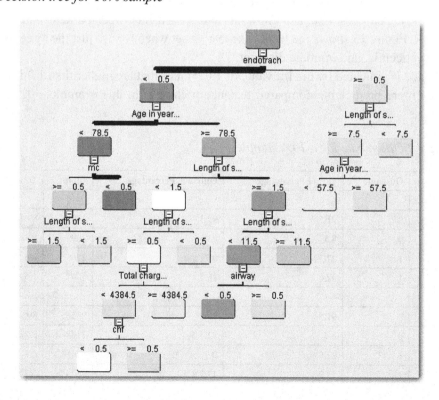

Figure 15. Lift function for three-variable input

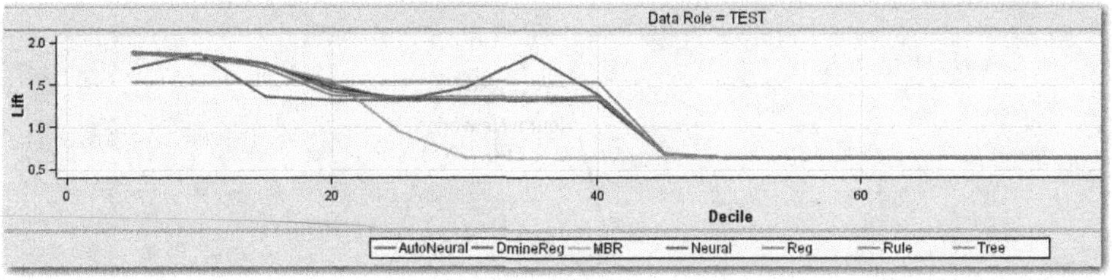

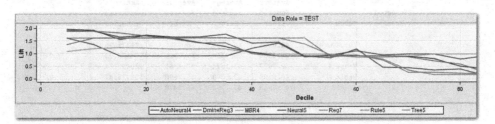

records have a higher level of prediction than just chance. Therefore, we can concentrate on these 4 deciles of patients. If we use the expanded model that includes patient demographic information plus additional diagnosis and procedure codes for COPD, we get the lift shown in Figure 16. The model can now predict the first 5 deciles of patient outcomes.

Therefore, we can predict accurately those patients most at risk for death; we can determine which patients can benefit from more aggressive treatment to reduce the likelihood that this outcome will occur.

PREDICTIVE MODELING OF CONTINUOUS OUTCOMES

We next turn our attention to predictive models using length of stay, cost, or charges as the outcome variable. In this case, we are trying to determine whether patients of similar severity have similar outcomes. Not all of the available predictive models will work with interval outcomes, so we will reduce the model choices to neural networks, memory based reasoning, regression, and decision trees.

Because we are no longer concerned with a rare occurrence as a target, we do not have to sample before the analysis. Therefore, we use the predictive model as given in Figure 17. It is not necessary to use the entire sample; a subsample will give nearly the same results and reduce the computational time, which can be considerable if the data set is extremely large. We will use different subsamples to examine the data. We use length of stay as the target variable, and limit our analysis to pneumonia, septicemia, and immune disorder. We also include mortality as an input variable. We start with a 1% sample. According to the model comparison, the optimal model is a decision tree with the smallest average error (Figure 18).

The reporting results will be different compared to a binary model. There is no misclassification rate reported, nor is there lift. Instead, the focus is on the average error of the model.

Figure 16. Lift function for complete model

125

Figure 17. Predictive model for length of stay

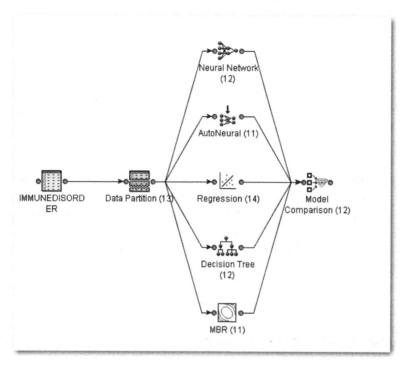

Figure 19 gives the decision tree.
The English rules are given below:

```
IF 0.5 <= septicemia
THEN
  NODE: 3
  N: 717
  AVE: 11.9609
  SD: 13.1085
```

Figure 18. Model comparison for length of stay

Fit Statistics
Model selection based on _TASE_

Selected Model	MODEL	Test: Average Squared Error	Train: Average Squared Error	Valid: Average Squared Error	Train: Akaike's Information Criterion
	AutoNeural11	42.0925	44.3105	56.7396	121271.76
	MBR11	54.5305	26.7366	69.8921	188.73
	Neural12	40.7977	43.1674	55.2365	120400.24
	Reg14	40.9100	43.3070	55.3690	120475.47
Y	Tree12	40.7913	43.1752	55.2478	.

Figure 19. Decision tree for length of stay

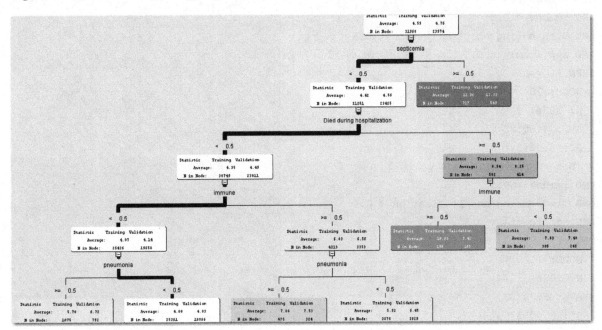

The first split occurs based upon the value of septicemia; if the value is equal to one, then the average length of stay is predicted to be almost 12 days.

```
IF immune < 0.5
AND 0.5 <= Died during hospitalization
AND septicemia < 0.5
THEN
   NODE: 8
   N: 306
   AVE: 7.8268
   SD: 13.8321
IF 0.5 <= immune
AND 0.5 <= Died during hospitalization
AND septicemia < 0.5
THEN
   NODE: 9
   N: 196
   AVE: 10.6837
   SD: 15.0706
```

The second split occurs for a value of immune disorder and mortality. If the patient died, the value of septicemia is positive and the value of immune disorder is negative, then the average length of stay is almost 8 days; if immune disorder is positive and the patient died (and has septicemia), then the average length of stay is almost 11 days.

```
IF pneumonia < 0.5
AND immune < 0.5
AND Died during hospitalization < 0.5
AND septicemia < 0.5
THEN
  NODE: 10
  N: 25361
  AVE: 4.00122
  SD: 5.98604
IF 0.5 <= pneumonia
AND immune < 0.5
AND Died during hospitalization < 0.5
AND septicemia < 0.5
THEN
  NODE: 11
  N: 1075
  AVE: 5.70233
  SD: 5.00537
IF pneumonia < 0.5
AND 0.5 <= immune
AND Died during hospitalization < 0.5
AND septicemia < 0.5
THEN
  NODE: 12
  N: 3878
  AVE: 5.91594
  SD: 7.19594
IF 0.5 <= pneumonia
AND 0.5 <= immune
AND Died during hospitalization < 0.5
AND septicemia < 0.5
THEN
  NODE: 13
  N: 435
  AVE: 7.07586
  SD: 6.33627
```

The final split occurs for pneumonia, given different values of immune disorder, septicemia, and mortality. If the patient has pneumonia and immune disorder, but not septicemia, then the average stay is 7 days. If the patient has immune disorder and septicemia but not pneumonia, then the stay is slightly longer at 7.2 days. Figure 20 gives the regression results.

All of the variables are statistically significant, but the r^2 value is less than 5%, indicating that most of the variability in length of stay is not accounted for by these variables. If we cut the size of the sample in half, the results are virtually the same as in the larger sample (Figure 21).

Figure 20. Regression results for length of stay

```
                         Analysis of Variance

                              Sum of
Source              DF       Squares    Mean Square   F Value   Pr > F

Model                4         64853         16213    374.32   <.0001
Error            31963       1384438     43.313776
Corrected Total  31967       1449291


                      Model Fit Statistics

R-Square      0.0447    Adj R-Sq        0.0446
AIC       120475.4721    BIC        120477.4737
SBC       120517.3346    C(p)            5.0000


              Analysis of Maximum Likelihood Estimates

                              Standard
Parameter    DF    Estimate     Error    t Value    Pr > |t|

Intercept     1      4.0432     0.0408      99.06     <.0001
DIED          1      3.1844     0.2684      11.86     <.0001
immune        1      1.7859     0.1043      17.12     <.0001
pneumonia     1      1.3155     0.1641       8.02     <.0001
septicemia    1      6.2236     0.2554      24.37     <.0001
```

Figure 21. Results of predictive modeling for length of stay with a 0.5% sample

```
Fit Statistics
Model selection based on _TASE_

                        Test:      Train:     Valid:
                       Average    Average    Average
Selected               Squared    Squared    Squared
Model       MODEL       Error      Error      Error

          AutoNeural11  41.1477    29.834    32.0370
          MBR11         55.0735   128.983    44.3662
          Neural12      40.4087    29.461    31.4543
          Reg14         40.4808    29.669    31.9930
    Y     Tree12        40.2800    29.657    32.1527
```

Figure 21 shows the results limited to just 1000 random observations. The average squared error is slightly smaller (Figure 22). Otherwise, the decision tree remains the best model, with regression having just a slightly larger error rate.

The regression model increases the r^2 slightly to 0.06; however, not all of the variables are statistically significant with this small dataset (Figure 23).

Note that mortality, immune disorder, and pneumonia are no longer statistically significant. The remaining significant variable is septicemia. This result again demonstrates that a sample that is too large will indicate that all variables are statistically significant, but with an r^2 that is so low as to make the model meaningless. Reflecting that smaller sample size and lack of significance in the model, the decision tree is simpler as well (Figure 24); pneumonia is not used at all in the tree.

We can also include the interactions in the model, to include consideration of patients with 2 or 3 of the diseases we are using in the model. However, that change does not alter the results terribly much. We

Figure 22. Results of predictive modeling for length of stay with 1000 random observations

```
Fit Statistics
Model selection based on _TASE_

                            Test:       Train:      Valid:
                            Average     Average     Average
         Selected          Squared     Squared     Squared
         Model    MODEL     Error       Error       Error

                  AutoNeural11  40.0401     31.510      21.6310
                  MBR11         40.9281     120.646     21.4760
                  Neural12      38.2763     30.011      20.0929
                  Reg14         38.9176     31.510      20.9170
         Y        Tree12        38.0370     31.507      20.9850
```

Figure 23. Results of regression using 1000 observations

```
                        Analysis of Variance

                             Sum of
Source              DF       Squares     Mean Square   F Value   Pr > F

Model               4        865.215537  216.303884    6.78      <.0001
Error               395      12604       31.909271
Corrected Total     399      13469


                Model Fit Statistics

R-Square      0.0642    Adj R-Sq      0.0548
AIC           1390.1271 BIC           1392.2534
SBC           1410.0844 C(p)          5.0000


           Analysis of Maximum Likelihood Estimates

                            Standard
Parameter    DF   Estimate  Error     t Value   Pr > |t|

Intercept    1    4.4433    0.3115    14.26     <.0001
DIED         1    2.8333    2.4131    1.17      0.2410
immune       1    1.0333    0.8254    1.25      0.2114
pneumonia    1    -1.0882   1.1825    -0.92     0.3580
septicemia   1    8.2087    1.9147    4.29      <.0001
```

do, however, want to add more information about patient diagnoses, using the diagnoses and procedures listed in Tables 2 and 3 in the preceding section. We use the same sample size to examine the target value of length of stay for patients with COPD (1% of the patients with COPD). The only change we make to the diagram process is to change the target variable to length of stay, and to include mortality as an input variable. We also remove rule induction as a potential model. We change the sampling method to random rather than to stratify since there is no categorical outcome on which to base the stratification. Figure 25 shows that Dmine regression (where the interval variables are categorized) is the best model, and that there is considerable variability in the average error for the testing set.

Figure 24. Decision tree for length of stay using 1000 observations

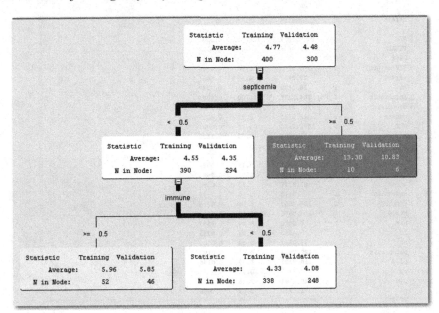

Figure 25. Results for COPD and length of stay

Fit Statistics
Model selection based on _TASE_

Selected Model	MODEL	Test: Average Squared Error	Train: Average Squared Error	Valid: Average Squared Error
	AutoNeural12	20.0664	24.7004	20.8968
Y	DmineReg7	14.5243	17.5501	15.3507
	MBR12	21.1796	23.8999	22.1213
	Neural13	16.4288	19.8373	17.1540
	Reg15	15.8810	19.0674	16.6686
	Tree13	15.0973	18.0821	16.0617

The tree has a larger error, but it is reasonably close to regression so that we can examine it and compare it to Dmine regression and standard regression. Figure 27 gives the summary table for the standard regression, with a 28% r² value. The standard regression indicates that age, race, and income quartile are statistically significant. In addition, there are procedures, including ventilation, the use of a venous catheter, ultrasound, and antibiotic use that are statistically significant for length of stay. There are also patient diagnoses that are significant, including congestive heart failure, cerebral vascular event, and dementia. However, diabetes, HIV, and peripheral vascular disease are not significant.

Figure 26 gives the decision tree; Figure 28 gives the results for the Dmine regression, which does a stepwise procedure as well.

Many of the patient conditions are statistically significant, including age, race, and income quartile as well as the use of antibiotics, congestive heart failure, and dementia. Diabetes is not significant. The decision tree indicates that prolonged use of a ventilator is of first importance in making the split.

Figure 26. Regression results

Effect	DF	Squares	F Value	Pr > F
AGE	1	2337.5297	125.85	<.0001
FEMALE	1	11.9536	0.64	0.4225
RACE	5	301.2745	3.24	0.0063
ZIPInc_Qrtl	3	165.8230	2.98	0.0303
airway	1	78.2683	4.21	0.0401
ami	1	26.2172	1.41	0.2349
antibiotic	1	204.2272	11.00	0.0009
biopbronc	1	707.5975	38.10	<.0001
cancer	1	12.0283	0.65	0.4210
chf	1	1562.9613	84.15	<.0001
ctd	1	37.7909	2.03	0.1538
cva	1	288.2956	15.52	<.0001
dc	1	22.0866	1.19	0.2755
dementia	1	170.0337	9.15	0.0025
diabetes	1	1.6059	0.09	0.7687
endo	1	67.8377	3.65	0.0560
endotrach	1	1.4772	0.08	0.7779
esophag	1	184.4860	9.93	0.0016
hemod	1	294.7856	15.87	<.0001
hiv	1	0.0480	0.00	0.9595
ld	1	0.4562	0.02	0.8755
mc	1	71.3327	3.84	0.0501
paraplegia	1	122.7853	6.61	0.0102
pd	1	110.9305	5.97	0.0146
pu	1	17.6725	0.95	0.3294
pvd	1	40.4594	2.18	0.1400
rd	1	1.6371	0.09	0.7666

Figure 27. Decision tree for length of stay

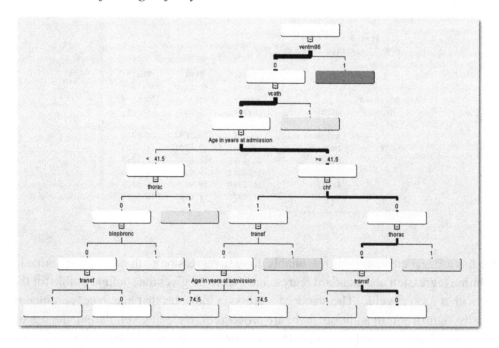

Note the similarity between Figures 27 and 28. The variables in the decision tree are in a similar order to those in the Dmine regression. These two show that both procedures and diagnoses are important to length of stay, with prolonged use of ventilation having the greatest contribution followed by the use of a venous catheter, the patient's age, and the use of a blood transfusion.

Figure 28. Dmine regression results for length of stay

```
The DMINE Procedure

                           Effects Chosen for Target: LOS

                                                              Sum of      Error Mean
Effect                 DF     R-Square    F Value   p-Value   Squares       Square

Class: venta96          1     0.148446  1604.821073  <.0001     33004      20.565731
Class: vcath            1     0.033285   374.429109  <.0001   7400.228117  19.764030
AOV16: AGE             15     0.031939    24.885088  <.0001   7101.057464  19.023595
Class: transf           1     0.018516   221.591563  <.0001   4116.654322  18.577667
Class: thorac           1     0.014099   171.867847  <.0001   3134.616022  18.238525
Class: chf              1     0.011695   144.792175  <.0001   2600.104093  17.957490
Class: biopbronc        1     0.009488   118.981914  <.0001   2109.525485  17.729800
Class: esophag          1     0.001873    23.540705  <.0001    416.350339  17.686400
Class: hemod            1     0.001509    19.009959  <.0001    335.559789  17.651789
Class: ultrasound       1     0.001241    15.658793  <.0001    275.965226  17.623659
Class: endo             1     0.000992    12.532250   0.0004   220.587088  17.601555
```

We reduce the sample size to 1000 to see if the results are similar. Results indicate that the tree model is now the best (Figure 29).

The r^2 value increases to 42% with the smaller set of observations compared to the previous value of 28%. The decision tree, too, becomes simpler (Figure 30). In this result, the use of venous catheterization, congestive heart failure, and the patient's age are the only three variables used. None of the procedures are significant. This r^2 value appears to be much more reasonable compared to models in Chapter 3.

We consider one last series of models. We categorize length of stay and define the target variable as ordinal. We use quantiles and define the target as ordinal. Note that a misclassification rate has been added to the average error (Figure 31). Standard regression is the optimcal model.

The decision tree results are almost identical. Both procedures and diagnoses are statistically significant in the tree (Figure 32). However, many of the branches to the tree are related to age. It suggests that we should also have categorized age.

We will show in the next section how a predictive model can be used to rank the quality of providers. This can be done with binary outcomes such as mortality, and with continuous outcomes such as length of stay. Most commonly, the outcome used to define quality is that of mortality.

Figure 29. Model comparison for length of stay for 1000 observations

```
Fit Statistics
Model selection based on _TASE_

                          Test:      Train:     Valid:
                          Average    Average    Average
              Selected    Squared    Squared    Squared
              Model   MODEL   Error      Error      Error

                      AutoNeural12   19.1456    24.5106    21.8871
                      DmineReg7      15.2629    13.5409    19.7408
                      MBR12          14.0877    23.1638    20.8020
                      Neural13       15.1135    16.8712    18.7502
                      Reg15          17.1121    13.8266    21.9313
              Y       Tree13         13.9606    17.0963    18.0887
```

Figure 30. Decision tree for 1000 observations

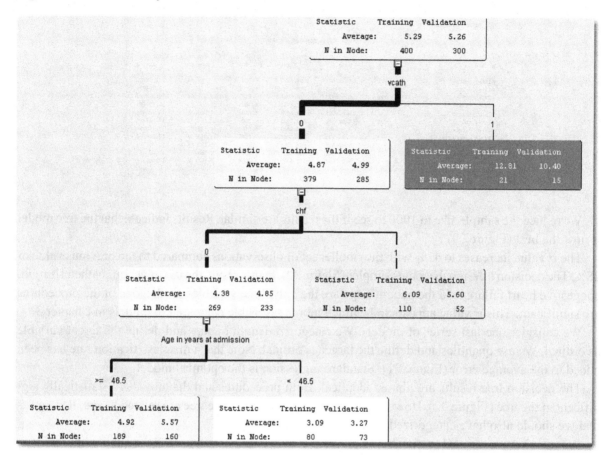

Figure 31. Predictive models with ordinal target for length of stay

```
Fit Statistics
Model selection based on _TMISC_

                                        Train:      Valid:      Test:
                             Test:      Average     Average     Average
Selected                     Misclassification  Squared     Squared     Squared
Model       MODEL            Rate       Error       Error       Error

            AutoNeural13     0.59812    0.17412     0.17509     0.17466
            MBR13            0.66310    0.19005     0.20595     0.20904
            Neural14         0.57713    0.16753     0.16921     0.16934
   Y        Reg16            0.57149    0.16612     0.16831     0.16856
            Tree14           0.57410    0.16770     0.16847     0.16850
```

Figure 32. Decision tree results for ordinal target

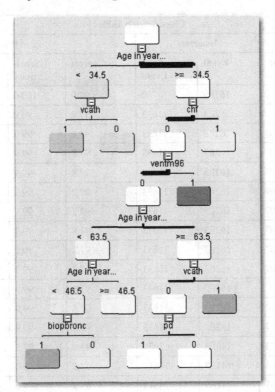

PREDICTIVE MODELING TO RANK THE QUALITY OF PROVIDERS

Ultimately, the definition of a patient severity index is used in a model to rank the quality of healthcare providers. Unlike the standard logistic regression investigation of mortality, what we want to do to predict the quality of providers is to look not at the similarity between actual and predicted values, but to look at the difference between them. Quality rankings assume that if a provider does better than predicted, then it must be because the provider is delivering better care compared to a provider who does worse than predicted. This approach assumes that the predicted value is the established norm for a patient with a certain level of severity and demographics, and any deviation from that norm is a result of the quality of care. This assumption has not yet been validated.

We first look at the logistic regression model defined in Chapter 3. We reproduce Table 15 from Chapter 3 (here as Table 7) that gives the threshold values when we consider just the three patient conditions of pneumonia, septicemia, and immune disorder. Any choice of a threshold value will have a high false negative rate. It we use a threshold value of 0.720 or less, then the predicted value of mortality is equal to $4907/(782 \times 10^4)$. This is approximately 0.06% of the time overall. If we choose a threshold value above 0.760, the predicted mortality level becomes 0.034%. The only change in determining quality rankings when changing the threshold value will be to change the predicted value but not the order of the ranking of the providers. This is because the predicted mortality level is not really determined by the patient's actual severity; rather, it is defined uniformly for all patients.

This table together with a defined threshold value will determine the rankings of providers. Then, the worse the model is in predicting a provider's true mortality, the better that provider will appear in

Table 7. Classification table for logistic regression (Table 15 from Chapter 3)

	Classification Table								
Prob Level	**Correct**		**Incorrect**		**Percentages**				
	Event	**Non-Event**	**Event**	**Non-Event**	**Correct**	**Sensi-tivity**	**Speci-ficity**	**False POS**	**False NEG**
0.480	782E4	0	167E3	0	97.9	100.0	0.0	2.1	.
0.500	781E4	4907	162E3	11633	97.8	99.9	2.9	2.0	70.3
0.520	781E4	4907	162E3	11633	97.8	99.9	2.9	2.0	70.3
0.540	781E4	4907	162E3	11633	97.8	99.9	2.9	2.0	70.3
0.560	781E4	4907	162E3	11633	97.8	99.9	2.9	2.0	70.3
0.580	781E4	4907	162E3	11633	97.8	99.9	2.9	2.0	70.3
0.600	781E4	4907	162E3	11633	97.8	99.9	2.9	2.0	70.3
0.620	781E4	4907	162E3	11633	97.8	99.9	2.9	2.0	70.3
0.640	781E4	4907	162E3	11633	97.8	99.9	2.9	2.0	70.3
0.660	781E4	4907	162E3	11633	97.8	99.9	2.9	2.0	70.3
0.680	781E4	4907	162E3	11633	97.8	99.9	2.9	2.0	70.3
0.700	781E4	4907	162E3	11633	97.8	99.9	2.9	2.0	70.3
0.720	781E4	4907	162E3	11633	97.8	99.9	2.9	2.0	70.3
0.740	776E4	21322	146E3	65076	97.4	99.2	12.8	1.8	75.3
0.760	775E4	26363	141E3	78618	97.3	99.0	15.8	1.8	74.9
0.780	775E4	26363	141E3	78618	97.3	99.0	15.8	1.8	74.9
0.800	775E4	26363	141E3	78618	97.3	99.0	15.8	1.8	74.9
0.820	775E4	26363	141E3	78618	97.3	99.0	15.8	1.8	74.9
0.840	775E4	26363	141E3	78618	97.3	99.0	15.8	1.8	74.9
0.860	775E4	26363	141E3	78618	97.3	99.0	15.8	1.8	74.9
0.880	775E4	26363	141E3	78618	97.3	99.0	15.8	1.8	74.9
0.900	768E4	41608	126E3	149E3	96.6	98.1	24.9	1.6	78.1
0.920	757E4	51297	116E3	258E3	95.3	96.7	30.7	1.5	83.4
0.940	757E4	51297	116E3	258E3	95.3	96.7	30.7	1.5	83.4
0.960	757E4	51297	116E3	258E3	95.3	96.7	30.7	1.5	83.4
0.980	634E4	103E3	64219	149E4	80.6	81.0	61.6	1.0	93.5
1.000	0	167E3	0	782E4	2.1	0.0	100.0	.	97.9

terms of quality. A model that can define a ranking will be "good" regardless of its ability to actually predict mortality.

Given that the three conditions of pneumonia, septicemia, and immune disorder all have higher mortality rates compared to patients generally, and patients with two of the three conditions can have a higer rate still, it is clear that hospitals with higher proportions of such patients will have higher mortality rates. We will examine a random selection of ten hospitals in detail. We will compare their rates of the three diseases, their overall actual mortality rate in comparison to the predicted value, and how the ten hospitals would be ranked by this model. Table 8 gives the proportion of death by hospital. The

Table 8. Mortality (all causes) by hospital

Table of DSHOSPID by DIED			
Hospital Code	**DIED**		**Total**
Frequency Row Pct Col Pct	**0**	**1**	
1	2795 97.12 9.21	83 2.88 12.56	2878
2	1460 96.95 4.81	46 3.05 6.96	1506
3	884 97.46 2.91	23 2.54 3.48	907
4	7652 97.76 25.21	175 2.24 26.48	7827
5	2369 97.89 7.80	51 2.11 7.72	2420
6	5237 96.84 17.25	171 3.16 25.87	5408
7	1476 98.07 4.86	29 1.93 4.39	1505
8	938 100.00 3.09	0 0.00 0.00	938
9	5370 98.62 17.69	75 1.38 11.35	5445
10	2172 99.63 7.16	8 0.37 1.21	2180
Total	30353	661	31014

mortality rate ranges from a low of 0 to a high of 3.16. We want to know if the hospital with zero deaths has patients that are as severe as the hospital with 3.16% deaths.

Table 9 gives the proportion of patients with septicemia by hospital. Note that hospital #8 with zero deaths also has zero patients with septicemia. Hospital #6 with the highest death rate has almost 7% patients with septicemia, which is the highest of the ten hospitals. This hospital should probably be investigated to determine whether this high rate of septicemia is a result of nosocomial infection, or whether patients enter the hospital with it. Table 10 gives the rate of pneumonia. Does this hospital take in sicker patients compared to the other nine hospitals?

Hospital #6 again has the highest rate of pneumonia to go with the highest death rate; hospital #8 has the lowest rate of pneumonia; in fact, it is the only hospital with a rate of less than 1%. Table 11 gives the

Table 9. Patients with septicemia by hospital

Table of DSHOSPID by septicemia			
Hospital Code	**septicemia**		**Total**
Frequency **Row Pct** **Col Pct**	**0**	**1**	
1	2782 96.66 9.24	96 3.34 10.49	2878
2	1444 95.88 4.80	62 4.12 6.78	1506
3	892 98.35 2.96	15 1.65 1.64	907
4	7628 97.46 25.34	199 2.54 21.75	7827
5	2347 96.98 7.80	73 3.02 7.98	2420
6	5035 93.10 16.73	373 6.90 40.77	5408
7	1498 99.53 4.98	7 0.47 0.77	1505
8	938 100.00 3.12	0 0.00 0.00	938
9	5360 98.44 17.81	85 1.56 9.29	5445
10	2175 99.77 7.23	5 0.23 0.55	2180
Total	30099	915	31014

rate for immune disorder. The trend is similar; hospital #8 has the lowest rate, hospital #6 has the highest.

These three tables suggest that hospital #6 has a very good reason to have a higher mortality rate. For this reason, we compare the expected mortality to the actual mortality. We use a predictive model with hospital, septicemia, immune disorder, and pneumonia as the input variables and mortality as the output variable. Figure 33 gives the results, indicating that Dmine regression gives the best fit.

The best misclassification rate is still almost 30%. We partition the data to define the model; we then score the entire dataset so that we can examine the difference between the predicted and actual values. Figure 34 shows the datasets generated by the score node in Enterprise Miner.

The dataset EMWS3.Score_Score contains the predicted values as well as the actual values. We can use PROC FREQ in SAS to examine the relationship to hospital. Table 12 gives the actual and predicted values by hospital.

By this process, hospitals #8 and #10 have the smallest differential between the actual and predicted

Table 10. Patients with pneumonia by hospital

Table of DSHOSPID by pneumonia			
Hospital Code	**pneumonia**		**Total**
Frequency Row Pct Col Pct	**0**	**1**	
1	2638 91.66 9.14	240 8.34 11.23	2878
2	1382 91.77 4.79	124 8.23 5.80	1506
3	830 91.51 2.87	77 8.49 3.60	907
4	7416 94.75 25.68	411 5.25 19.22	7827
5	2273 93.93 7.87	147 6.07 6.88	2420
6	4802 88.79 16.63	606 11.21 28.34	5408
7	1416 94.09 4.90	89 5.91 4.16	1505
8	932 99.36 3.23	6 0.64 0.28	938
9	5149 94.56 17.83	296 5.44 13.84	5445
10	2038 93.49 7.06	142 6.51 6.64	2180
Total	28876	2138	31014

values. Therefore, they would be ranked the lowest even though they both have very low mortality values. In contrast, hospital #6 with the highest actual mortality would rank the highest because the difference between the actual and predicted mortality rates is the greatest. However, a hospital with 0 actual mortality has very little room for an increase in the predicted mortality; a hospital with a higher actual mortality is more likely to "game" the system by increasing the predicted mortality.

Our second example is restricted to the treatment of patients with a primary diagnosis of COPD. We use a predictive model that is similar to that in the previous section, but now we add a hospital identifier. The results are given in Figure 35 with the ROC curve in Figure 36. Note that the minimum error rate is still 32%.

The ROC curves indicate that accuracy decreases considerably on the test data compared to the train-

Table 11. Patients with immune disorder by hospital

Table of DSHOSPID by immune			
Hospital Code	**immune**		**Total**
Frequency Row Pct Col Pct	**0**	**1**	
1	2198 76.37 8.84	680 23.63 11.05	2878
2	1164 77.29 4.68	342 22.71 5.56	1506
3	638 70.34 2.57	269 29.66 4.37	907
4	6324 80.80 25.44	1503 19.20 24.42	7827
5	1928 79.67 7.76	492 20.33 7.99	2420
6	3599 66.55 14.48	1809 33.45 29.40	5408
7	1362 90.50 5.48	143 9.50 2.32	1505
8	878 93.60 3.53	60 6.40 0.97	938
9	4868 89.40 19.58	577 10.60 9.38	5445
10	1901 87.20 7.65	279 12.80 4.53	2180
Total	24860	6154	31014

ing data. Table 13 gives the actual and predicted mortality levels by hospital.

The provider that has the largest difference between actual and predicted mortality is #7. The overall ranking is 1>3>9>2>4>6>5>1>10; again, a hospital with zero mortality is penalized using this system. Usually, zero mortality would be considered good. In fact, regardless of the actual mortality, a hospital with zero predicted morality will rank low in comparison to other providers.

In a third example, we will restrict attention to ten hospitals, and examine patients undergoing just one procedure, that of cardiovascular bypass surgery. We will compare actual mortality rates across these hospitals, and look at the relationship of patient diagnosis to prediction of mortality. We discussed this example briefly in Chapter 3. We will discuss it in more detail here.

We will use a different set of hospitals from the ones in the COPD example since not all of those

Figure 33. Model comparison to predict mortality

```
Fit Statistics
Model selection based on _TMISC_

                                        Train:    Valid:    Test:
                              Test:     Average   Average   Average
Selected              Misclassification Squared   Squared   Squared
 Model    Model Node        Rate        Error     Error     Error

          AutoNeural       0.41206      0.24282   0.26105   0.25049
          DMNeural         0.29899      0.20388   0.21929   0.18838
   Y      DmineReg         0.29397      0.20973   0.22101   0.19603
          MBR              0.41206      0.33253   0.27731   0.27399
          Neural           0.30653      0.20294   0.21838   0.19115
          Reg              0.30402      0.20854   0.22038   0.19452
          Rule             0.29899         .         .         .
          Tree             0.29899      0.21273   0.22793   0.20109
```

Figure 34. Datasets generated by score node

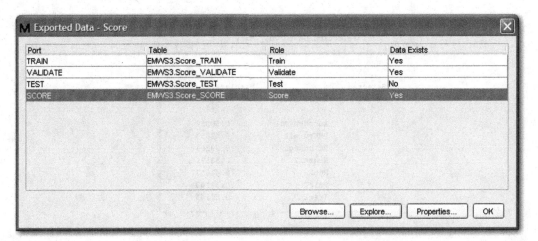

hospitals perform bypass surgery. Then we will examine the ranking that the model gives to the hospitals. Cardiovascular bypass (or CABG) is assigned an ICD9 procedure code of 36.1. We will restrict attention to patients for whom 36.1 is the primary procedure. In this example, we will use the list of patient conditions as given in Table 3 to define a patient severity level. We will use a stratified sample to define the predicted value of mortality. Then, we will compare the predicted results to the actual results by patient and by hospital. Note that the list in Table 3 contains a condition for congestive heart failure and for myocardial infarction. However, it does not include a code for congested arteries. As we will show in subsequent chapters, patients undergoing bypass surgery already have considerable severity in their conditions. However, not all severity indices will identify that severity level.

This example differs from the previous example because the patient condition will be considered in defining the predicted value. This example was previously discussed in Chapter 2, and the code to extract the data was listed in that chapter. Figure 37 gives the results of the predictive model, with hospital included as one of the input variables. The best misclassification rate is 26%.

The lift function indicates that the top half of the data can be predicted easily (Figure 38). However,

Table 12. Actual versus predicted mortality values by hospital

Hospital	Actual Mortality	Predicted Mortality	Difference
1	2.88	30.06	27.18
2	3.05	29.68	26.63
3	2.54	35.06	32.52
4	2.24	23.89	21.65
5	2.11	25.95	23.84
6	3.16	39.87	36.71
7	1.93	14.49	12.56
8	0	0	0
9	1.38	15.76	14.38
10	0.37	0.23	-0.14

Figure 35. Mortality prediction for patients with COPD

```
Fit Statistics
Model selection based on _TMISC_


                                      Test:
          Selected              Misclassification
           Model    Model Node        Rate

                    AutoNeural2      0.50000
                    DMNeural2        0.42857
                    DmineReg2        0.39286
                    Neural2          0.53571
                    Reg2             0.42857
              Y     Rule2            0.32143
                    Tree2            0.32143
```

the test data are much less predictable compared to the training set.

The decision tree indicates that prediction is based largely upon the occurrence of congestive heart failure in the model (Figure 39). For this reason, a provider that can increase the proportion of patients identified as having congestive heart failure will rank higher compared to those who do not inflate the proportion. This condition is loosely defined as a disease that weakens the heart muscle, or weakens the ability of the heart to pump. The definition tends to be vague, and the condition can be assigned differently by different providers.

We translate procedures in Table 14; Table 15 gives the number of procedures by hospital. In both cases, the total sample size is restricted to the ten hospitals with the given procedures.

We compare the difference between the actual and predicted mortality by hospital (Table 16). Table 17 gives the actual and predicted values by procedure.

Table 15 shows the relationship of hospital to procedure. It shows that there is a considerable difference in the procedures performed across the hospitals. For example, #1 has over 50% in 3615, Single internal mammary-coronary artery bypass. The remaining hospitals are more divided in their procedures. Hospital #4 has almost 30% in 3614, (Aorto)coronary bypass of four or more coronary arteries, sug-

Figure 36. ROC curves for predicted results

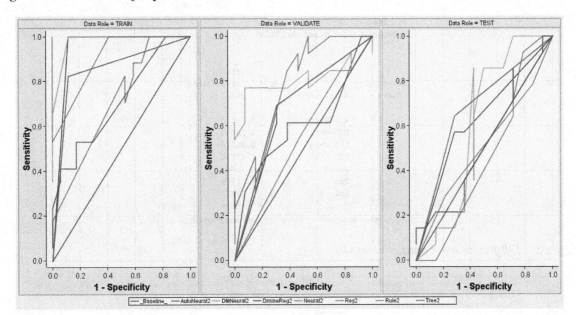

Table 13. Actual versus predicted mortality values by hospital for patients with COPD

Hospital		Actual Mortality	Predicted Mortality	Difference
	1	3.94	23.62	19.68
	2	7.94	33.33	25.39
	3	2.13	44.68	42.55
	4	4.78	29.57	24.79
	5	4.65	29.07	24.42
	6	3.21	27.98	24.77
	7	3.85	50.00	46.15
	8	No COPD Patients		
	9	4.11	43.84	39.73
	10	0	0	0

gesting that it treats patients with very severe blockage in the coronary vessels. The same hospital has approximately 20% of its procedures in 3611, 3612, and 3613.

Table 15 shows that there is considerable difference in the procedures performed across the hospitals. For example, #1 has over 50% in 3615, Single internal mammary-coronary artery bypass. The remaining hospitals are more divided in their procedures. Hospital #4 has almost 30% in 3614, (Aorto)coronary bypass of four or more coronary arteries, suggesting that it treats patients with very severe blockage in the coronary vessels. The same hospital has approximately 20% of the procedures in 3611, 3612, and 3613.

Note that the difference between the predicted mortality and the actual value is considerable, both by

Figure 37. Results of predictive model

```
Fit Statistics
Model selection based on _TMISC_


                                  Test:
          Selected          Misclassification
          Model    Model Node      Rate

                   AutoNeural     0.63158
                   DMNeural       0.36842
             Y     DmineReg       0.26316
                   MBR            0.47368
                   Neural         0.36842
                   Reg            0.31579
                   Rule           0.31579
                   Tree           0.31579
```

Figure 38. Lift function for predictive model

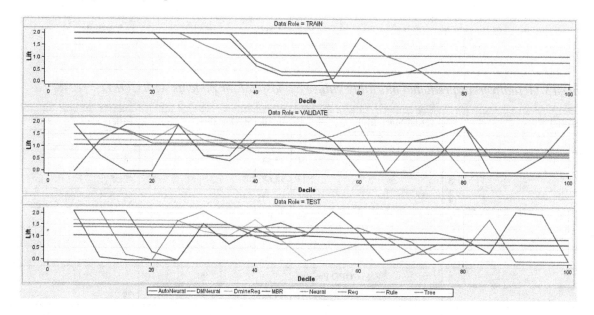

Table 14. Procedures related to cardiovascular surgery

Procedure	Translation	Frequency	Percent
3610	Aortocoronary bypass for heart revascularization, not otherwise specified	8	0.02
3611	(Aorto)coronary bypass of one coronary artery	5112	11.14
3612	(Aorto)coronary bypass of two coronary arteries	13449	29.30
3613	(Aorto)coronary bypass of three coronary arteries	13176	28.70
3614	(Aorto)coronary bypass of four or more coronary arteries	7208	15.70
3615	Single internal mammary-coronary artery bypass	6419	13.98
3616	Double internal mammary-coronary artery bypass	508	1.11
3617	Abdominal - coronary artery bypass	3	0.01
3619	Other bypass anastomosis for heart revascularization	24	0.05

Table 15. Procedures by hospital

	\multicolumn{7}{c}{Table of DSHOSPID by PR1}	
HOSPID	\multicolumn{7}{c}{**PR1(Principal procedure)**}	**Total**
Frequency Row Pct Col Pct	**3611**	**3612**	**3613**	**3614**	**3615**	**3616**	**3619**	
1	16 4.92 14.81	37 11.38 12.85	47 14.46 11.69	24 7.38 9.09	193 59.38 51.47	8 2.46 28.57	0 0.00 0.00	325
2	3 27.27 2.78	4 36.36 1.39	1 9.09 0.25	0 0.00 0.00	2 18.18 0.53	1 9.09 3.57	0 0.00 0.00	11
3	5 4.46 4.63	10 8.93 3.47	19 16.96 4.73	7 6.25 2.65	69 61.61 18.40	2 1.79 7.14	0 0.00 0.00	112
4	22 8.70 20.37	59 23.32 20.49	82 32.41 20.40	75 29.64 28.41	15 5.93 4.00	0 0.00 0.00	0 0.00 0.00	253
5	2 2.27 1.85	14 15.91 4.86	34 38.64 8.46	29 32.95 10.98	9 10.23 2.40	0 0.00 0.00	0 0.00 0.00	88
6	5 2.86 4.63	23 13.14 7.99	51 29.14 12.69	36 20.57 13.64	58 33.14 15.47	2 1.14 7.14	0 0.00 0.00	175
7	21 7.42 19.44	79 27.92 27.43	95 33.57 23.63	60 21.20 22.73	15 5.30 4.00	12 4.24 42.86	1 0.35 100.00	283
8	7 15.56 6.48	11 24.44 3.82	17 37.78 4.23	9 20.00 3.41	1 2.22 0.27	0 0.00 0.00	0 0.00 0.00	45
9	15 19.23 13.89	23 29.49 7.99	23 29.49 5.72	7 8.97 2.65	9 11.54 2.40	1 1.28 3.57	0 0.00 0.00	78
10	12 12.50 11.11	28 29.17 9.72	33 34.38 8.21	17 17.71 6.44	4 4.17 1.07	2 2.08 7.14	0 0.00 0.00	96
Total	108	288	402	264	375	28	1	1466

procedure and by hospital. Therefore, the ability of this model to rank hospitals is highly questionable. There is a considerable difference between the average and the maximum values of outcomes (Table 18). In particular, at least one patient stayed 150 days or more for 3611, 3612, 3613, and 3614. How should these outliers be considered when ranking quality? We use the following code to find the kernel density estimation functions.

```
proc sort data=nis.cardiovascular out=work.cardiovascular2;
by pr1;
proc kde data=work.cardiovascular2;
univar los/gridl=0 gridu=15 out=nis.kdecardlos;
univar totchg/gridl=20000 gridu=100000 out=nis.kdecardchg bwm=.9;
```

Figure 39. Decision tree to predict mortality for patients undergoing cardiovascular bypass surgery

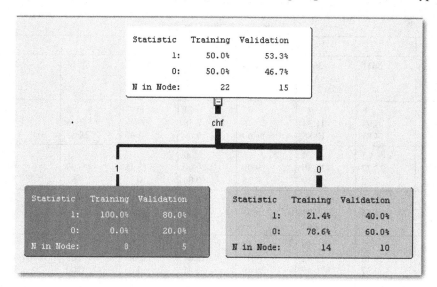

Table 16. Percent of predicted versus actual mortality by procedure

Procedure	Actual Mortality	Predicted Mortality
3610	2.78	42.59
3611	2.78	42.36
3612	2.49	39.55
3613	1.14	39.02
3614	1.07	40.53
3615	0	32.14
3616	0	32.14
3617	0	0
3619	0	100

```
by pr1;
run;
```

Figure 40 shows the length of stay by hospital. As shown in Table 18, stay differed considerably by procedure. It also differs considerably by hospital. Hospital #6 has the greatest probability of a shorter length of stay compared to the other hospitals. Hospital #2 has the highest probability of a longer length of stay. Hospital #7 tends to be in the middle in probability for both a high and low length of stay, as does hospital #1.

Figure 41 shows the total charges compared to hospital. There is a definite shift in the curves, indicating that some hospitals charge far more compared to other hospitals, especially hospitals #3 and #9. Hospital #1 has the least charges, reinforcing the fact that it more generally performs a procedure that is less risky compared to the other procedures. Interestingly, hospital #7, while performing higher risk

Table 17. Predicted versus actual mortality by hospital (given as percent)

Hospital	Actual Mortality	Predicted Mortality
1	1.23	15.08
2	0	0
3	4.46	25.89
4	0.79	11.86
5	1.14	15.91
6	0.57	16.00
7	3.53	26.15
8	2.22	20.00
9	1.28	15.38
10	3.13	16,67

Table 18. Length of stay and total charges by procedure

Principal procedure	N Obs	Variable	Mean	Std Dev	Minimum	Maximum
3610	8	TOTCHG	65496.75	20519.46	39277.00	99584.00
		LOS	5.8750000	1.3562027	3.0000000	7.0000000
3611	5112	TOTCHG	90656.52	68257.93	84.0000000	829195.00
		LOS	8.9047340	7.5870299	0	161.0000000
3612	13449	TOTCHG	96585.12	73855.08	534.0000000	997836.00
		LOS	9.3835973	7.4754109	0	153.0000000
3613	13176	TOTCHG	101269.45	75537.11	2029.00	998991.00
		LOS	9.5980571	7.3233339	0	188.0000000
3614	7208	TOTCHG	103371.69	74343.53	839.0000000	918286.00
		LOS	9.6594062	7.4100765	0	155.0000000
3615	6419	TOTCHG	92813.63	66991.61	484.0000000	898653.00
		LOS	8.7963857	6.6919820	0	114.0000000
3616	508	TOTCHG	89716.19	56349.01	20786.00	461205.00
		LOS	8.1909449	6.1948121	1.0000000	78.0000000
3617	3	TOTCHG	78057.33	56807.84	43820.00	143632.00
		LOS	6.3333333	2.3094011	5.0000000	9.0000000
3619	24	TOTCHG	88172.17	56691.47	20741.00	282273.00
		LOS	8.0833333	7.6437907	1.0000000	32.0000000

procedures, also tends to charge a lower amount.

Next, we examine the length of stay by procedure for a specific hospital. We contrast hospital #7 to hospital #6. For hospital #6, there is a natural hierarchy in the kernel density estimators, demonstrating the severity of each of the procedures. Procedure 3613 has the highest probability of a long length of stay; Procedures 3611 and 3616 have the highest probability of a short length of stay. Figure 42 shows the length of stay for hospital #7. Figures 43 and 44 show additional hospitals.

First, hospital #6 does only four of the procedures. In contrast to hospital #7, procedure 3611 has the lowest probability of a short length of stay for hospital #6; procedure 3613 has the highest probability of a short length of stay. The ordering of the procedures is completely different for the two hospitals.

Figure 40. Length of stay by hospital for cardiovascular surgery

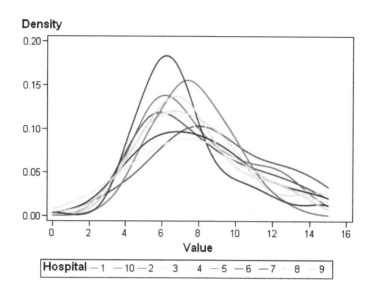

Figure 41. Total charges by hospital for cardiovascular surgery

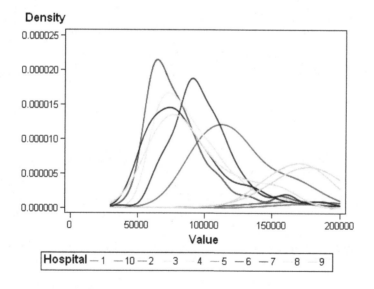

We do a final examination in Figure 42 for hospital #1.

In this figure, it is clear that procedure 3612 has the highest probability of a long length of stay while 3611 has a high probability of a short length of stay. In other words, we have three different hospitals and they have three very different graphs, indicating that there is almost no relationship between procedure and length of stay when comparing the different hospitals.

We use predictive modeling to determine whether length of stay and total charges can be predicted. Dmine regression gives the best estimate (Figure 45).

It shows that hospital, patient demographic factors, and patient conditions are significant in the

Figure 42. Length of stay for hospital #6 by procedure

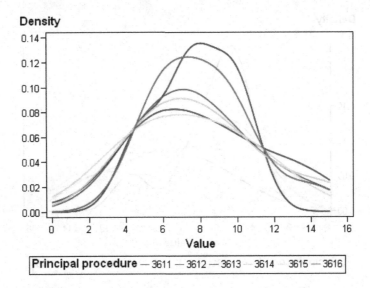

Figure 43. Length of stay for hospital #7 by procedure

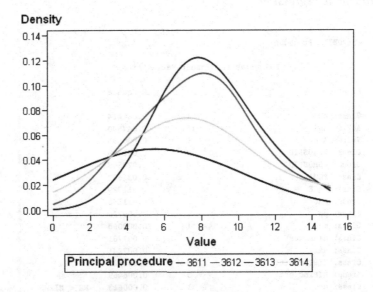

model. Of the patient demographic factors, race, gender, and age are significant in the model. Hospital is also high on the list, indicating that length of stay can depend upon the choice of hospitals as well as on patient condition. As to patient condition, congestive heart failure is the one of highest importance. Figure 46 gives the results with total charges as the target variable. With this target variable, the Dmine regression is also the optimal model.

For total charges, the hospital is of primary importance, which is reasonable since hospitals set their own charges, which are then modified by payers. The most important patient condition is still congestive heart failure.

Figure 44. Length of stay for hospital #1 by procedure

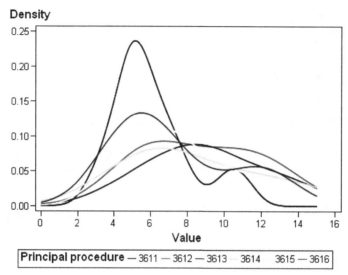

Figure 45. Results of Dmine regression

```
The DMINE Procedure

              R-Squares for Target Variable: LOS

Effect                    DF        R-Square

Class: chf                 1        0.088414
AOV16: AGE                15        0.044500
Var:   AGE                 1        0.030685
Class: DSHOSPID            9        0.023798
Group: DSHOSPID            4        0.023586
Class: FEMALE              1        0.023507
Class: RACE                6        0.011729
Group: RACE                2        0.011553
Class: pd                  1        0.009796
Class: mc                  1        0.008090
Class: diabetes            1        0.007781
Class: ami                 1        0.007241
Class: ZIPInc_Qrtl         4        0.006520
Group: ZIPInc_Qrtl         3        0.006469
Class: dc                  1        0.000613     R2 < MINR2
Class: ctd                 1        0.000611     R2 < MINR2
Class: DIED                1        0.000534     R2 < MINR2
Class: pvd                 1        0.000477     R2 < MINR2
Class: cva                 1        0.000439     R2 < MINR2
Class: paraplegia          1        0.000042316  R2 < MINR2
Class: cancer              1        0.000023262  R2 < MINR2
Class: pu                  1        0.000012459  R2 < MINR2
Class: hiv                 0               0     R2 < MINR2
Class: dementia            0               0     R2 < MINR2
```

Figure 46. Results for total charges as target

```
The DMINE Procedure

            R-Squares for Target Variable: TOTCHG

Effect                          DF        R-Square

Class: DSHOSPID                  9        0.444874
Group: DSHOSPID                  5        0.444713
Class: RACE                      6        0.116278
Group: RACE                      4        0.116035
Class: DIED                      1        0.065598
AOV16: AGE                      15        0.044787
Class: chf                       1        0.030534
Var:   AGE                       1        0.026700
Class: ZIPInc_Qrtl               4        0.013427
Class: diabetes                  1        0.011510
Class: FEMALE                    1        0.010728
Class: ami                       1        0.006690
Class: cancer                    1        0.002099    R2 < MINR2
Class: paraplegia                1        0.001558    R2 < MINR2
Class: pd                        1        0.000802    R2 < MINR2
Var:   ld                        1        0.000597    R2 < MINR2
AOV16: ld                        1        0.000597    R2 < MINR2
Class: pu                        1        0.000398    R2 < MINR2
Class: pvd                       1        0.000331    R2 < MINR2
Class: dc                        1     0.000043281    R2 < MINR2
Class: cva                       1     0.000012564    R2 < MINR2
Class: mc                        1     0.000004881    R2 < MINR2
Class: ctd                       1     0.000000920    R2 < MINR2
Class: hiv                       0               0    R2 < MINR2
Class: dementia                  0               0    R2 < MINR2
```

FUTURE TRENDS

Predictive modeling already includes all regression models. Therefore, it will be used much more often when analyzing health outcomes than it has been used in the past. It needs to be brought more commonly into the curriculum for students specializing in health outcomes research before predictive modeling will become more common. Departments of Biostatistics and Informatics need to recognize the availability of data mining tools and their use in health outcomes research. The process of predictive modeling should be substituted for the now common use of regression models. Misclassification and cost should be used instead of p-values and odds ratios to have more accurate results generally in health outcomes research.

DISCUSSION

The process of data mining automatically incorporates important components that are not generally a part of more traditional statistical methods. These components include sampling, partitioning, and model comparison. In addition, they include a component for scoring new data and defining a more meaningful definition of a "best" model. Best does not always mean the most accurate. Often in healthcare, we can sacrifice some accuracy in the false positive prediction to greatly reduce the false negative rate. However, as predictive modeling automatically incorporates regression models, the process of predictive modeling is essential to health outcomes research.

In addition, the common practice of using the difference between observed and predicted outcomes to rank the quality of providers should be reconsidered. As it is now, providers with low mortality can be penalized compared to providers with high mortality since the differential between actual and predicted can be much larger for providers with higher adverse outcomes.

REFERENCES

Cerrito, P. (2008). *Data Mining Healthcare and Clinical Databases with SAS*. Cary, NC: SAS Institute.

Cerrito, P. B. (2007). *Introduction to Data Mining with Enterprise Miner.* Cary, NC: SAS Press.

Gamito, E. J., & Crawford, D. E. (2004). Artificial neural networks for predictive modeling in prostate cancer. *Current Oncology Reports, 6*(3), 216–221.

Hodgman, S. B. (2008). Predictive modeilng & outcomes. *Professional Case Management, 13*(1), 19–23.

Powers, C. A., Meyer, C. M., Roebuck, M. C., & Vaziri, B. (2005). Predictive modeling of total healthcare costs using pharmacy claims data: a comparison of alternative econometric cost modeling techniques. *Medical Care, 43*(11), 1065–1072.

Sylvia, M. L., Shadmi, E., Hsiao, C.-J., Boyd, C. M., Schuster, A. B., & Boult, C. (2006). Clinical features of high risk older person identified by predictive modeling. *Disease Management, 9*(1), 56–62.

Tewari, A., Porter, C., Peabody, J., Crawford, E., Demers, R., & Johnson, C. (2001). Predictive modeling techniques in prostate cancer. *Molecular Urology, 5*(4), 147–152.

Tropsha, A., & Golbraikh, A. (2007). Predictive QSAR modeling workflow, model applicability domains, and virtual screening. *Current Pharmaceutical Design, 13*(34), 3494–3504.

Weber, C., & Neeser, K. (2006). Using individualized predictive disease modeling to identify patients with the potential to benefit from a disease management program for diabetes mellitus. *Disease Management, 9*(4), 242–256.

Whitlock, T., & Johnston, K. (2006). Using predictive modeling to evaluate the financial effect of disease management. *Managed Care Interface, 19*(9), 29–34.

Chapter 5
The Charlson Comorbidity Index

INTRODUCTION

In this chapter, we consider the Charlson Comorbidity Index (CCI). This index is published, and the weights used to define risk adjustment in the logistic regression model are clearly identified as well. (Sundararajan et al., 2004) Therefore, we are able to examine this index in detail, and to see if the index is meaningful in terms of adjusting risk based upon patient condition. We will suggest an alternative to the Charlson Index in Chapter 8 that gives improvements in terms of its relationship to outcomes.

In Chapters 6 and 7, we will discuss other commonly used severity index measures. We will compare their results to those computed using the Charlson Index. We will also continue to discuss the examples given in Chapter 4 of patients having cardiovascular bypass surgery and COPD (chronic obstructive pulmonary disease) in addition to other examples introduced in this chapter.

Since the Charlson Index is published, it is not used by payers to rank the quality of providers. If it were used, the providers could focus on this minimal set of patient conditions. There is, of course, a similar danger if the developers of proprietary indices released, or sold, their model to healthcare providers who could use the values to focus on specific diagnosis codes. Therefore, in order to reduce the problem of upcoding, providers should not know the details of the model used.

DOI: 10.4018/978-1-60566-752-2.ch005

BACKGROUND

The Charlson Index was developed to provide risk adjustment and to predict patient mortality or other outcomes in the hospital.(Charlson, Pompei, Ales, & MacKenzie, 1987) It was tested and validated on a general population.(Romano, Roos, & Jollis, 1993a, 1993b) Other data have modified the Charlson Index for specific patient populations.(Ghali, Hall, Rosen, Ash, & Moskowitz, 1996) It is representative of many different indices. (Iezzoni, 2003)

The problems with the Charlson Index show some of the problems generally with risk adjustment measures.(Melfi, Holleman, Arthur, & Katz, 1995) In any index that limits the choice of the diseases used to define the index, there will be omitted diseases that can have as much importance in relationship to patient outcomes as the ones in the model. As a result, the indices tend to be poor predictors of actual outcomes.

One of the problems with using the Charlson Index is that information is not uniformly entered by healthcare providers. In one study, hospitals consistently under-coded for diabetes and for diabetes with complications compared to physicians. In contrast, physicians tended to under-code on myocardial infarction and cerebral vascular disease.(Klabunde, Potosky, Legler, & Warren, 2000) Similarly, there is under-coding in the billing data, usually discovered through a review of patient charts.(Doorn et al., 2001; Kieszak, Flanders, Kosinski, Shipp, & Karp, 1999) Under-coded patients will show a reduced risk compared to what they should normally be assigned, and their predicted risk will be reduced as well.

Since providers are measured in terms of quality based upon the difference between predicted outcomes and actual outcomes, providers that have a high proportion of patients with the diseases listed in the index will have a greater difference between predicted and actual values compared to providers that have patients with severe problems that are not in the index list. A different list of diseases can completely change the risk adjustment and the rank order of providers. We will demonstrate how such a different list compares to the Charlson Index.

STATISTICAL EXAMINATION OF THE CHARLSON INDEX

Table 1 gives the patient condition, the related ICD9 codes, and the associated weights for the Charlson Index.(Sundararajan et al., 2004)

The score is the sum of the weights of the nonzero indicators of categories 1-17 in Table 1. Other references give a weight of 3 to metastatic cancer as well in spite of the high risk of mortality.(Gettman et al., 2003) For our purposes, the actual weights are not important; the methodology remains the same regardless of the assigned weights.

However, there is a clear problem of multicollinearity given the relationship between diabetes and diabetes with complications, and so on. Consider, for example, diabetes with complications. This can include diabetes if both 2501 and 2504 are listed as secondary patient conditions. Approximately 9% of those with complications of diabetes are also identified as having diabetes. A higher 14% of those with diabetes complications also have renal disease. To avoid the issue of collinearity, only the score is used in a logistic regression to examine mortality, or in a linear regression to examine costs and utilization.

First, we define the Charlson Index on the 2005 National Inpatient Sample using the SAS code listed below. We use the SUBSTR function to reduce the ICD9 codes to 3-digits. Next, we concatenate the 15 columns of ICD9 codes into one column. Then, the rxmatch function is used to find the relevant codes for

Table 1. Definition of Charlson index

Condition	ICD9 Codes	Weights
Acute myocardial infarction	410, 412	1
Congestive heart failure	428	1
Peripheral vascular disease	441,4439,7854,V434	1
Cerebral vascular accident	430-438	1
Dementia	290	1
Pulmonary disease	490,491,492,493,494,495,496,500,501,502,503,504,505	1
Connective tissue disorder	7100,7101,7104,7140,7141,7142,7148,5171,725	1
Peptic ulcer	531,532,533,534	1
Liver disease	5712,5714,5715,5716	1
Diabetes	2500,2501,2502,2503,2507	1
Diabetes complications	2504,2505,2506	2
Paraplegia	342,3441	2
Renal disease	582,5830,5831,5832,5833,5835,5836,5837,5834,585,586,588	2
Cancer	14,15,16,17,18,170,171,172,174,175,176,179,190,191,193, 194,1950,1951,1952,1953,1954,1955,1958,200,201,202,203, 204,205,206,207,208	2
Metastatic cancer	196,197,198,1990,1991	3
Severe liver disease	5722,5723,5724,5728	6
HIV	042,043,044	6

the Charlson Index. Once found, an indicator function is defined for each of the 17 Charlson categories, with a code of zero if the category is absent for the patient; otherwise a code of one is assigned. Then the Charlson Index is defined by a combination sum of weights times the indicator function value. If the Charlson Index is zero, then the patient has none of the codes for the Charlson Index; the largest sum defined in this dataset is a value of 13.

```
data nis.charlson;
set nis.nis_2005_core;
    DX11=substr(DX1,1,3);
    DX12=substr(DX2,1,3);
    DX13=substr(DX3,1,3);
    DX14=substr(DX4,1,3);
    DX15=substr(DX5,1,3);
    DX16=substr(DX6,1,3);
    DX17=substr(DX7,1,3);
    DX18=substr(DX8,1,3);
    DX19=substr(DX9,1,3);
    DX110=substr(DX10,1,3);
    DX111=substr(DX11,1,3);
    DX112=substr(DX12,1,3);
```

```
DX113=substr(DX13,1,3);
DX114=substr(DX14,1,3);
DX115=substr(DX15,1,3);
```

The first part of this code reduces each of the 15 diagnosis columns to 3 digits. The next part reduces each code to 4 digits and the combination of new variables is used to define the index.

```
DX21=substr(DX1,1,4);
DX22=substr(DX2,1,4);
DX23=substr(DX3,1,4);
DX24=substr(DX4,1,4);
DX25=substr(DX5,1,4);
DX26=substr(DX6,1,4);
DX27=substr(DX7,1,4);
DX28=substr(DX8,1,4);
DX29=substr(DX9,1,4);
DX210=substr(DX10,1,4);
DX211=substr(DX11,1,4);
DX212=substr(DX12,1,4);
DX213=substr(DX13,1,4);
DX214=substr(DX14,1,4);
DX215=substr(DX15,1,4);
ami=0; chf=0; pvd=0; cva=0; dementia=0; pd=0; ctd=0; pu=0; ld=0; diabetes=0; dc=0; para-
plegia=0;
rd=0; cancer=0; mc=0; sld=0; hiv=0;
```

The indicator functions for each of the 17 Charlson categories is set equal to zero.

```
diagnoses3digits=catx(' ',dx11,dx12,dx13, dx14,dx15,dx16,dx17,dx18,dx19,dx110,
dx111,dx112,dx113,dx114,dx115);
diagnoses4digits=catx(' ', dx21,dx22, dx23,dx24,dx25, dx26,dx27,dx28,dx29,dx210,dx211,d
x212, dx213,dx214, dx215);
```

The 15 columns of 3 digit codes are concatenated followed by the 15 columns of 4 digit codes. The concatenation just makes the remaining code easier to do, allowing us to examine just one column of data instead of all 15.

```
if (rxmatch('410',diagnoses3digits)>0 or rxmatch('412',diagnoses3digits)>0) then ami=1;
```

The above if...then statement defines the indicator function for an acute myocardial infarction.

```
if (rxmatch('428',diagnoses3digits)>0) then chf=1;
if (rxmatch('441',diagnoses3digits)>0 or rxmatch('4439',diagnoses4digits)>0 or
rxmatch('7854',diagnoses4digits)>0 or rxmatch('V434',diagnoses4digits)>0) then pvd=1;
```

These codes, 4439-V434, define the condition of peripheral vascular disease. The remaining code needed to define the index is provided below:

```
if (rxmatch('430',diagnoses3digits)>0 or rxmatch('431',diagnoses3digits)>0 or rxmatch('4
32',diagnoses3digits)>0 or
rxmatch('433',diagnoses3digits)>0 or rxmatch('434',diagnoses3digits)>0 or rxmatch('435',
diagnoses3digits)>0 or
rxmatch('436',diagnoses3digits)>0 or rxmatch('437',diagnoses3digits)>0 or rxmatch('438',
diagnoses3digits)>0) then cva=1;
if (rxmatch('290',diagnoses3digits)>0) then dementia=1;
if (rxmatch('490',diagnoses3digits)>0 or rxmatch('491',diagnoses3digits)>0 or rxmatch('4
92',diagnoses3digits)>0 or
rxmatch('493',diagnoses3digits)>0 or rxmatch('494',diagnoses3digits)>0 or rxmatch('495',
diagnoses3digits)>0 or
rxmatch('496',diagnoses3digits)>0 or rxmatch('500',diagnoses3digits)>0 or rxmatch('501',
diagnoses3digits)>0 or
rxmatch('502',diagnoses3digits)>0 or rxmatch('503',diagnoses3digits)>0 or rxmatch('504',
diagnoses3digits)>0 or
rxmatch('505',diagnoses3digits)>0) then pd=1;
if (rxmatch('7100',diagnoses4digits)>0 or rxmatch('7101',diagnoses4digits)>0 or rxmatch(
'7104',diagnoses4digits)>0 or
rxmatch('7140',diagnoses4digits)>0 or rxmatch('7141',diagnoses4digits)>0 or rxmatch('714
2',diagnoses4digits)>0 or
rxmatch('7148',diagnoses4digits)>0 or rxmatch('725',diagnoses3digits)>0) then ctd=1;
if (rxmatch('531',diagnoses3digits)>0 or rxmatch('532',diagnoses3digits)>0 or rxmatch('5
33',diagnoses3digits)>0 or
rxmatch('534',diagnoses3digits)>0) then pu=1;
if (rxmatch('5712',diagnoses4digits)>0 or rxmatch('5714',diagnoses4digits)>0 or rxmatch(
'5715',diagnoses4digits)>0 or
rxmatch('5716',diagnoses4digits)>0) then ld=1;
if (rxmatch('2500',diagnoses4digits)>0 or rxmatch('2501',diagnoses4digits)>0 or rxmatch(
'2502',diagnoses4digits)>0 or
rxmatch('2503',diagnoses4digits)>0 or rxmatch('2507',diagnoses4digits)>0) then diabe-
tes=1;
if (rxmatch('2504',diagnoses4digits)>0 or rxmatch('2505',diagnoses4digits)>0 or rxmatch(
'2506',diagnoses4digits)>0)
then dc=1;
if (rxmatch('342',diagnoses3digits)>0 or rxmatch('3441',diagnoses4digits)>0) then para-
plegia=1;
if (rxmatch('582',diagnoses3digits)>0 or rxmatch('5830',diagnoses4digits)>0 or rxmatch('
5831',diagnoses4digits)>0 or
rxmatch('5832',diagnoses4digits)>0 or rxmatch('5833',diagnoses4digits)>0 or rxmatch('583
5',diagnoses4digits)>0 or
rxmatch('5836',diagnoses4digits)>0 or rxmatch('5837',diagnoses4digits)>0 or rxmatch('583
```

```
4',diagnoses4digits)>0 or

rxmatch('585',diagnoses3digits)>0 or rxmatch('586',diagnoses3digits)>0 or rxmatch('588',
diagnoses3digits)>0) then rd=1;

if (rxmatch('014',diagnoses3digits)>0 or rxmatch('015',diagnoses3digits)>0 or rxmatch('0
16',diagnoses3digits)>0 or

rxmatch('018',diagnoses3digits)>0 or rxmatch('170',diagnoses3digits)>0 or rxmatch('171',
diagnoses3digits)>0 or

rxmatch('172',diagnoses3digits)>0 or rxmatch('174',diagnoses3digits)>0 or rxmatch('175',
diagnoses3digits)>0 or

rxmatch('176',diagnoses3digits)>0 or rxmatch('179',diagnoses3digits)>0 or rxmatch('190',
diagnoses3digits)>0 or

rxmatch('191',diagnoses3digits)>0 or rxmatch('192',diagnoses3digits)>0 or rxmatch('193',
diagnoses3digits)>0 or

rxmatch('194',diagnoses3digits)>0 or rxmatch('1950',diagnoses4digits)>0 or rxmatch('1951
',diagnoses4digits)>0 or

rxmatch('1952',diagnoses4digits)>0 or rxmatch('1953',diagnoses4digits)>0 or rxmatch('195
4',diagnoses4digits)>0 or

rxmatch('1955',diagnoses4digits)>0 or rxmatch('1958',diagnoses4digits)>0 or rxmatch('200
',diagnoses3digits)>0 or

rxmatch('201',diagnoses3digits)>0 or rxmatch('202',diagnoses3digits)>0 or rxmatch('203',
diagnoses3digits)>0 or

rxmatch('204',diagnoses3digits)>0 or rxmatch('205',diagnoses3digits)>0 or rxmatch('206',
diagnoses3digits)>0 or

rxmatch('206',diagnoses3digits)>0 or rxmatch('207',diagnoses3digits)>0 or rxmatch('208',
diagnoses3digits)>0) then cancer=1;

if (rxmatch('196',diagnoses3digits)>0 or rxmatch('197',diagnoses3digits)>0 or rxmatch('1
98',diagnoses3digits)>0 or

rxmatch('1990',diagnoses4digits)>0 or rxmatch('1991',diagnoses4digits)>0) then mc=1;

if (rxmatch('5722',diagnoses4digits)>0 or rxmatch('5723',diagnoses4digits)>0 or rxmatch(
'5724',diagnoses4digits)>0 or

rxmatch('5728',diagnoses4digits)>0) then sld=1;

if (rxmatch('042',diagnoses3digits)>0 or rxmatch('043',diagnoses3digits)>0 or rxmatch('0
44',diagnoses3digits)>0) then hiv=1;
```

Once the indicator functions are defined, the Charlson Index is defined as a sum of indicators times weights.

```
charlson=ami+chf+pvd+cva+dementia+pd+ctd+pu+ld+diabetes+2*(dc+paraplegia+rd+cancer)+3*mc
+6*(sld+hiv);
run;
```

Given the weights for the index, those with a weight of one should have similar mortality rates, and the mortality should increase with the weighting. Table 2 gives the mortality by Charlson Index. Table 3 gives the mortality by each of the 17 conditions.

Table 2. Mortality by Charlson index

Charlson Index	DIED		Total
Frequency Row Pct Col Pct	0	1	
0	4506290 99.30 57.59	31815 0.70 19.03	4538105
1	1664508 97.43 21.27	43878 2.57 26.25	1708386
2	890356 96.08 11.38	36325 3.92 21.73	926681
3	446533 94.12 5.71	27891 5.88 16.69	474424
4	181510 92.40 2.32	14938 7.60 8.94	196448
5	76798 91.69 0.98	6962 8.31 4.17	83760
6	39256 92.14 0.50	3347 7.86 2.00	42603
7	12066 91.49 0.15	1122 8.51 0.67	13188
8	5134 90.34 0.07	549 9.66 0.33	5683
9	1600 90.14 0.02	175 9.86 0.10	1775
10	557 85.17 0.01	97 14.83 0.06	654
11	187 86.18 0.00	30 13.82 0.02	217
12	52 73.24 0.00	19 26.76 0.01	71
13	10 83.33 0.00	2 16.67 0.00	12

Note that there are only 12 patients with a Charlson value of 13. However, patients with a Charlson value of 12 have a mortality of 27%, higher than an index value of 13.

Table 3. Mortality by patient condition

Patient Condition	# Patients With Condition	# Patients Who Died in the Hospital	Proportion of Patients Who Died
Acute Myocardial Infarction	407,376	22,842	5.56
Congestive Heart Failure	859,327	54,599	6.35
Peripheral Vascular Disease	190,961	7100	3.72
Cerebral Vascular Accident	373,049	20,689	5.55
Dementia	52,247	2258	4.32
Pulmonary Disease	1,294,183	43,921	3.39
Connective Tissue Disorder	119,542	2502	2.09
Peptic Ulcer	89,582	2530	2.82
Liver Disease	83,672	6490	7.76
Diabetes	1,052,854	22,785	2.16
Diabetes Complications	177.179	3579	2.02
Paraplegia	52,769	2936	5.56
Renal Disease	163,674	10,974	6.70
Cancer	182,145	10,010	5.50
Metastatic Cancer	206,543	21,625	10.47
Severe Liver Disease	38,920	4911	12.62
HIV	33,034	1683	5.09

Figure 1 gives the percentage of mortality by the computed Charlson Index value. It shows that a higher value of the index does not always result in a higher rate of mortality. In particular, an index value of 13 has a mortality rate 10% lower compared to an index value of 12. However, the purpose of the weighting is to have a higher risk of mortality as the index value increases. Clearly, there are some problems with the index since this ordering of mortality does not occur.

Figure 1. Percentage of mortality by Charlson index

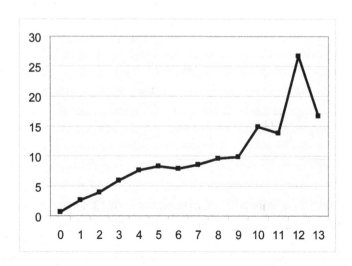

Note that there is a steady decrease in the number of patients as the Charlson Index increases in value. Table 3 gives the total number and proportion of patients who died while inpatients compared to the total number of patients in each of the Charlson categories.

There are some obvious problems with these results. The death rates for all conditions with weight 1 range from a low of 2.09 to a high of 7.76 while those with weight of 2 range from a low of 2.02 to a high of 6.70, lower than the higher values for weight 1. Moreover, the mortality rate for diabetes with complications is lower than the rate for diabetes without complications, indicating that the Charlson Index favors the under-coding of diabetes complications. Some patients with diabetes complications are under-coded as diabetes with no complications as indicated by the mortality rates.

Weight 3 seems fairly consistent with rates of 10.47 and 12.62 for metastatic cancer and severe liver disease respectively, but the death rate for HIV with the highest weight of 6 is only 5.09. Moreover, some very high risk diagnoses are omitted completely from this score. Consider, for example, pneumonia (ICD9 code 486, Table 4) with a mortality rate as high or higher than all conditions with weights 1 and 2.

As a result, patients with pneumonia and no other co-morbidities will receive a Charlson Index of 0 while having a fairly high risk of mortality. Therefore, a hospital with a community flu epidemic that

Table 4. Mortality for pneumonia

Table of Pneumonia by DIED				
Pneumonia		DIED		Total
Frequency Row Pct Col Pct		0	1	
0		7431129 98.21 94.97	135419 1.79 81.02	7566548
1		393728 92.54 5.03	31731 7.46 18.98	425459
Total		7824857	167150	7992007

Table 5. Mortality by TB

Table of TB by DIED				
tb		DIED		Total
Frequency Row Pct Col Pct		0	1	
0		7821310 97.91 99.95	166964 2.09 99.89	7988274
1		3547 95.02 0.05	186 4.98 0.11	3733
Total		7824857	167150	7992007
Frequency Missing = 3041				

results in high rates of pneumonia will have patient risk seriously under-coded. While not as high, the mortality rate for tuberculosis approaches that of the diseases contained within the Charlson index (Table 5). Its mortality rate is certainly comparable to a weight of one.

Anemia also has a mortality rate that fits in with a Charlson weight of 1 (Table 6).

It is expected that the higher the score, the higher the mortality level. However, this is not the case in that a Score of 13 has a much lower mortality rate compared to a score of 12. In addition, a score of 11 has a lower mortality rate than a score of 10. These unexpected results suggest that the weights should be revised, as well as the list of diseases that are included within the index.

In fact, the weights should probably be adjusted on a regular basis, and the set of codes should be considered as well; this presents another problem. A severity index that keeps changing does not allow for longitudinal comparisons. It would be better to develop an index that uses all of the available diagnosis codes instead of a subset of them.

Now suppose we consider a logistic regression comparing mortality to the Charlson Index as well as the available patient demographics of age, sex, race, and income level as provided in the National Inpatient Sample. The odds ratios for the regression are given in Table 7. For this analysis, the Charlson Index is considered a quantitative variable. Generally, as the index increases, so does the level of mortality (as indicated by the odds ratio). However, as we saw previously, the mortality is not always higher for higher levels of the Index.

The logistic regression has a c-statistic of 76%. Consider also the small width of the Wald confidence limits for the odds ratios. When the sample size is so large, the results can be statistically significant, but of no real practical importance. In addition, mortality overall represents only 2% of the patient base. Therefore, we must consider where the misclassifications occur. Table 8 gives the predicted versus actual value from the logistic regression when no sampling is used. Note that almost none of the actual mortality is predicted in the model. All of the error comes from incorrect predicting of non-mortality as mortality.

Table 8 shows that the model does not predict the occurrence of mortality accurately. We also show the decision tree in Figure 2, and decision rules to show how the input variables are used to define the predictions.

Table 6. Mortality by anemia

Table of anemia by DIED			
anemia	**DIED**		**Total**
Frequency **Row Pct** **Col Pct**	**0**	**1**	
0	6653023 98.17 85.02	124048 1.83 74.21	6777071
1	1171834 96.45 14.98	43102 3.55 25.79	1214936
Total	7824857	167150	7992007
Frequency Missing = 3041			

Note that age is the first variable split followed by the Charlson Index, and then age again. We give the English rules to accompany the decision tree. First, if the patient's age is less than 47.5 and the Charlson Index is less than 2.5, then the prediction is for non-mortality, which comprises 86% of the prediction.

```
IF charlson < 2.5
AND Age in years at admission < 47.5
THEN
  NODE: 4
  N: 36470
  1: 14.2%
  0: 85.8%
```

Next, if the Charlson Index is 3 or greater with an age of less than 47.5, the mortality in the subgroup is almost 70%.

```
IF 2.5 <= charlson
AND Age in years at admission < 47.5
THEN
```

Table 7. Odds ratios for logistic regression for mortality outcome

Odds Ratio Estimates			
Effect	Point Estimate	95% Wald Confidence Limits	
charlson	0.673	0.666	0.679
AGE	0.955	0.953	0.956
FEMALE 0 vs 1	0.862	0.836	0.889
RACE 1 vs 6	1.024	0.923	1.136
RACE 2 vs 6	0.965	0.863	1.079
RACE 3 vs 6	0.960	0.858	1.075
RACE 4 vs 6	0.721	0.626	0.829
RACE 5 vs 6	0.882	0.690	1.127
Income quartile 1 vs 4	1.008	0.964	1.054
Income quartile 2 vs 4	1.017	0.972	1.064
Income quartile 3 vs 4	1.077	1.029	1.128

Table 8. Predicted versus actual outcome

Predicted Value	Actual Value	Count
0	0	5477484
0	1	15
1	0	117002
1	1	2

Figure 2. Decision tree to predict mortality

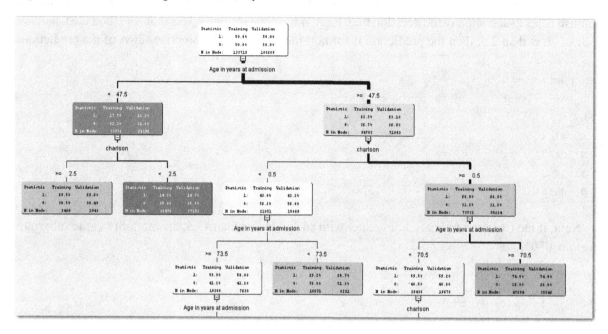

```
NODE: 5
N: 2466
1: 69.5%
0: 30.5%
```

If the patient's age is between 47.5 and 73.5 with a Charlson Index of zero, the probability of non-mortality is 71%.

```
IF 47.5 <= Age in years at admission < 73.5
AND charlson < 0.5
THEN
  NODE: 12
  N: 10671
  1: 29.2%
  0: 70.8%
```

The probability increases to 74% for mortality if the age is greater than 70.5 years and the Charlson Index is greater than 0.

```
IF 70.5 <= Age in years at admission
AND 0.5 <= charlson
THEN
  NODE: 15
  N: 47294
```

```
1: 74.0%
0: 26.0%
```

It is clear from the remaining part of the decision tree that the prediction is based largely upon the age and the level of the Charlson Index.

```
IF 86.5 <= Age in years at admission
AND charlson < 0.5
THEN
  NODE: 27
  N: 3397
  1: 69.0%
  0: 31.0%
IF 2.5 <= charlson
AND 47.5 <= Age in years at admission < 70.5
THEN
  NODE: 29
  N: 10808
  1: 74.6%
  0: 25.4%
```

This next node is one of two where sex plays a role. If the patient is male, between 73.5 and 86.5 years of age with a 0 Charlson Index, then the mortality in the subgroup is almost 60%.

```
IF Indicator of sex EQUALS 0
AND 73.5 <= Age in years at admission < 86.5
AND charlson < 0.5
THEN
  NODE: 42
  N: 2915
  1: 58.8%
  0: 41.2%
IF 47.5 <= Age in years at admission < 57.5
AND 0.5 <= charlson < 2.5
THEN
  NODE: 46
  N: 5349
  1: 43.1%
  0: 56.9%
```

The next node is the second one where sex plays a role. If the patient is between 72.5 and 80.5 years of age, is female, and has a Charlson Index greater than zero, then the subgroup has a 46% mortality rate.

```
IF 73.5 <= Age in years at admission < 80.5
AND Indicator of sex EQUALS 1
AND charlson < 0.5
THEN
  NODE: 60
  N: 2030
  1: 46.3%
  0: 53.7%
IF 80.5 <= Age in years at admission < 86.5
AND Indicator of sex EQUALS 1
AND charlson < 0.5
THEN
  NODE: 61
  N: 2038
  1: 54.4%
  0: 45.6%
IF 0.5 <= charlson < 1.5
AND 57.5 <= Age in years at admission < 70.5
THEN
  NODE: 64
  N: 5913
  1: 48.4%
  0: 51.6%
IF 1.5 <= charlson < 2.5
AND 57.5 <= Age in years at admission < 70.5
THEN
  NODE: 65
  N: 4368
  1: 57.2%
  0: 42.8%
```

When testing for a rare occurrence, it is better to use a random sample of the non-occurrences, although this is rarely done.(D'Hoore, Bouckaert, & Tilquin, 1996) Logistic regression works most effectively when the group sizes are fairly equal. In addition, given the size of the dataset, we can split the data into a training set and a holdout sample. Table 9 gives the results on the holdout sample using a 50/50 split of mortality to non-mortality. Note the difference in accuracy compared to that given in Table 8.

With this split, the model accurately predicts a much higher percentage of the actual mortality in the dataset. As the disparity between the groups increases, the accuracy of predicting actual mortality decreases. Consider the holdout sample with mortality decreased to 25% of the whole; the actual mortality predicted is less than 6% of the 25% (Table 10).

When mortality is reduced to 10%, the prediction of actual mortality decreases to less than 0.2% (Table 11).

Without considering the fact that mortality is a rare occurrence, the results will look exceptionally good.(D'Hoore et al., 1996) However, such results are very misleading. Similarly, if we look at the pre-

Table 9. Predicted versus actual mortality with a 50/50 split in the data

Predicted Value	Actual Value	Count	Percentage
0	0	23393	23.2%
0	1	6747	6.6%
1	0	26751	26.7%
1	1	43398	43.3%

Table 10. Predicted versus actual mortality with a 75/25 split in the data

Predicted Value	Actual Value	Count	Percentage
0	0	190073	71.1%
0	1	51922	19.4%
1	0	10507	3.9%
1	1	14937	5.6%

Table 11. Predicted versus actual mortality with a 90/10 split in the data

Predicted Value	Actual Value	Count	Percentage
0	0	450265	89.8%
0	1	49339	9.8%
1	0	1039	0.2%
1	1	806	0.16%

diction of length of hospital stay, use of the Charlson Index in a linear regression yields a 3% r^2 value (even though all of the variables are statistically significant).

However, in studies with small samples and small levels of mortality, the correlation to the Charlson Index is not necessarily statistically significant.(Gettman et al., 2003) Other indices can be substituted if they increase the level of the R^2, or of the c-statistic in a logistic regression.(Colinet et al., 2005; Holman, Preen, Baynham, Finn, & Semmens, 2005) Figure 3 gives the average length of stay by level of the Charlson Index. Note the considerable decrease for patients with an Index value of 13. Similarly, there are drops at the Index value of 5 and 11. Again, an index of patient risk should be increasing as the index increases.

It is clear that the highest level of the index has reduced risk and mortality compared to the previous level. As there are only 12 patients in this group with an Index of 13, we can look at them in detail. All 12 have a diagnosis of HIV with a weight of 6. These results suggest that the weight for HIV should be reconsidered; it is probably too high.(Zavascki & Fuchs, 2007) Figure 4 gives a comparison of the Index to total charges. It again shows that the charges can decrease as the level of the Index increases.

Yet validation of an Index typically is declared by comparing the Index to patient outcomes, including mortality, or by comparing it to another index.(Byles, D'Este, Parkinson, O'Connell, & Treloar, 2005; Fried, Bernardini, & Piraino, 2003; Goldstein, Samsa, Matchar, & Horner, 2004; Groll, Heyland, Caeser, & Wright, 2006; Lesens et al., 2003) While many factors can be correlated with mortality, the Charlson

Figure 3. Average length of stay by Charlson index value

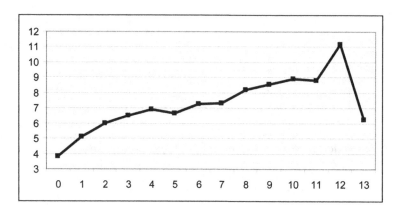

Figure 4. Total charges by Charlson index value

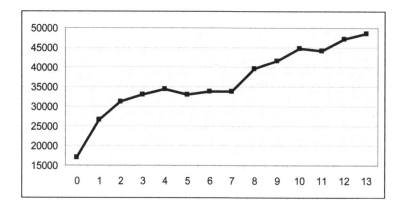

index should be examined for its predictive ability to see if decisions on patient care can be based upon prediction, or whether the quality of care can be measured by comparing actual to predicted values. (Birim et al., 2003; Matteo et al., 2007; McGregor et al., 2005; Rius et al., 2004; Senni et al., 2006; Volk, Hernandez, Lok, & Marrero, 2007) It is clear that the Index cannot be truly predictive unless it can accurately predict the outcomes of incoming patients; statistical significance alone is not sufficient.

We next look to the length of stay and total charges as outcomes. Table 12 gives basic summary statistics. Again, we should expect the average value to increase as the Charlson index value increases. Unfortunately, this is not the case. In addition, the magnitude of the difference from one Charlson value to the next is not consistent.

Using just a 10% random sample, we drill down into the data to examine the entire distribution of length of stay with the following code. Proc KDE estimates the entire population distribution. In this example, we write multiple Proc KDE procedures so that we can view a partial list of indices on the same graph.

```
proc kde data=nis.charlsonsample;
univar los/gridl=0 gridu=20 out=nis.kdelos3 method=srot bwm=4;
```

Table 12. Summary statistics for length of stay and total charges

charlson	N Obs	Variable	Mean	Std Dev	Minimum	Maximum	N
0	4538105	LOS	3.8132948	6.4827794	0	365.0000000	4537934
		TOTCHG	16946.36	33463.31	25.0000000	999720.00	4457967
1	1708386	LOS	5.0914773	6.7995739	0	364.0000000	1708259
		TOTCHG	26524.86	41152.46	25.0000000	999926.00	1685723
2	926681	LOS	5.9793568	7.3538667	0	364.0000000	926601
		TOTCHG	31218.01	46997.48	29.0000000	998514.00	913823
3	474424	LOS	6.5102839	7.4676395	0	335.0000000	474383
		TOTCHG	33083.38	47701.57	25.0000000	998508.00	467085
4	196448	LOS	6.9255654	7.5988107	0	308.0000000	196441
		TOTCHG	34317.32	48332.13	29.0000000	998461.00	193419
5	83760	LOS	6.6702365	7.4820287	0	314.0000000	83757
		TOTCHG	32904.84	45877.64	29.0000000	986244.00	82342
6	42603	LOS	7.2759050	8.6108387	0	233.0000000	42598
		TOTCHG	33847.22	51960.12	35.0000000	991975.00	42003
7	13188	LOS	7.3181680	8.6143188	0	311.0000000	13188
		TOTCHG	33837.62	51531.71	32.0000000	950447.00	13012
8	5683	LOS	8.2118599	10.3810108	0	206.0000000	5683
		TOTCHG	39683.73	60616.23	58.0000000	893263.00	5608
9	1775	LOS	8.5729577	9.4393066	0	89.0000000	1775
		TOTCHG	41507.33	58197.17	660.0000000	865888.00	1740
10	654	LOS	8.9188361	10.5716006	0	107.0000000	653
		TOTCHG	44892.91	62465.84	1181.00	691096.00	644
11	217	LOS	8.8202765	10.1210248	0	108.0000000	217
		TOTCHG	44177.88	79898.36	2322.00	877351.00	213
12	71	LOS	11.1690141	15.4836189	0	88.0000000	71
		TOTCHG	47114.89	57476.33	2400.00	256315.00	70
13	12	LOS	6.2500000	4.8453352	1.0000000	18.0000000	12
		TOTCHG	48569.75	84774.64	3246.00	307731.00	12

```
univar totchg/gridl=0 gridu=50000 out=nis.kdetotchg3 method=srot bwm=4;
by charlson;
where charlson=0;
run;
proc kde data=nis.charlsonsample;
univar los/gridl=0 gridu=20 out=nis.kdelos method=srot bwm=2;
univar totchg/gridl=0 gridu=50000 out=nis.kdetotchg method=srot bwm=2;
by charlson;
where charlson<3 and charlson>0;
run;
proc kde data=nis.charlsonsample;
univar los/gridl=0 gridu=20 out=nis.kdelos2 method=srot bwm=2;
univar totchg/gridl=0 gridu=50000 out=nis.kdetotchg2 method=srot bwm=2;
by charlson;
where charlson>2 and charlson<9;
```

```
run;
proc kde data=nis.charlsonsample;
univar los/gridl=0 gridu=20 out=nis.kdelos4 method=srot ;
univar totchg/gridl=0 gridu=50000 out=nis.kdetotchg4 method=srot ;
by charlson;
where charlson>8 ;
run;
```

Figure 5 gives the probability density graph for a Charlson Index of 0, and for indices of 1 and 2.

Note that the average length of stay for patients with a Charlson code of zero occurs at 2 days; for an index of 1, it peaks at 2.1 days and at 2.6 days for an index of two. There is more variability in the distribution for indices 2 and 3 compared to an index of zero. Figure 6 gives the probability density for indices 3-12.

For values 3-8, there is a clear order to the distribution with 3>4>5>6>7>8 in terms of the probability in the peak of the curve at less than five days. There is also a cutpoint at about 6 days where the probabilities reverse and 3<4<5<6<7<8. There is some confusion in that the peak for index 3 is at 2.85, for 4 at 3.2, for 5 at 3.1, for 6 at 3.25, for 7 at 3.75 and for 8 at 4.15. These values indicate that there is some ambiguity between indices 4 and 5 that could result from moving the patient from one class into the other. However, the cutpoints are reasonably clustered compared to those for Index values 9-12.

This confusion between indices increases when we consider 9-12. For index 9, the peak occurs at 3.25 with a crossover at day 7.5. There is a second crossover at 15.6, where index 9 again has the highest

Figure 5. Probability density for a Charlson index of 0,1,2

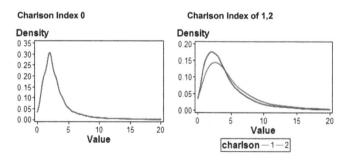

Figure 6. Probability density for a Charlson index of 3-12

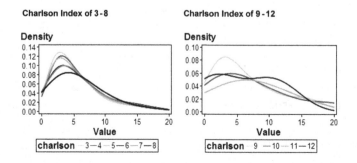

probability. Index 10 follows the pattern with a first peak at 3.9 and a crossover at day 7.5. However, the second crossover occurs at day 13.3. Index 11 has just one peak at day 7.2; Index 12 has two peaks, one at day 2.25 and a second at day 10.8 with a crossover at day 15.6. Figure 7 gives the probability density for a Charlson Index of 13.

For index 13, the peak value occurs at day 4.15, again, indicating that HIV is now over-weighted in the model. We show the similar distributions for total charges. Figure 8 gives the probability functions for indices 0-2.

The peak for index 0 occurs at $8625. It is at $8000 for index value 1 and at $9875 for index 2. There is a crossover point between 1 and 2 at $14,500. These values indicate ambiguity between code 0 and code 1 in terms of charges. Figure 9 gives the Index values for 3-12.

The pattern for indices 3-8 is fairly regular with peak values of $10,750<$11,500<$12,125<$12,750=$12,750<$16,375 as the index increases from 3 to 8. In addition, there is a crossover point for all indices at $27,375. However, there is no regular pattern for indices 9-12 with a peak of $12,750 for index 9, which is much lower than the $16,375 for index 8. While the peak for index 10 is $13,750, it decreases to a peak of $12,750 before increasing to $25,125 for index 12. The crossover point between index 10 and 11 occurs at $30,375. Figure 10 has the Charlson Index of 13.

For index 13, the peak occurs at $8750, which is very close to what it is for index zero.

Figure 7. Probability density for Charlson index 13

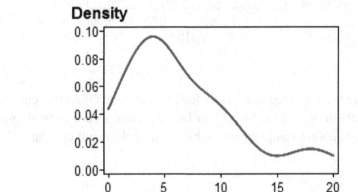

Figure 8. Probability density for total charges for Charlson index of 0-2

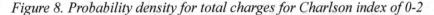

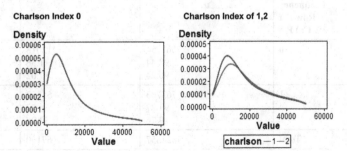

Figure 9. Probability density for total charges for Charlson index of 3-12

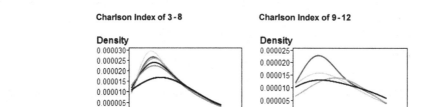

Figure 10. Probability density for total charges for Charlson index of 13

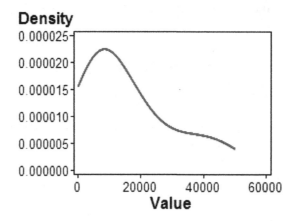

One way of eliminating these discrepancies is to define a cutpoint. Often that cutpoint is defined at index 2 or 3, so that all patients with an index of 2 or less are given a code of 0; all others are given a code of 1. We use the code to define a cutpoint at 2. Table 13 gives the resulting relationship to mortality.

Table 13. Mortality by Charlson code with a cutpoint at 2

Table of charlsoncode by DIED				
charlsoncode		DIED		Total
Frequency Row Pct Col Pct	**0**	**1**	
0	7061154 98.44 90.24	112018 1.56 67.02	7173172
1	763703 93.27 9.76	55132 6.73 32.98	818835
Total	7824857	167150	7992007

```
data nis.modifiedcharlson;
set nis.charlson_regression;
if (charlson<3) then charlsoncode=0;
if (charlson>2) then charlsoncode=1;
run;
```

Note that there is now a considerable difference in the mortality rate between those with a code of 0 and those with a code of 1; all discrepancies have disappeared. We can just as easily make a different cutpoint, say at the index value of 5 (Table 14). The difference is approximately 6% between mortality for code 0 and mortality for code 1.

Similarly, if we restrict our attention to averages, we can show that patients with code 0 use fewer resources compared to code 1 (Table 15).

There is a difference of 2 days in the length of stay between the two subgroups, and a difference of $11,000 as well. For a cutpoint of 5 (Table 16), this difference increases slightly with a difference of just under 3 days in length of stay and a difference of $12,000.

Table 14. Mortality by Charlson code with a cutpoint at 5

Table of charlsoncode by DIED			
charlsoncode	DIED		Total
Frequency Row Pct Col Pct	0	1	
0	7765995 97.96 99.25	161809 2.04 96.80	7927804
1	58862 91.68 0.75	5341 8.32 3.20	64203
Total	7824857	167150	7992007

Table 15. Use of resources for Charlson code with a cutpoint at 2

charlsoncode	N Obs	Variable	Mean	Std Dev	Minimum	Maximum	N
0	7173172	LOS TOTCHG	4.3975221 21082.16	6.7260265 37802.33	0 25.0000000	365.0000000 999926.00	7172794 7057513
1	818835	LOS TOTCHG	6.6983407 33491.09	7.6227648 48127.72	0 25.0000000	335.0000000 998508.00	818778 806148

Table 16. Use of resources for Charlson code with a cutpoint at 5

charlsoncode	N Obs	Variable	Mean	Std Dev	Minimum	Maximum	N
0	7927804	LOS TOTCHG	4.6106097 22253.78	6.8357345 39017.86	0 25.0000000	365.0000000 999926.00	7927375 7800359
1	64203	LOS TOTCHG	7.4293503 34737.46	8.8511050 53172.30	0 32.0000000	311.0000000 991975.00	64197 63302

The definition of a cutpoint just serves to mask the problem of assigning weights that are too high for specific diseases. If we consider the entire distribution, there is considerable overlap between the subgroups in the population by the Charlson Code. Figure 11 gives the probability functions for length of stay and total charges for a cutpoint of 2; Figure 12 gives them for a cutpoint of 5.

Note that while the peak for length of stay is at 2 days for code zero (and $10,000 for total charges), it shifts to 4 days and $11,000 for code one. However, almost the entire curve for cutpoint one is in the area of the cutpoint zero, suggesting that there will be little predictive ability when a cutpoint is used.

Similarly, the area for code one is in the area for code zero, suggesting that there will be little predictive ability except at the high end of the scale beyond day 20 and $50,000 in cost.

CHANGE IN DISEASES TO DEFINE NEW INDEX

We want to suggest an alternative set of diseases to create a new index. One of the biggest problems with such a list of diseases is what should be included, and what should be excluded. We can consider the patient conditions most associated with mortality (Table 17). In order to find these patient conditions, we need to investigate all fifteen columns of diagnosis codes that are available in the NIS. We limit the codes to the first three digits. The following SAS code will give us the necessary values.

```
data nis.died;
set nis.sort;
where died=1;
```

Figure 11. Probability density of length of stay and total charges for a cutpoint at 2

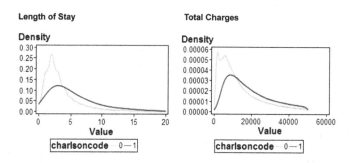

Figure 12. Probability density of length of stay and total charges for a cutpoint at 5

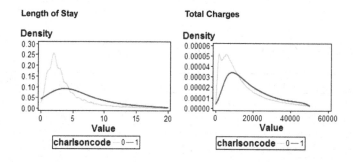

This part of the code filters the data down to just the patients who died so we can see which diagnosis codes are the most closely affiliated with mortality.

```
data nis.code1;
set nis.died;
    DX=substr(DX1,1,3);
    data nis.code2;
    set nis.died;
    DX=substr(DX2,1,3);
    data nis.code3;
set nis.died;
    DX=substr(DX3,1,3);
    data nis.code4;
set nis.died;
    DX=substr(DX4,1,3);
```

Table 17. Diagnosis codes most frequently associated with mortality

ICD9 Code	Code Translation	Frequency with Mortality	Percentage With Mortality
276	Disorders involving the immune mechanism	142494	6.3828186101
427	Cardiac dysrhythmias	123230	5.5199147847
518	Other diseases of lung	118320	5.2999782303
428	Heart failure	99826	4.4715654735
038	Septicemia	75987	3.4037309482
584	Acute renal failure	64743	2.9000717593
486	Pneumonia, organism unspecified	56844	2.5462471478
401	Essential hypertension	51696	2.3156497177
496	Chronic airway obstruction, not elsewhere classified	44370	1.9874918364
599	Other disorders of urethra and urinary tract	43501	1.9485662018
995	Certain adverse effects not elsewhere classified	42203	1.8904241147
785	Symptoms involving cardiovascular system	40523	1.8151708741
250	Diabetes	39668	1.7768723499
414	Other forms of chronic ischemic heart disease	37612	1.6847767174
410	Acute myocardial infarction	35847	1.6057160211
197	Secondary malignant neoplasm of respiratory and digestive systems	33655	1.5075284596
780	General symptoms	32084	1.4371577209
507	Pneumonitis due to solids and liquids	29470	1.3200672621
403	Hypertensive kidney disease	28268	1.2662253602
198	Secondary malignant neoplasm of other specified sites	25279	1.1323373029
285	Other and unspecified anemias	25033	1.1213180784
707	Chronic ulcer of skin	24874	1.1141958967

```
   data nis.code5;
set nis.died;
   DX=substr(DX5,1,3);
   data nis.code6;
set nis.died;
   DX=substr(DX6,1,3);
   data nis.code7;
set nis.died;
   DX=substr(DX7,1,3);
   data nis.code8;
set nis.died;
   DX=substr(DX8,1,3);
   data nis.code9;
set nis.died;
   DX=substr(DX9,1,3);
   data nis.code10;
set nis.died;
   DX=substr(DX10,1,3);
   data nis.code11;
set nis.died;
   DX=substr(DX11,1,3);
   data nis.code12;
set nis.died;
   DX=substr(DX12,1,3);
   data nis.code13;
set nis.died;
   DX=substr(DX13,1,3);
   data nis.code14;
set nis.died;
   DX=substr(DX14,1,3);
   data nis.code15;
set nis.died;
   DX=substr(DX15,1,3);
   run;
```

This next part of the code creates a new dataset for each column of diagnosis code. In addition, it relabels the column to be consistent across each of these datasets. The purpose is so that the columns can be stacked (ie, easily appended).

```
PROC SQL;
CREATE TABLE SASUSER.APPEND_TABLE_0009 AS
SELECT * FROM NIS.CODE1
 OUTER UNION CORR
SELECT * FROM NIS.CODE10
```

```
 OUTER UNION CORR
SELECT * FROM NIS.CODE11
 OUTER UNION CORR
SELECT * FROM NIS.CODE12
 OUTER UNION CORR
SELECT * FROM NIS.CODE13
 OUTER UNION CORR
SELECT * FROM NIS.CODE14
 OUTER UNION CORR
SELECT * FROM NIS.CODE15
 OUTER UNION CORR
SELECT * FROM NIS.CODE2
 OUTER UNION CORR
SELECT * FROM NIS.CODE3
 OUTER UNION CORR
SELECT * FROM NIS.CODE4
 OUTER UNION CORR
SELECT * FROM NIS.CODE5
 OUTER UNION CORR
SELECT * FROM NIS.CODE6
 OUTER UNION CORR
SELECT * FROM NIS.CODE8
 OUTER UNION CORR
SELECT * FROM NIS.CODE9
 OUTER UNION CORR
SELECT * FROM NIS.CODE7
;
Quit;
```

This next part of the code appends the 15 datasets just created; each dataset with just one of the 15 columns of diagnosis codes.

```
PROC FREQ DATA=WORK.SORT
    ORDER=FREQ
    NOPRINT
;
    TABLES DX /
    OUT=NIS.ONEWAYFREQOFDXINAPPEND_TABLE_000(LABEL="Cell statistics for DX analysis of
SASUSER.APPEND_TABLE_0009") SCORES=TABLE;
RUN;
```

This last part finds a frequency count for each of the diagnosis codes in the appended dataset. Instead of printing, we collect the values into a dataset. They are listed in descending order so that we can find the ones with the greatest frequency. The codes that have a mortality percentage greater than 1 are collected and shown in Table 17. This gives us a new list to define a new index code.

We consider some of the codes listed in Table 17. Table 18 shows the relationship of code 038, Septicemia by mortality. It shows a 25% mortality rate, higher than any of the mortality levels listed in Table 1 that define the Charlson Index. There is no question that the occurrence of this disease puts a patient at high risk of death; yet, the risk will not be counted at all in the Charlson Index. If investigating hospital quality, it can be argued that Septicemia is most likely nosocomial; that is, the infection was acquired in the hospital and should, therefore, not count when predicting the likelihood of mortality. However, it misses the issue of predicting the patients most at risk. Moreover, Septicemia does occur in the community and the patient can arrive at the hospital with the condition.

While heart failure and COPD are in the Charlson Index, urinary tract disorders are not included, nor is the code '780' representing general symptoms, meaning that the patient's condition does not yet have a diagnosis.

Table 19 gives the mortality level for code 197, Secondary malignant neoplasm of respiratory and digestive systems. It has a mortality rate of 8%, which has a probability sufficiently high to warrant a weight of two by the Charlson Index standard; it is given a weight of 3 according to Table 1.

Table 20 gives the mortality for code 707, Chronic ulcer of skin. As the lowest associated level of mortality given in Table 17, it still has a probability higher than those for a Charlson Index weight of 1.

Table 18. Mortality by occurrence of septicemia

Table of code038 by DIED			
code038	**DIED**		**Total**
Frequency **Col Pct**	**0**	**1**	
0	7676279 98.10	125542 75.11	7801821
1	148578 1.90	41608 24.89	190186
Total	7824857	167150	7992007
Frequency Missing = 3041			

Table 19. Mortality by secondary malignant neoplasm

Table of code197 by DIED			
code197	**DIED**		**Total**
Frequency **Col Pct**	**0**	**1**	
0	7728732 98.77	153351 91.74	7882083
1	96125 1.23	13799 8.26	109924
Total	7824857	167150	7992007
Frequency Missing = 3041			

The following code is used to define an Index where all of the codes are given equal weight.

```
data nis.code3digits;
set nis.charlson;
code276=0; code427=0; code518=0; code428=0; code038=0;
code584=0; code486=0; code401=0; code496=0; code599=0;
code995=0; code785=0; code250=0; code414=0; code410=0; code197=0; code780=0; code507=0;
code403=0; code198=0; code285=0; code707=0;
if (rxmatch('276',diagnoses)>0) then code276=1;
if (rxmatch('427',diagnoses)>0) then code427=1;
if (rxmatch('518',diagnoses)>0) then code518=1;
if (rxmatch('428',diagnoses)>0) then code428=1;
if (rxmatch('038',diagnoses)>0) then code038=1;
if (rxmatch('584',diagnoses)>0) then code584=1;
if (rxmatch('486',diagnoses)>0) then code486=1;
if (rxmatch('401',diagnoses)>0) then code401=1;
if (rxmatch('496',diagnoses)>0) then code496=1;
if (rxmatch('599',diagnoses)>0) then code599=1;
if (rxmatch('995',diagnoses)>0) then code995=1;
if (rxmatch('785',diagnoses)>0) then code785=1;
if (rxmatch('250',diagnoses)>0) then code250=1;
if (rxmatch('414',diagnoses)>0) then code414=1;
if (rxmatch('410',diagnoses)>0) then code410=1;
if (rxmatch('197',diagnoses)>0) then code197=1;
if (rxmatch('780',diagnoses)>0) then code780=1;
if (rxmatch('507',diagnoses)>0) then code507=1;
if (rxmatch('403',diagnoses)>0) then code403=1;
if (rxmatch('198',diagnoses)>0) then code198=1;
if (rxmatch('285',diagnoses)>0) then code285=1;
if (rxmatch('707',diagnoses)>0) then code707=1;
newindex=code276+code427+code518+code428+code038+code584+code486+code401+code496+code599
```

Table 20. Mortality by chronic ulcer of skin

Table of code707 by DIED			
code707	DIED		Total
Frequency Col Pct	0	1	
0	7658437 97.87	153879 92.06	7812316
1	166420 2.13	13271 7.94	179691
Total	7824857	167150	7992007
Frequency Missing = 3041			

```
+code995
+code785+code250+code414+code197+code780+code507+code403+code198+code285+code707;
run;
```

We could also have defined cutpoint levels in the frequency of mortality to define a series of weights for this New Index. Table 21 shows the relationship of this new index to mortality.

Note that as the index increases, so does the level of mortality to a peak at index level 10. Figure 13 show the relationship. Note that the curve is very smooth, with each higher index level having a correspondingly higher mortality rate. Moreover, the rate accelerates as the index increases. It follows a natural curve that can be modeled.

Table 21. Mortality by new index code

Table of newindex by DIED			
newindex	DIED		Total
Frequency Row Pct Col Pct	0	1	
0	3121856 99.77 39.90	7189 0.23 4.30	3129045
1	1420115 99.24 18.15	10921 0.76 6.53	1431036
2	1221538 98.42 15.61	19558 1.58 11.70	1241096
3	955517 97.16 12.21	27925 2.84 16.71	983442
4	609314 94.93 7.79	32536 5.07 19.47	641850
5	315583 91.20 4.03	30444 8.80 18.21	346027
6	129128 85.46 1.65	21964 14.54 13.14	151092
7	40966 77.89 0.52	11626 22.11 6.96	52592
8	9395 69.43 0.12	4136 30.57 2.47	13531
9	1346 63.22 0.02	783 36.78 0.47	2129
10	99 59.28 0.00	68 40.72 0.04	167

Figure 13. Mortality by new index

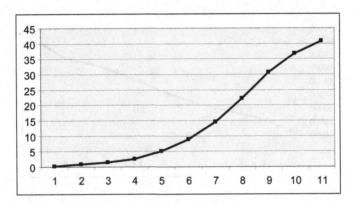

Table 22. Length of stay and total charges by new index

newindex	N Obs	Variable	Mean	Std Dev	Minimum	Maximum	N
0	3129583	LOS	3.2428094	5.4167516	0	364.0000000	3129525
		TOTCHG	12302.79	23539.62	25.0000000	999710.00	3066669
1	1431567	LOS	4.2416399	6.5166212	0	364.0000000	1431473
		TOTCHG	21116.97	32688.84	25.0000000	998317.00	1411635
2	1241687	LOS	4.8663472	6.5674068	0	365.0000000	1241575
		TOTCHG	25750.44	37562.91	25.0000000	997707.00	1224680
3	983962	LOS	5.6671874	7.1677542	0	365.0000000	983872
		TOTCHG	29850.70	44159.59	25.0000000	999926.00	970517
4	642297	LOS	6.7287520	8.2115352	0	361.0000000	642250
		TOTCHG	34921.58	53050.54	27.0000000	999720.00	633893
5	346270	LOS	7.9652441	9.3912188	0	341.0000000	346243
		TOTCHG	41731.68	63744.23	28.0000000	998554.00	341986
6	151208	LOS	9.2747138	10.5047496	0	308.0000000	151201
		TOTCHG	49817.70	73879.86	29.0000000	997836.00	149465
7	52635	LOS	10.4419851	11.4814388	0	282.0000000	52633
		TOTCHG	57487.55	79616.93	64.0000000	997590.00	52103
8	13541	LOS	11.3076582	12.4802009	0	268.0000000	13541
		TOTCHG	63405.66	86361.05	29.0000000	944763.00	13419
9	2131	LOS	11.7550446	13.0429794	0	197.0000000	2131
		TOTCHG	67360.56	87828.53	244.0000000	737108.00	2111
10	167	LOS	13.9221557	16.2343508	0	127.0000000	167
		TOTCHG	79270.05	108184.58	2055.00	693193.00	167

Since mortality was used to define the index, we want to validate it by comparing length of stay to total charges (Table 22). Unlike the Charlson Index, the values increase as the New Index level increases. This is depicted graphically in Figures 14 and 15 for total charges and in Figures 16-18 for length of stay.

Note that the increase by the New Index level is almost completely linear. The kernel density in Figure 15 shows that the transition from one index level to another is very regular compared to the transitions of the Charlson Index. The transition from one Index level to another is very smooth with very natural cutpoints.

Figure 14. Average total charges by new index

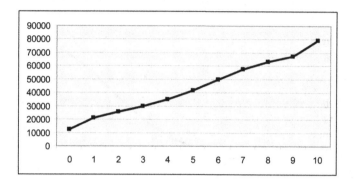

Figure 15. Probability density of total charges by new index

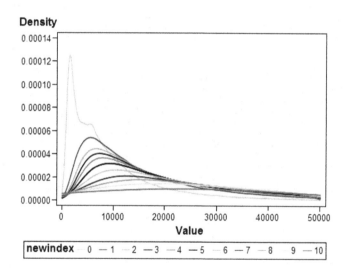

Figure 16. Average length of stay by new index

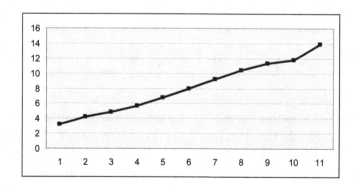

Again, the pattern is almost totally linear with an increase for every index level. Figure 17 gives the probability density for a New Index of 0. It shows a very sharp peak at a length of stay of approximately 2 days with smaller peaks at 1 and 3 days. The probability of a stay beyond 5 days is virtually zero. Figure 18 gives the length of stay distribution for an index of 1-10.

The pattern displayed is again very regular, showing a similar change in magnitude from one index level to the next. Table 23 compares the two indices directly. It appears that this new index gives a better result generally; it is not yet known how well it will work with new data. However, NIS data from a previous year can be used to demonstrate reliability in the Index.

Table 22 shows that there is no real correspondence between the two indices. For example, while 62% of the Charlson Index values also have zero value for the new index, fully 20% are shifted to new

Figure 17. Length of stay for new index zero

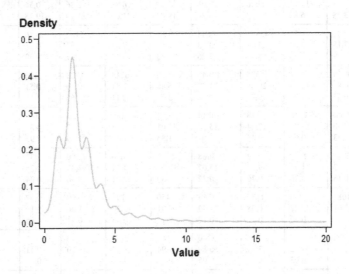

Figure 18. Length of stay for new index 1-10

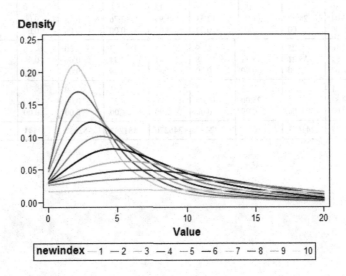

Table 23. Comparison of Charlson index to new index

Table of charlson by newindex

charlson	newindex											Total
Frequency Row Pct Col Pct	0	1	2	3	4	5	6	7	8	9	10	
0	2827794 62.29 90.36	888447 19.57 62.06	466248 10.27 37.55	216606 4.77 22.01	88110 1.94 13.72	33238 0.73 9.60	13138 0.29 8.69	4537 0.10 8.62	1077 0.02 7.95	161 0.00 7.56	6 0.00 3.59	4539362
1	217927 12.75 6.96	361979 21.18 25.29	445779 26.08 35.90	351018 20.54 35.67	193528 11.32 30.13	87032 5.09 25.13	35064 2.05 23.19	12655 0.74 24.04	3561 0.21 26.30	601 0.04 28.20	44 0.00 26.35	1709188
2	53633 5.78 1.71	99516 10.73 6.95	188757 20.36 15.20	231620 24.98 23.54	181912 19.62 28.32	104529 11.27 30.19	45573 4.92 30.14	16241 1.75 30.86	4532 0.49 33.47	787 0.08 36.93	74 0.01 44.31	927174
3	12404 2.61 0.40	46920 9.88 3.28	84628 17.83 6.82	110415 23.26 11.22	104463 22.01 16.26	68798 14.49 19.87	32793 6.91 21.69	11208 2.36 21.29	2638 0.56 19.48	400 0.08 18.77	28 0.01 16.77	474695
4	5502 2.80 0.18	14122 7.18 0.99	30155 15.34 2.43	45342 23.07 4.61	46644 23.73 7.26	33062 16.82 9.55	15314 7.79 10.13	5164 2.63 9.81	1136 0.58 8.39	132 0.07 6.19	10 0.01 5.99	196583
5	4278 5.10 0.14	9068 10.82 0.63	13794 16.46 1.11	17305 20.65 1.76	17848 21.30 2.78	12909 15.40 3.73	6214 7.41 4.11	1928 2.30 3.66	426 0.51 3.15	35 0.04 1.64	4 0.00 2.40	83809
6	5895 13.83 0.19	7630 17.90 0.53	7578 17.78 0.61	7348 17.24 0.75	6514 15.28 1.01	4691 11.01 1.35	2197 5.15 1.45	627 1.47 1.19	129 0.30 0.95	14 0.03 0.66	1 0.00 0.60	42624
7	1258 9.53 0.04	2312 17.52 0.16	2799 21.21 0.23	2552 19.34 0.26	2068 15.67 0.32	1357 10.28 0.39	626 4.74 0.41	190 1.44 0.36	33 0.25 0.24	1 0.01 0.05	0 0.00 0.00	13196
8	702 12.35 0.02	1082 19.03 0.08	1289 22.67 0.10	1142 20.08 0.12	763 13.42 0.12	450 7.91 0.13	191 3.36 0.13	60 1.06 0.11	7 0.12 0.05	0 0.00 0.00	0 0.00 0.00	5686
9	115 6.48 0.00	300 16.89 0.02	432 24.32 0.03	411 23.14 0.04	300 16.89 0.05	141 7.94 0.04	59 3.32 0.04	16 0.90 0.03	2 0.11 0.01	0 0.00 0.00	0 0.00 0.00	1776
10	63 9.62 0.00	124 18.93 0.01	145 22.14 0.01	142 21.68 0.01	98 14.96 0.02	49 7.48 0.01	27 4.12 0.02	7 1.07 0.01	0 0.00 0.00	0 0.00 0.00	0 0.00 0.00	655
11	9 4.15 0.00	50 23.04 0.00	54 24.88 0.00	45 20.74 0.00	38 17.51 0.01	13 5.99 0.00	6 2.76 0.00	2 0.92 0.00	0 0.00 0.00	0 0.00 0.00	0 0.00 0.00	217
12	2 2.82 0.00	16 22.54 0.00	25 35.21 0.00	13 18.31 0.00	9 12.68 0.00	1 1.41 0.00	5 7.04 0.00	0 0.00 0.00	0 0.00 0.00	0 0.00 0.00	0 0.00 0.00	71
13	1 8.33 0.00	1 8.33 0.00	4 33.33 0.00	3 25.00 0.00	2 16.67 0.00	0 0.00 0.00	1 8.33 0.00	0 0.00 0.00	0 0.00 0.00	0 0.00 0.00	0 0.00 0.00	12
Total	3129583	1431567	1241687	983962	642297	346270	151208	52635	13541	2131	167	7995048

index level one. However, Charlson Index 3 is scattered across all values of the new index with a peak of just 23%. Moreover, the Charlson Index of 12 has most of its values at a new index value of 4 or below.

VALIDATION

We want to validate these indices by using another dataset. In this case, we use the Medical Expenditure Panel Survey (MEPS). We use the inpatient dataset to look at the costs involved in treatment. Unfortunately, the MEPS truncates the ICD9 codes to 3 digits. Therefore, it is not possible to use the MEPS datasets to compute the Charlson Index. However, there is a modification of the Charlson Index developed by D'Hoore that only uses 3 digit ICD9 codes. Therefore, we will consider this adaptation after we validate the New Index. (Schneeweiss & Maclure, 2000)

Since the New Index uses the 3 digit truncation, we can compute it on MEPS data. Table 24 shows the results. Since the MEPS inpatient dataset limits the number of ICD9 diagnosis codes to 4, the highest the index can go is to a value of 4. It also shows that there will be diagnosis codes that are part of the New Index that will be omitted from the computation just for lack of space. In the table, mdtotal=total payment to physician, fcpayment=total payment to hospital. Total charges represent the total charged for treatment; totalexpenditure is the total reimbursed to the providers. The value NUMNIGHTX represents the length of stay.

Table 24. New index for MEPS inpatient data for 2003-2005

newindex	N Obs	Variable	Mean	Std Dev	Minimum	Maximum	N
0	8252	mdtotal	3565.89	5910.45	0	198416.00	8252
		fcpayment	8381.05	17536.86	0	637900.13	8252
		totalcharge	25542.01	50220.27	10.0000000	1546859.16	8252
		totalexpenditure	9729.83	18437.73	0	645378.22	8252
		NUMNIGHX	5.4634028	10.6935358	0	365.0000000	8252
1	1705	mdtotal	2309.32	4586.37	0	76777.34	1705
		fcpayment	8125.71	22306.17	0	628631.24	1705
		totalcharge	24454.16	48659.21	34.0000000	869502.46	1705
		totalexpenditure	8998.66	23090.35	0	648408.48	1705
		NUMNIGHX	6.3601173	12.5818654	0	300.0000000	1705
2	209	mdtotal	2161.17	3267.31	0	26462.87	209
		fcpayment	8958.48	12960.77	0	90633.69	209
		totalcharge	26465.19	34836.55	374.7100000	264901.98	209
		totalexpenditure	9777.35	13591.35	0	93908.21	209
		NUMNIGHX	7.9282297	12.3346610	0	133.0000000	209
3	17	mdtotal	1959.16	3031.05	0	11582.90	17
		fcpayment	12493.18	17787.87	0	62770.70	17
		totalcharge	35518.08	43059.24	632.3200000	148754.40	17
		totalexpenditure	13265.28	18696.60	0	67023.64	17
		NUMNIGHX	12.7058824	21.7966876	1.0000000	90.0000000	17
4	2	mdtotal	4380.75	6195.32	0	8761.50	2
		fcpayment	21881.30	8135.83	16128.40	27634.20	2
		totalcharge	52052.35	10003.52	44978.79	59125.90	2
		totalexpenditure	23053.11	6478.65	18472.01	27634.20	2
		NUMNIGHX	7.0000000	1.4142136	6.0000000	8.0000000	2

The total expenditure increases as the value of the New Index increases except for the value of zero. This could occur because many of the ICD9 codes included in the New Index may not be defined in the inpatient dataset, resulting in a code of zero. Fortunately, there is a dataset in the MEPS files containing all possible patient conditions. We will use this dataset combined with the inpatient costs to examine the New Index. To set up the conditions, we use the following code to transpose the patient conditions so that each patient has just one observation in the dataset:

```
proc sort data=nis.patientconditions
out=work.patientconditions;
by dupersid;
proc Transpose data=work.patientconditions
out=work.tran (drop=_name_ _label_)
             prefix=med_ ;
      var icd9codx ;
      by dupersid;
run;
```

Next, we concatenate the patient conditions into one column in the dataset.

```
data work.concat(keep= dupersid icd9codx) ;
   length icd9codx $32767 ;
   set work.tran ;
   array chconcat {*} med_: ;
   icd9codx = left(trim(med_1)) ;
   do i = 2 to dim(chconcat) ;
      icd9codx = left(trim(icd9codx)) || ` ` || left(trim(chconcat[i])) ;
   end ;
run ;
```

Because it is unknown just how many variables need to be concatenated, the maximum possible length was used. Proc SQL is used to reduce the length of the text string to its minimum possible.

```
proc sql ;
   select max(length(icd9codx)) into:icd9codx_LEN from work.concat ;
quit ;
%put icd9codx_LEN=&icd9codx_LEN ;
data icd9.icd9codes ;
   length icd9codx $ &icd9codx_LEN ;
   set work.concat ;
run ;
```

The next step is to merge the dataset of patient conditions with the dataset of inpatient data:

```
PROC SQL;
CREATE TABLE NIS.inpatientandconditions AS SELECT inpatient.DUID,
    ICD9CODES.icd9codx,
    ICD9CODES.DUPERSID AS DUPERSID1,
    inpatient.PID,
    inpatient.DUPERSID,
    inpatient.EVNTIDX,
    inpatient.EVENTRN,
    inpatient.ERHEVIDX,
    inpatient.FFEEIDX,
    inpatient.MPCDATA,
    inpatient.IPBEGYR,
    inpatient.IPBEGMM,
    inpatient.IPBEGDD,
    inpatient.IPENDYR,
    inpatient.IPENDMM,
    inpatient.IPENDDD,
    inpatient.NUMNIGHX,
    inpatient.NUMNIGHT,
    inpatient.EMERROOM,
    inpatient.SPECCOND,
    inpatient.RSNINHOS,
    inpatient.ANYOPER,
    inpatient.VAPLACE,
    inpatient.IPICD1X,
    inpatient.IPICD2X,
    inpatient.IPICD3X,
    inpatient.IPICD4X,
    inpatient.IPPRO1X,
    inpatient.IPPRO2X,
    inpatient.IPCCC1X,
    inpatient.IPCCC2X,
    inpatient.IPCCC3X,
    inpatient.IPCCC4X,
    inpatient.DSCHPMED,
    inpatient.FFIPTYPE,
    inpatient.IMPFLAG,
    inpatient.PERWT03F,
    inpatient.VARSTR,
    inpatient.VARPSU,
    inpatient.year,
    inpatient.mdmedicaid,
    inpatient.mdmedicare,
    inpatient.mdotherfed,
```

```
        inpatient.mdotherpv,
        inpatient.mdotherinsur,
        inpatient.mdotherpub,
        inpatient.mdprivateins,
        inpatient.mdselfpaid,
        inpatient.mdstate,
        inpatient.mdtotal,
        inpatient.mdtricare,
        inpatient.mdveterans,
        inpatient.mdworkcomp,
        inpatient.mdpayment,
        inpatient.fcmedicaid,
        inpatient.fcmedicare,
        inpatient.fcotherfed,
        inpatient.fcotherpv,
        inpatient.fcotherinsur,
        inpatient.fcotherpub,
        inpatient.fcprivateins,
        inpatient.fcselfpaid,
        inpatient.fcstate,
        inpatient.fctotal,
        inpatient.fctricare,
        inpatient.fcveterans,
        inpatient.fcworkcomp,
        inpatient.fcpayment,
        inpatient.totalcharge,
        inpatient.totalexpenditure,
        inpatient.PERWT04F,
        inpatient.PANEL,
        inpatient.PERWT05F
FROM NIS.INPATIENT AS inpatient
    LEFT JOIN NIS.ICD9CODES AS ICD9CODES ON (inpatient.DUPERSID = ICD9CODES.DUPERSID);
QUIT;
```

Table 25 gives the results of this combination to define the New Index on the MEPS dataset.

Index 6 has slightly lower expenditures as well as charges compared to index 5, with a considerable reduction for index 7, while increasing back for index 8. Figure 19 gives a kernel density comparison for total charges; Figure 20 gives it for length of stay.

While not as regular for Figure 15, it still has a regular hierarchy. There is a small crossover between NewIndex levels 5 and 7 that makes it slightly irregular. The same pattern is visible for the length of stay in Figure 20.

These results show that the New Index can be transferred to other datasets. However, it also shows that there is room for improvement in the development of a risk adjustment index. It shows the limitations in the use of the Charlson Index when the ICD9 codes are incomplete.

Table 25. New index for MEPS inpatient data for 2003-2005 with patient condition files

newindex	N Obs	Variable	Mean	Std Dev	Minimum	Maximum	N
1	2623	mdtotal	3377.95	6521.21	0	198416.00	2623
		fcpayment	8533.57	18429.56	0	628631.24	2623
		totalcharge	24482.67	38611.66	10.0000000	869502.46	2623
		totalexpenditure	9835.77	19319.22	0	648408.48	2623
		NUMNIGHX	5.4510103	11.8639545	0	365.0000000	2623
2	1928	mdtotal	3423.74	6436.70	0	94628.11	1928
		fcpayment	8749.98	14891.03	0	360361.35	1928
		totalcharge	28335.80	54127.87	21.7500000	1546859.16	1928
		totalexpenditure	9954.87	16180.14	0	403439.83	1928
		NUMNIGHX	6.4221992	13.3005326	0	300.0000000	1928
3	1173	mdtotal	3285.27	5474.32	0	45335.61	1173
		fcpayment	9874.08	21482.06	0	399396.38	1173
		totalcharge	31748.64	60792.41	10.0000000	888660.70	1173
		totalexpenditure	11044.67	22522.57	0	402036.64	1173
		NUMNIGHX	7.2199488	11.8110571	0	133.0000000	1173
4	571	mdtotal	3169.70	4774.59	0	43493.02	571
		fcpayment	10046.23	22858.37	0	453475.25	571
		totalcharge	29483.19	67996.88	92.0000000	1386326.55	571
		totalexpenditure	11178.54	23639.67	0	463118.67	571
		NUMNIGHX	6.8336252	9.8884297	0	122.0000000	571
5	218	mdtotal	3455.85	4426.52	0	25409.50	218
		fcpayment	11799.17	19265.95	0	170410.61	218
		totalcharge	34998.45	60857.97	632.3200000	552498.97	218
		totalexpenditure	12987.43	19889.30	0	171126.35	218
		NUMNIGHX	8.7889908	14.3687920	0	120.0000000	218
6	133	mdtotal	2816.81	4367.51	0	28598.00	133
		fcpayment	11462.41	20544.11	0	169745.27	133
		totalcharge	25492.32	38576.84	1215.00	312955.83	133
		totalexpenditure	12448.93	21386.27	73.9200000	171325.46	133
		NUMNIGHX	6.8721805	14.4113873	0	152.0000000	133
7	25	mdtotal	2771.13	4178.09	0	17478.91	25
		fcpayment	5214.05	4287.26	0	15511.79	25
		totalcharge	21675.75	17434.72	374.7100000	59454.36	25
		totalexpenditure	6050.42	4847.68	0	19034.18	25
		NUMNIGHX	4.3600000	5.6412174	1.0000000	30.0000000	25
8	10	mdtotal	5037.35	6313.74	513.0000000	20930.00	10
		fcpayment	13248.55	10506.79	2329.44	32674.92	10
		totalcharge	59745.14	58970.40	7011.00	174415.85	10
		totalexpenditure	15231.12	12564.53	2576.92	38562.08	10
		NUMNIGHX	9.9000000	13.1946959	1.0000000	44.0000000	10

For the D'Hoore Charlson Index, we use the same merged dataset. Table 26 defines this modified index. Note that in the modification, HIV has been eliminated completely. Table 27 gives the results of the analysis for the modified Charlson Index. Compared to the New Index, the decrease in value as the level increases is even more pronounced.

We also look at the kernel density estimations for total charges and for length of stay (Figures 21,22). Note that the graphs are much more irregular compared to Figure 19 for total charges; however, the graph for length of stay in Figure 22 retains a regular pattern. Since charges are not reimbursed by providers at the same rate across hospitals, it is possible that there is a confounding factor for charges that is not

Figure 19. Probability density for total charges

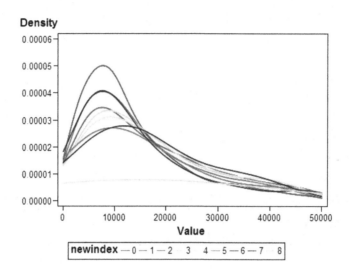

Figure 20. Probability density for length of stay

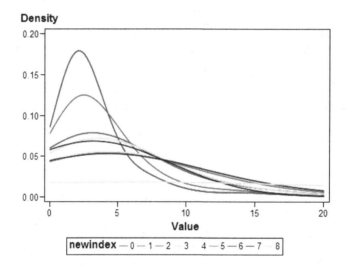

present for length of stay.

USE OF THE CHARLSON INDEX TO RANK PROVIDERS

We again want to look at the difference between actual and expected mortality to rank the quality of providers when treating patients with COPD, and then to rank patients undergoing cardiovascular by-pass surgery (procedure 36.1). We compare our results here to those found in chapter 4 when a severity index was not used.

Using the Charlson Index along with patient demographics, we have the results in Figure 23. The

Table 26. D'Hoore Charlson index using 3 digits of ICD9 codes

Condition	ICD9 Codes	Weights
Myocardial infarction	410,411	1
Congestive heart failure	398,402,428	1
Peripheral vascular disease	440-447	1
Dementia	290,291,294	1
Cerebrovascular disease	430-433,435	1
Chronic Pulmonary disease	491-493	1
Connective tissue disorder	710,714,725	1
Ulcer disease	531-534	1
Mild Liver disease	571,573	1
Diabetes	250	2
Hemiplegia	342,434,436,437	2
Moderate or severe renal disease	403,404,580-586	2
Any tumor	140-195	2
Leukemia	204-208	2
Lymphoma	200,202,203	2
Moderate or severe liver disease	070,570,572	3
Metastatic solid tumor	196-199	6

Figure 21. Probability density for total charges for the D'Hoore Charlson index

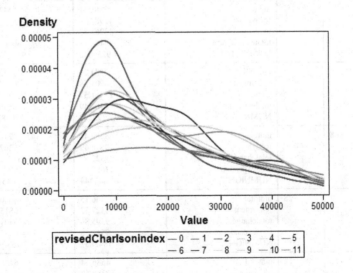

smallest misclassification rate is equal to 21% from a neural network model. The lift indicates that the model is better than chance through the 6th decile in the training set, but only through the third decile in the testing set (Figure 24). The high misclassification rate demonstrates that the model has difficulty in actual prediction.

Ultimately, we want to compare the predicted and actual values by hospital. Table 28 lists these values,

Table 27. Summary statistics for modified Charlson index

revisedCharlsonindex	N Obs	Variable	Mean	Std Dev	Minimum
0	5214	mdtotal	3250.68	5714.98	0
		fcpayment	6964.22	16422.59	0
		totalcharge	20563.61	36919.11	10.0000000
		totalexpenditure	8244.86	17203.21	0
		NUMNIGHX	4.6691600	9.3460888	0
1	1341	mdtotal	3029.54	5203.35	0
		fcpayment	8256.75	16291.78	0
		totalcharge	24735.72	40219.24	21.7500000
		totalexpenditure	9372.89	17080.99	0
		NUMNIGHX	5.3780761	9.4697206	0
2	1771	mdtotal	3680.68	6487.12	0
		fcpayment	9962.57	16661.71	0
		totalcharge	31666.69	63193.74	30.0000000
		totalexpenditure	11310.70	17958.09	0
		NUMNIGHX	6.9446640	12.9649806	0
3	827	mdtotal	3293.15	4783.87	0
		fcpayment	11160.11	31286.59	0
		totalcharge	32871.78	67155.26	99.0000000
		totalexpenditure	12333.69	31941.19	0
		NUMNIGHX	7.1305925	15.9030011	0
4	465	mdtotal	3613.56	5292.84	0
		fcpayment	10662.15	16173.17	0
		totalcharge	35911.85	81562.96	10.0000000
		totalexpenditure	11858.37	17085.54	0
		NUMNIGHX	8.1440860	14.0177955	0
5	236	mdtotal	3145.31	5041.46	0
		fcpayment	9612.51	14964.47	0
		totalcharge	33623.69	65098.20	34.0000000
		totalexpenditure	10820.54	16639.80	0
		NUMNIGHX	7.0000000	10.7469936	0
6	152	mdtotal	3882.11	6542.69	0
		fcpayment	12984.98	28246.97	0
		totalcharge	33265.82	47339.31	1135.79
		totalexpenditure	14482.12	30373.32	0
		NUMNIGHX	7.9736842	9.9807413	0
7	37	mdtotal	2884.26	2332.85	230.0000000
		fcpayment	6908.68	6094.51	0
		totalcharge	23251.57	17405.10	3287.85
		totalexpenditure	8167.49	6556.64	11.9300000
		NUMNIGHX	7.7297297	12.8098240	0
8	90	mdtotal	3289.47	4240.33	0
		fcpayment	10546.69	19362.78	0
		totalcharge	29323.87	37925.57	374.7100000
		totalexpenditure	11662.66	19602.24	0
		NUMNIGHX	8.3444444	13.3645188	0
9	28	mdtotal	3466.15	4670.12	0
		fcpayment	8327.32	10815.02	1177.62
		totalcharge	29595.80	36301.15	1177.62
		totalexpenditure	9517.58	10956.82	1177.62
		NUMNIGHX	7.4642857	7.7530503	1.0000000
10	19	mdtotal	4636.64	6428.45	0
		fcpayment	12348.50	15124.69	724.9100000
		totalcharge	49777.15	88196.79	1346.57
		totalexpenditure	13517.97	15655.34	724.9100000
		NUMNIGHX	7.5789474	9.9906389	0
11	5	mdtotal	537.1160000	129.4973640	359.0000000
		fcpayment	2716.31	2792.08	0
		totalcharge	17141.50	13698.51	3945.75
		totalexpenditure	3032.57	2798.71	0
		NUMNIGHX	4.2000000	3.4928498	1.0000000

Figure 22. Probability density for length of stay for the D'Hoore Charlson index

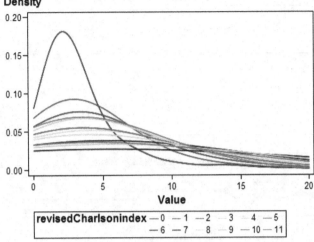

Figure 23. Predicted mortality with risk adjustment by Charlson index

```
Fit Statistics
Model selection based on _TMISC_


                                    Test:
Selected                     Misclassification
Model        Model Node           Rate

             AutoNeural3         0.42857
   Y         DMNeural3           0.21429
             DmineReg3           0.35714
             Neural3             0.42857
             Reg3                0.42857
             Rule3               0.32143
             Tree3               0.32143
```

and the difference for ranking purposes. We use the same list of hospitals as were used in Chapter 4.

This table is in fact identical to Table 12 defined in Chapter 4 using a number of diagnosis and procedure indicator functions. This is not unexpected since the Charlson Index was defined using the diagnosis codes in the indicator functions listed in the previous chapter.

In our next example, we limit the patients to those undergoing procedure 36.1, and use the list of ten hospitals that do perform cardiovascular bypass surgery.

We first want to examine the relationship between procedure and Charlson Index. Table 29 compares the Index to each of the procedures. Note that even though every one of the patients has serious heart conditions that require bypass surgery, there are still some patients with a code of 0 in the index; none have an index higher than 9. It indicates that many of these patients are not identified as having any level

Figure 24. Lift function for risk adjustment by Charlson index

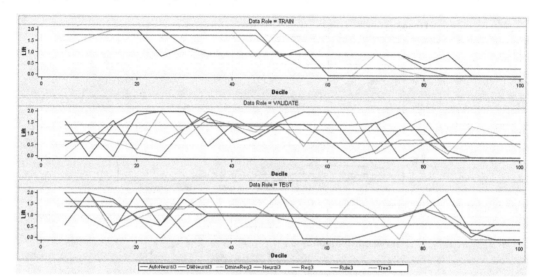

Table 28. Actual versus predicted mortality values by hospital for patients with COPD using Charlson index for risk adjustment

Hospital		Actual Mortality	Predicted Mortality	Difference
	1	3.94	23.62	19.68
	2	7.94	33.33	25.39
	3	2.13	44.68	42.55
	4	4.78	29.57	24.79
	5	4.65	29.07	24.42
	6	3.21	27.98	24.77
	7	3.85	50.00	46.15
	8	No COPD Patients		
	9	4.11	43.84	39.73
	10	0	0	0

of severity. However, as we review the Charlson Index codes, it is clear that severe heart disease is not included in the definition of severity, unless it is diagnosed as congestive heart failure.

We look at the ten hospitals performing cardiovascular surgery to examine their Charlson Index levels (Table 30). Hospital #1, with 50% of procedure number 3615, has almost 45% of its patients in Charlson category #1; hospital #4 with its divided procedures, has 36% of its patients in Charlson categories #2 and #3. It is hospital #10 that appears to have shifted its patients into higher Charlson catgories, with 1% in category #5. It, too, has its procedures relatively divided between 3611-3614. We use predictive modeling to investigate the patient outcomes. The results with the Charlson Index should be very similar to those found in Chapter 4, since the patient conditions that are used to define the Charlson Index were used in the models in Chapter 4. The optimal model for mortality is a neural network model. The lift

Table 29. Charlson index by procedure

Table of charlson by PR1										
charlson	PR1(Principal procedure)									Total
Frequency Row Pct Col Pct	3610	3611	3612	3613	3614	3615	3616	3617	3619	
0	2	1497	3174	2983	1591	1684	181	0	8	11120
	0.02	13.46	28.54	26.83	14.31	15.14	1.63	0.00	0.07	
	25.00	29.28	23.60	22.64	22.07	26.23	35.63	0.00	33.33	
1	4	1887	4969	4874	2655	2376	190	0	9	16964
	0.02	11.12	29.29	28.73	15.65	14.01	1.12	0.00	0.05	
	50.00	36.91	36.95	36.99	36.83	37.02	37.40	0.00	37.50	
2	2	1124	3388	3355	1818	1504	85	3	4	11283
	0.02	9.96	30.03	29.73	16.11	13.33	0.75	0.03	0.04	
	25.00	21.99	25.19	25.46	25.22	23.43	16.73	100.00	16.67	
3	0	416	1346	1407	814	605	35	0	3	4626
	0.00	8.99	29.10	30.42	17.60	13.08	0.76	0.00	0.06	
	0.00	8.14	10.01	10.68	11.29	9.43	6.89	0.00	12.50	
4	0	139	411	442	251	186	10	0	0	1439
	0.00	9.66	28.56	30.72	17.44	12.93	0.69	0.00	0.00	
	0.00	2.72	3.06	3.35	3.48	2.90	1.97	0.00	0.00	
5	0	38	124	81	67	47	5	0	0	362
	0.00	10.50	34.25	22.38	18.51	12.98	1.38	0.00	0.00	
	0.00	0.74	0.92	0.61	0.93	0.73	0.98	0.00	0.00	
6	0	7	26	26	9	11	0	0	0	79
	0.00	8.86	32.91	32.91	11.39	13.92	0.00	0.00	0.00	
	0.00	0.14	0.19	0.20	0.12	0.17	0.00	0.00	0.00	
7	0	4	5	7	2	4	2	0	0	24
	0.00	16.67	20.83	29.17	8.33	16.67	8.33	0.00	0.00	
	0.00	0.08	0.04	0.05	0.03	0.06	0.39	0.00	0.00	
8	0	0	6	0	1	1	0	0	0	8
	0.00	0.00	75.00	0.00	12.50	12.50	0.00	0.00	0.00	
	0.00	0.00	0.04	0.00	0.01	0.02	0.00	0.00	0.00	
9	0	0	0	1	0	1	0	0	0	2
	0.00	0.00	0.00	50.00	0.00	50.00	0.00	0.00	0.00	
	0.00	0.00	0.00	0.01	0.00	0.02	0.00	0.00	0.00	
Total	8	5112	13449	13176	7208	6419	508	3	24	45907

function (Figure 25) shows that the model can predict up through the 50th decile.

We look at the predicted versus actual values for mortality (Table 31). Given the values in Table 31, four hospitals have a predictive mortality of zero. Therefore, these hospitals will rank lower than any of the other hospitals. The two hospitals with the greatest differential are #10 and #3, so they will rank high in quality even though hospital #3 also has the highest actual mortality. Yet it is hospital 5 that has the greatest proportion of patients in the highest Charlson level; yet it has a moderate actual mortality level.

We also examine length of stay by hospital and Charlson Index. The optimal predictive model is a decision tree (Figure 26). The first split is on sex followed by age, and then by level of Charlson Index. The hospital code is not included in the tree model. The average error is given in Figure 27.

Considering that the average stay is equal to 9.7, the average squared error is approximately 64, or

Table 30. Charlson index by hospital

Table of charlson by DSHOSPID											
charlson	HOSPID										Total
Frequency Row Pct Col Pct	1	2	3	4	5	6	7	8	9	10	
0	66 18.64 20.31	4 1.13 36.36	25 7.06 22.32	46 12.99 18.18	21 5.93 23.86	62 17.51 35.43	74 20.90 26.15	10 2.82 22.22	19 5.37 24.36	27 7.63 28.13	354
1	142 24.44 43.69	6 1.03 54.55	36 6.20 32.14	104 17.90 41.11	31 5.34 35.23	61 10.50 34.86	108 18.59 38.16	23 3.96 51.11	37 6.37 47.44	33 5.68 34.38	581
2	66 20.25 20.31	0 0.00 0.00	34 10.43 30.36	63 19.33 24.90	25 7.67 28.41	34 10.43 19.43	60 18.40 21.20	9 2.76 20.00	14 4.29 17.95	21 6.44 21.88	326
3	31 20.81 9.54	1 0.67 9.09	12 8.05 10.71	32 21.48 12.65	9 6.04 10.23	14 9.40 8.00	32 21.48 11.31	1 0.67 2.22	6 4.03 7.69	11 7.38 11.46	149
4	16 38.10 4.92	0 0.00 0.00	4 9.52 3.57	7 16.67 2.77	1 2.38 1.14	3 7.14 1.71	6 14.29 2.12	1 2.38 2.22	1 2.38 1.28	3 7.14 3.13	42
5	2 28.57 0.62	0 0.00 0.00	1 14.29 0.89	0 0.00 0.00	0 0.00 0.00	1 14.29 0.57	2 28.57 0.71	0 0.00 0.00	0 0.00 0.00	1 14.29 1.04	7
6	1 20.00 0.31	0 0.00 0.00	0 0.00 0.00	0 0.00 0.00	1 20.00 1.14	0 0.00 0.00	1 20.00 0.35	1 20.00 2.22	1 20.00 1.28	0 0.00 0.00	5
7	1 100.00 0.31	0 0.00 0.00	0 0.00 0.00	0 0.00 0.00	0 0.00 0.00	0 0.00 0.00	0 0.00 0.00	0 0.00 0.00	0 0.00 0.00	0 0.00 0.00	1
8	0 0.00 0.00	0 0.00 0.00	0 0.00 0.00	1 100.00 0.40	0 0.00 0.00	0 0.00 0.00	0 0.00 0.00	0 0.00 0.00	0 0.00 0.00	0 0.00 0.00	1
Total	325	11	112	253	88	175	283	45	78	96	1466

approximately 8 days, which is less than the value of the mean. As the regression model has approximately the same error value, we also examine that model (Figure 28).

The p-value is statistically significant, but the r^2 value is only 0.0979, indicating that the model remains a relatively poor fit. Note that age, race, and the Charlson index are statistically significant.

FUTURE TRENDS

In the past, measures of quality have been taken too much for granted. Now that reimbursements are becoming dependent upon these rankings, it is essential to scrutinize the methodology to ensure that the definition of ranking actually provides a ranking of quality that is reasonable and valid.

We will discuss additional risk adjustment methods in subsequent chapters before providing a technique that uses all of the diagnosis codes to define patient risk. This technique requires the use of text

Figure 25. Lift function for mortality prediction

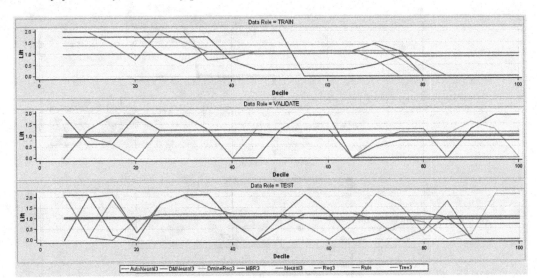

Table 31. Predicted versus actual mortality for cardiovascular surgery using the Charlson index to define patient severity

Hospital	Actual Mortality	Predictive Mortality
1	1.23	23.08
2	0	0
3	4.46	41.07
4	0.79	26.88
5	1.14	26.14
6	0.57	0
7	3.53	0
8	2.22	0
9	1.28	24.36
10	3.13	70.83

analysis. We will compare the Charlson Index to other severity indices in subsequent chapters.

DISCUSSION

A risk adjustment index can be defined through consensus or through statistical analysis or both. In this chapter, we discussed the Charlson Index in detail, and defined a new index that appears to have better features than the Charlson Index. One of the failings of the Charlson Index is that once it was defined, it was not updated. The need for an update is most apparent in the high weight given to HIV, which did not really have any effective treatment at the time the Charlson Index was initially defined, but which now

Figure 26. Predictive model for length of stay for cardiovascular surgery

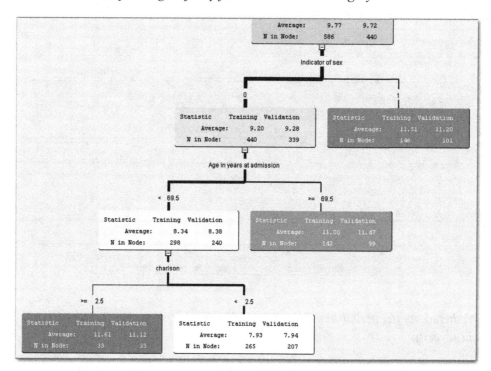

Figure 27. Average error to predict length of stay

Selected Model	MODEL	Test: Average Squared Error
	AutoNeural4	64.4248
	DMNeural4	61.1681
	DmineReg4	60.4748
	MBR4	63.5769
	Neural4	61.6583
	Reg4	61.6968
Y	Tree4	60.3972

has some treatments available so that patients are now living longer with HIV compared to previously.

The Charlson Index was defined through a consensus process. Its validity based upon evidence has yet to be established. The standard practice of taking the differential of the actual and predicted mortality, too, can result in low rankings for providers with very low or even zero mortality; hospitals with high mortality rates are better able to increase their defined predicted mortality. Therefore, great care must be taken before reimbursements are defined by these rankings.

Figure 28. Regression results to predict length of stay

```
                        Analysis of Variance

                            Sum of
    Source         DF       Squares      Mean Square    F Value    Pr > F

    Model          18     1303.300583     72.405588      2.05      0.0074
    Error          340       12014        35.335680
    Corrected Total 358      13317


               Model Fit Statistics

    R-Square     0.0979    Adj R-Sq      0.0501
    AIC        1298.2754   BIC        1302.3927
    SBC        1372.0585   C(p)         19.0000


               Type 3 Analysis of Effects

                        Sum of
    Effect         DF     Squares    F Value    Pr > F

    AGE            1      287.3412    8.13      0.0046
    DIED           1       38.5106    1.09      0.2972
    DSHOSPID       6      138.7362    0.65      0.6866
    FEMALE         1       57.3573    1.62      0.2035
    RACE           5      393.5320    2.23      0.0512
    ZIPInc_Qrtl    3       11.8215    0.11      0.9533
    charlson       1      206.0152    5.83      0.0163
```

REFERENCES

Birim, O., Maat, A., Kappetein, A., Meerbeeck, J. v., Damhuis, R., & Bogers, A. (2003). Validation of the Charlson comorbidity index in patients with operated primary non-small cell lung cancer. *European Journal of Cardio-Thoracic Surgery, 23,* 30–34.

Byles, J. E., D'Este, C., Parkinson, L., O'Connell, R., & Treloar, C. (2005). Single index of multimorbidity did not predict multiple outcomes. *Journal of Clinical Epidemiology, 58,* 997–1005.

Charlson, M., Pompei, P., Ales, K., & MacKenzie, C. (1987). A new method of classifying prognostic comorbidity in longitudinal studies: Development and validation. *Journal of Chronic Diseases, 40,* 373–383.

Colinet, B., Jacot, W., Bertrans, D., Lacombe, S., Bozonnat, M., & Daures, J. (2005). A new simplified comorbidity score as a prognostic factor in non-small-cell lung cancer patients: description and comparison with the Charlson's index. *British Journal of Cancer, 93,* 1098–1105.

D'Hoore, W., Bouckaert, A., & Tilquin, C. (1996). Practical considerations on the use of the Charlson comorbidity index with administrative data bases. *Journal of Clinical Epidemiology, 49*(12), 1429–1433.

Doorn, C. v., Bogardus, S. T., Williams, C. S., Concato, J., Towle, V. R., & Inouye, S. K. (2001). Risk adjustment for older hospitalized persons: a comparison of two methods of data collection for the Charlson index. *Journal of Clinical Epidemiology, 54,* 694–701.

Fried, L., Bernardini, J., & Piraino, B. (2003). Comparison of the Charlson comorbidity index and the Davies score as a predictor of outcomes in PD patients. *Peritoneal Dialysis International, 23*(6), 568–573.

Gettman, M. T., Boelter, C. W., Cheville, J. C., Zincke, H., Bryant, S. C., & Blute, M. L. (2003). Charlson co-morbidity index as a predictor of outcome after surgery for renal cell carcinoma with renal vein, vena cava or right atrium extension. *The Journal of Urology, 169*, 1282–1286.

Ghali, W. A., Hall, R. E., Rosen, A. K., Ash, A. S., & Moskowitz, M. A. (1996). Searching for an improved clinical comorbidity index for use with ICD-9-CM administrative data. *Journal of Clinical Epidemiology, 49*(3), 273–278.

Goldstein, L. B., Samsa, G. P., Matchar, D. B., & Horner, R. D. (2004). Charlson index comorbidity adjustment for ischemic stroke outcome studies. *Stroke, 35*, 1941–1945.

Groll, D., Heyland, D., Caeser, M., & Wright, J. (2006). Assessment of long-term physical function in acute respiratory distress syndrome (ARDS) patients. *American Journal of Physical Medicine & Rehabilitation, 85*(7), 574–581.

Holman, C. D., Preen, D. B., Baynham, N. J., Finn, J. C., & Semmens, J. B. (2005). A multipurpose comorbidity scoring system performed better than the Charlson index. *Journal of Clinical Epidemiology, 58*, 1006–1014.

Kieszak, S. M., Flanders, W. D., Kosinski, A. S., Shipp, C. C., & Karp, H. (1999). A comparison of the Charlson comorbidity index derived from medical record data and administrative billing data. *Journal of Clinical Epidemiology, 52*(2), 137–142.

Klabunde, C. N., Potosky, A. L., Legler, J. M., & Warren, J. L. (2000). Development of a comorbidity index using physician claims data. *Journal of Clinical Epidemiology, 53*, 1258–1267.

Lesens, O., Methlin, C., Hansmann, Y., Remy, V., Martinot, M., & Bergin, C. (2003). Role of comorbidity in mortality related to staphylococcus auerus bacteremia: a prospective study using the Charlson weighted index of comorbidity. *Infection Control and Hospital Epidemiology, 24*, 890–896.

McGregor, J. C., Kim, P. W., Perencevich, E. N., Bradham, D. D., Furuno, J. P., & Kaye, K. S. (2005). Utility of the chronic disease score and Charlson comorbidity index as comorbidity measures for use in epidemiologic studies of antibiotic-resistant organisms. *American Journal of Epidemiology, 161*(5), 483–493.

Melfi, C., Holleman, E., Arthur, D., & Katz, B. (1995). Selecting a patient characteristics index for the prediction of medical outcomes using administrative claims data. *Journal of Clinical Epidemiology, 48*(7), 917–926.

Monami, M., Lambertucci, L., Lamanna, C., Lotti, E., Marsili, A., & Masotti, G. (2007). Are comorbidity indices useful in predicting all-cause mortality in Type 2 diabetic patients? Comparison between Charlson index and disease count. *Aging Clinical and Experimental Research, 19*(6), 492–496.

Rius, C., Perez, G., Martinez, J. M., Bares, M., Schiaffino, A., & Gispert, R. (2004). An adaptation of Charlson comorbidity index predicted subsequent mortality in a health survey. *Journal of Clinical Epidemiology, 57*, 403–408.

Romano, P., Roos, L., & Jollis, J. (1993a). Adapting a clinical comorbidity index for use with ICD-9-CM administrative data: differing perspectives. *Journal of Clinical Epidemiology, 46*, 1075–1079.

Romano, P., Roos, L., & Jollis, J. (1993b). Further evidence concerning the use of a clinical comorbidity index with ICD-9-CM administrative data. *Journal of Clinical Epidemiology, 46*, 1085–1090.

Schneeweiss, S., & Maclure, M. (2000). Use of comorbidity scores for control of confounding in studies using administrative databases. *International Epidemiological Association, 29*, 891–898.

Senni, M., Santilli, G., Parrella, P., Maria, R. D., Alari, G., & Berzuini, C. (2006). A novel prognostic index to determine the impact of cardiac conditions and co-morbidities on one-year outcome in patients with heart failure. *The American Journal of Cardiology, 98*, 1076–1082.

Sundararajan, V., Henderson, T., Perry, C., Muggivan, A., Quan, H., & Ghali, W. A. (2004). New ICD-10 version of the Charlson comorbidity index predicted in-hospital mortality. *Journal of Clinical Epidemiology, 57*.

Volk, M. L., Hernandez, J. C., Lok, A. S., & Marrero, J. A. (2007). Modified Charlson comorbidity index for predicting survival after liver transplantation. *Liver Transplantation, 13*, 1515–1520.

Zavascki, A. P., & Fuchs, S. C. (2007). The need for reappraisal of AIDS score weight of Charlson comorbidity index. *Journal of Clinical Epidemiology, 60*, 867–868.

Chapter 6
The All Patient Refined Diagnosis Related Group

INTRODUCTION

In this chapter, we will discuss the APRDRG, or all patient refined diagnosis related group. It is another type of coding system that, unlike the Charlson Index, is proprietary and developed by the 3M Healthcare Company in 1990.(Anonymous-3M 2008) The APRDRG severity grouper is currently used by CMS (The Centers for Medicare and Medicaid) for severity adjusting all of Medicare's hospital discharges. The 3M Company is also responsible for maintaining, updating and creating new DRG's for CMS. Therefore, we cannot know what specific diagnosis codes are used to define the APRDRG severity index. In the APRDRG, patients are divided into one of four classes for severity of illness, and again divided into one of four classes for the risk of mortality.

The APRDRG differs from the Charlson Index in that all primary and secondary patient diagnoses are considered, usually within a specific procedure. Although the assignment of severity is proprietary, the resulting patient level APRDRG codes are publicly available in the National Inpatient Sample datasets. We will be using these publicly available results in this chapter. Procedures are also divided into medical versus surgical, and severity assignments are different for the two categories. Physician panels were used to define the categories of patient conditions, and the categories are periodically updated to ensure

DOI: 10.4018/978-1-60566-752-2.ch006

their timeliness. Unlike the Charlson Index, not all patients can be classified using the APRDRG index.

The National Inpatient Sample contains several risk adjustment coding methods, including the APRDRG severity and mortality indices. We will compare these indices to the Charlson Index discussed in Chapter 5. In addition, we will try to determine through data mining whether some codes are included or not included in computing the APRDRG indices. We will show how providers are ranked using the APRDRG index to compute the expected mortality rank.

BACKGROUND

Diagnosis related groups (DRG) are used throughout healthcare. Providers are paid a set fee for a patient treatment. However, they are limited in that they do not distinguish between patient conditions; sicker patients require more resources and health costs, but reimbursements are the same as they are for healthier patients. The DRGs were originally implemented by Medicare for billing purposes. However, relying only on the DRG without any reference to patient condition results in underpayments to those providers who treat patients with the most severe conditions.(Antioch, Ellis et al. 2007) Problems with DRG in relationship to patient condition were identified early on.(McNeil, Kominski et al. 1988) DRGs are not accurate predictors of either costs or outcomes.(Gross, et al. 1988) One of the reasons is that complications resulting from care need to be distinguished from pre-existing conditions, and DRG codes (and ICD9 codes) do a poor job of this.(Young, Macioce et al. 1990; Naessens and Huschka 2004)

One attempt to identify patient risk and identify those who need more resources was the development of the refined DRG codes (RDRG). The RDRG codes subdivide the DRGs into levels of complexity that describe the patient condition. There are four general classes for RDRG refinement: no comorbid conditions, moderate comorbid conditions, major comorbid conditions, and catastrophic comorbid conditions, although only surgical patients qualify for the catastrophic class.(Leary, Leary et al. 1993) Therefore, there are four severity classes for surgical patients, but only three for medical patients. Clearly then, a higher proportion of surgical to medical patients will result in a higher proportion of patients in the highest category. A number of analyses have been performed to validate the RDRG, although problems have occurred with it as well.(Cerrito 2007) Another system developed by Medicare (MS-DRG) uses three tiers of severity to assign payments for specific DRGs.(Maurici and Rosati 2007) There are also a number of attempts to define severity adjustment for specific groups of patients.(Barbash, Safran et al. 1987)

The all patient refined diagnostic related group (APRDRG) is another modification of the DRG with four classes of illness severity and four classes of mortality risk.(Pilotto, Scarcelli et al. 2005) Once the APRDRG is defined, a hospital case mix is defined as the sum of all relative weights divided by the number of Medicare cases where the weight is assigned based upon resource consumption in terms of diagnostics, therapeutics, bed services, and length of stay. The severity and mortality indices are defined as mild, moderate, severe, and extreme.(Lagman, Walsh et al. 2007) Thus, there is the base APRDRG value for the primary reason the patient is in the hospital along with the severity of illness subclass and the risk of mortality subclass. These subclasses are very specific to the value of the base DRG. Thus, patients with different DRG codes cannot be compared directly.

Details about the index are posted on the HCUP website (Healthcare Cost and Utilization Project) at http://www.hcup-us.ahrq.gov/db/nation/nis/APR-DRGsV20MethodologyOverviewandBibliography.pdf. The first step to defining the APRDRG values is to eliminate any and all secondary diagnoses that are already associated with the principal diagnosis. For example, a secondary diagnosis of urinary retention is eliminated from a primary diagnosis of prostate hypertrophy. The next step is to assign each secondary diagnosis to its standard severity of illness level. For example, uncomplicated diabetes is considered minor while diabetes with renal manifestations is considered moderate. Diabetes with ketoacidosis is major and diabetes with a coma is extreme. Next is to modify the severity of illness level based upon the patient's age. It may also be modified based upon the principal or secondary diagnosis. For example, renal failure increases the level of severity for patients with diabetes compared to patients with diabetes but no listed complications. Physician panels were used to decide upon the level of severity for each of the primary and secondary diagnoses.

While the predictive ability is small for patient outcomes and the APRDRG should not be used to compare the quality of providers, the APRDRG can be used to identify providers who routinely treat more severe patients.(Horn, Bulkley et al. 1985; Shen 2003) It can also be used to identify resource utilization by specific groups of patients.(Ciccone, Lorenzoni et al. 1999) Since the APRDRG is very sensitive to the assumption of the uniformity of data entry, it can be easily "gamed" by providers who want to upcode to demonstrate that they have more severe patients. Studies have been conducted to examine the relationship of the APRDRG to patient outcomes.(Shen 2003) It was discovered that the APRDRG is highly sensitive to the quality of the data, and that model results can change considerably with changes in the quality of data collection independent of the quality of patient outcomes.(Ciccone, Bertero et al. 1999) Unfortunately, the relationship is often statistically significant because of the large number of observations, but has very low predictive capabilities.(Rosen, Loveland et al. 2001; Naessens and Huschka 2004)

COMPARISON OF APRDRG INDEX TO PATIENT OUTCOMES

We would expect patients with a higher APRDRG index to have worse outcomes. Therefore, we examine the three basic outcomes of mortality, length of stay, and total charges. For length of stay and charges, we use kernel density estimation. Table 1 gives the relationship of mortality to the APRDRG severity index; Table 2 gives it for the APRDRG mortality index. Figures 1-4 give the relationship of the APRDRG index to the continuous outcomes. Table 3 compares the severity index to the mortality index.

Tables 1 and 2 do show an increase in mortality as the index increases, to a proportion of 32% in mortality level four. The level of mortality for the severity index is lower compared to that of the mortality index. A higher proportion of patients are in levels 3 and 4 for mortality compared to severity. Also, approximately 4000 or 0.05% of the patients cannot be classified into any level of the APRDRG index.

For those patients who can be classified, most of the patients are classified as mild followed by moderate. Only a very small number are classified as extreme. As suggested in Chapter 3, one of these values has to act as a threshold in a logistic regression. Very likely, the threshold that will be used is level 4. However, these indices will predict mortality at a much higher rate compared to actual mortality since the overall mortality is under 4%, but there are 32% of the patients in this category.

A code of zero indicates that the patient cannot be classified. Otherwise, the actual mortality increases as the APRDRG index level increases as well. Therefore, before we examine a logistic regression, we should eliminate all patients with an index level of zero. We filter these patients out of the model. Then we will get an equation such that

Table 1. APRDRG mortality index versus mortality

APRDRG Mortality Risk		DIED		Total
	Frequency Row Pct Col Pct	0	1	
0		3821 95.64 0.05	174 4.36 0.10	3995
1		5205132 99.91 66.52	4836 0.09 2.89	5209968
2		1803412 98.48 23.05	27877 1.52 16.68	1831289
3		650621 92.03 8.31	56328 7.97 33.70	706949
4		161871 67.50 2.07	77935 32.50 46.63	239806
Total		7824857	167150	7992007

Table 2. APRDRG severity versus mortality

APRDRG Mortality Risk		DIED		Total
	Frequency Row Pct Col Pct	0	1	
0		3821 95.64 0.05	174 4.36 0.10	3995
1		3279190 99.84 41.91	5294 0.16 3.17	3284484
2		2941762 99.24 37.60	22520 0.76 13.47	2964282
3		1335490 95.87 17.07	57568 4.13 34.44	1393058
4		264594 76.43 3.38	81594 23.57 48.81	346188
Total		7824857	167150	7992007

Table 3. Odds ratios for logistic regression to predict mortality

Odds Ratio Estimates			
Effect	**Point Estimate**	**95% Wald Confidence Limits**	
AGE	0.988	0.988	0.988
FEMALE 0 vs 1	0.971	0.959	0.984
Income Quartile 1 vs 4	0.914	0.898	0.931
Income Quartile 2 vs 4	0.954	0.937	0.971
Income Quartile 3 vs 4	1.036	1.018	1.055
RACE 1 vs 6	0.999	0.958	1.042
RACE 2 vs 6	1.121	1.072	1.174
RACE 3 vs 6	1.122	1.070	1.175
RACE 4 vs 6	0.951	0.896	1.009
RACE 5 vs 6	0.973	0.870	1.087
APRDRG_Risk_Mortalit 1 vs 4	170.865	163.037	179.068
APRDRG_Risk_Mortalit 2 vs 4	16.977	16.563	17.401
APRDRG_Risk_Mortalit 3 vs 4	3.939	3.869	4.010
APRDRG_Severity 1 vs 4	2.450	2.345	2.560
APRDRG_Severity 2 vs 4	2.333	2.273	2.394
APRDRG_Severity 3 vs 4	1.735	1.704	1.767

Figure 1. ROC curve for logistic regression

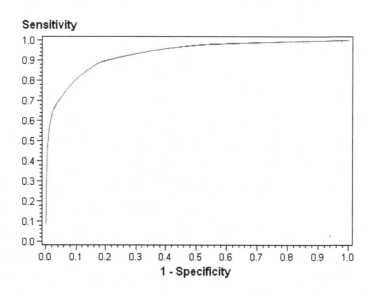

Figure 2. Optimal model to predict mortality using APRDRG indices

```
Fit Statistics
Model selection based on _TMISC_


                                        Test:
           Selected                  Misclassification
           Model      Model Node          Rate


                      AutoNeural14       0.26514
                      DmineReg8          0.14710
                      MBR14              0.34431
                      Neural15           0.24952
                      Reg17              0.24951
              Y       Rule9              0.14454
                      Tree15             0.14454
```

Figure 3. Decision tree for mortality

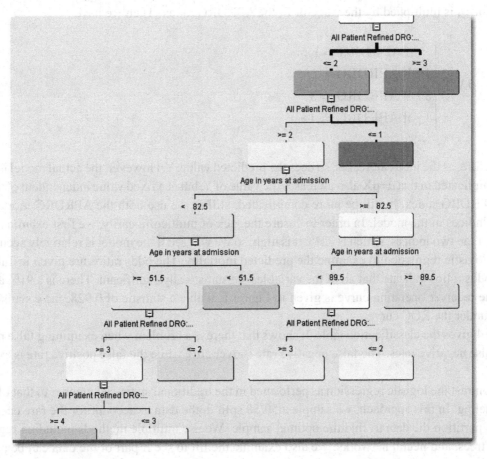

Figure 4. Results of Dmine regression

```
The DMINE Procedure

                    R-Squares for Target Variable: DIED

Effect                                    DF        R-Square

Class: APRDRG_Risk_Mortality              3         0.576932
Group: APRDRG_Risk_Mortality              2         0.566166
Class: APRDRG_Severity                    3         0.449720
AOV16: AGE                               15         0.210796
Var:   AGE                                1         0.195434
Class: RACE                               6         0.008890
Group: RACE                               2         0.008828
Class: FEMALE                             2         0.008028
Class: ZIPInc_Qrtl                        4         0.000374    R2 < MINR2
```

$$Y = \alpha + \beta X + \gamma Z$$

where α is equal to the intercept and β is the coefficient of the patient demographic information. The coefficient, γ, is multiplied by the value of Z, the APRDRG index. Then we have

$$Y = \alpha + \beta X + \begin{cases} \gamma \text{ if APRDRG} = 1 \\ 2\gamma \text{ if APRDRG} = 2 \\ 3\gamma \text{ if APRDRG} = 3 \\ 4\gamma \text{ if APRDRG} = 4 \end{cases}$$

Therefore, as the index increases, so does the predicted value, Y. However, the actual model is slightly more complicated in that α+βX also increases the value of Y, but at a fixed value independent of the value of the APRDRG index. It will be more complicated, still, if we use both the APRDRG mortality and severity indices in the model. In order to ensure the lack of multicollinearity, we first examine the correlation of the two indices, which is 72%. It is high, so we will see if the model is relatively accurate. We first use logistic regression to examine the predicted mortality. The odds ratios are given in Table 3.

The odds ratios indicate that all of the variables are statistically significant. There is a 91% accuracy level. The receiver operating curve is given in Figure 1, with a c statistic of 0.928; the c statistic gives the area under the ROC curve.

Table 4 gives the classification table. It shows that there is a problem when examining false positives versus false negative rates. The false negative rate is over 50% while the false positive rate is extremely small.

We contrast the logistic regression as performed in the traditional statistical manner to that of predictive modeling. In this approach, we sample a 50/50 split in the data to account for the rare occurrence. Then we partition the data to find the optimal sample. We use multiple methods including regression, decision trees, and neural networks. We also examine the lift to see if part of the data can be predicted

Table 4. Classification table for logistic regression

Classification Table										
Prob Level	Correct		Incorrect		Percentages					
	Event	Non-Event	Event	Non-Event	Correct	Sensi-tivity	Speci-ficity	False POS	False NEG	
0.500	556E4	0	124E3	0	97.8	100.0	0.0	2.2	.	
0.520	556E4	1	124E3	0	97.8	100.0	0.0	2.2	0.0	
0.540	556E4	18	124E3	31	97.8	100.0	0.0	2.2	63.3	
0.560	556E4	384	123E3	490	97.8	100.0	0.3	2.2	56.1	
0.580	555E4	2669	121E3	3426	97.8	99.9	2.2	2.1	56.2	
0.600	554E4	9086	115E3	13074	97.8	99.8	7.4	2.0	59.0	
0.620	553E4	18925	105E3	29564	97.6	99.5	15.3	1.9	61.0	
0.640	551E4	28151	95451	47410	97.5	99.1	22.8	1.7	62.7	
0.660	55E5	34456	89146	60902	97.4	98.9	27.9	1.6	63.9	
0.680	549E4	39410	84192	70966	97.3	98.7	31.9	1.5	64.3	
0.700	548E4	43484	80118	79038	97.2	98.6	35.2	1.4	64.5	
0.720	547E4	47262	76340	87519	97.1	98.4	38.2	1.4	64.9	
0.740	546E4	50537	73065	96728	97.0	98.3	40.9	1.3	65.7	
0.760	545E4	52947	70655	105E3	96.9	98.1	42.8	1.3	66.5	
0.780	545E4	54430	69172	11E4	96.8	98.0	44.0	1.3	66.9	
0.800	544E4	55584	68018	113E3	96.8	98.0	45.0	1.2	67.0	
0.820	544E4	56788	66814	115E3	96.8	97.9	45.9	1.2	67.0	
0.840	544E4	57433	66169	117E3	96.8	97.9	46.5	1.2	67.1	
0.860	543E4	59906	63696	128E3	96.6	97.7	48.5	1.2	68.2	
0.880	541E4	63404	60198	15E4	96.3	97.3	51.3	1.1	70.3	
0.900	538E4	67450	56152	18E4	95.9	96.8	54.6	1.0	72.7	
0.920	522E4	83230	40372	335E3	93.4	94.0	67.3	0.8	80.1	
0.940	504E4	95693	27909	516E3	90.4	90.7	77.4	0.6	84.4	
0.960	497E4	99497	24105	583E3	89.3	89.5	80.5	0.5	85.4	
0.980	481E4	105E3	18986	749E3	86.5	86.5	84.6	0.4	87.7	
1.000	0	124E3	0	556E4	2.2	0.0	100.0	.	97.8	

more accurately. Figure 2 indicates that the optimal model is a rule induction, but also that the decision tree and the Dmine regression are nearly identical.

We next look at the decision tree (Figure 3). It shows that the APRDRG is of first importance when predicting mortality. The patient's age is important as well.

Because the Dmine regression had a similar outcome, we look at its results as shown in Figure 4. This result shows that the APRDRG mortality index is of first importance followed by the severity index. Patient demographics, including age, race, and sex, follow. The patient's income quartile is below the threshold and is not included in the model. Note that the mortality index has an r^2 value of 58%. The ROC curve is given in Figure 5, showing that the fit is reasonable for the training, validation, and testing

Figure 5. ROC curves for prediction of mortality

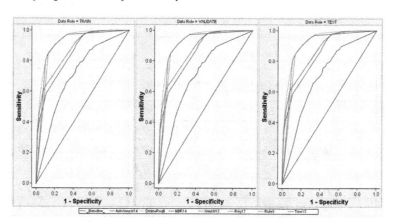

sets, with rule induction, decision tree, and dmine regression models showing very similar ROC curves. The ROC curves show that the model predicts better than random chance.

The lift curves show that the prediction is accurate to the sixth decile (Figure 6). The model does show different rates of false positive to false negative values (Figure 7. It shows that the chosen models have a much higer false negative rate compared to the models not chosen, which have a higher false positive rate. This difference can be troubling since the false negative is the more critical statistic.

For this reason, we also provide a decision weight to make the false negative more costly compared to the false positive rate (Figure 8).

The results suggest that the decision tree is the best model (Figure 9), with the tree given in Figure 10. Note that this tree is different compared to the one in Figure 2.

We next want to investigate length of stay and total charges in relationship to the APRDRG index. We use kernel density estimation. The code to find these graphs is equal to

Figure 6. Lift function for prediction of mortality

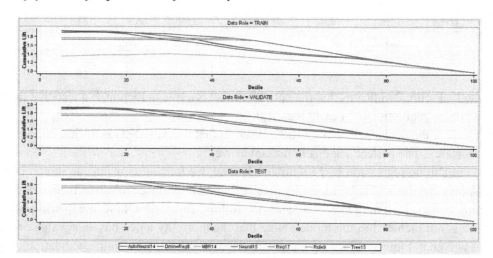

Figure 7. Classification table for mortality prediction

```
Event Classification Table
Model selection based on _TMISC_

                  Data                    False       True       False       True
MODEL             Role        Target    Negative    Negative    Positive    Positive

Reg17             TRAIN       DIED         7386       41032       25758       59403
Reg17             VALIDATE    DIED         5499       30829       19263       44594
Rule9             TRAIN       DIED        10243       58097        8693       56546
Rule9             VALIDATE    DIED         7552       43681        6411       42541
Neural15          TRAIN       DIED         6657       40297       26493       60132
Neural15          VALIDATE    DIED         4931       30282       19810       45162
Tree15            TRAIN       DIED        10234       58093        8697       56555
Tree15            VALIDATE    DIED         7547       43677        6415       42546
DmineReg8         TRAIN       DIED        11935       59265        7525       54854
DmineReg8         VALIDATE    DIED         8799       44544        5548       41294
MBR14             TRAIN       DIED        25806       46923       19867       40983
MBR14             VALIDATE    DIED        19322       35138       14954       30771
AutoNeural14      TRAIN       DIED         7349       39013       27777       59440
AutoNeural14      VALIDATE    DIED         5435       29373       20719       44658
```

Figure 8. Decision weights

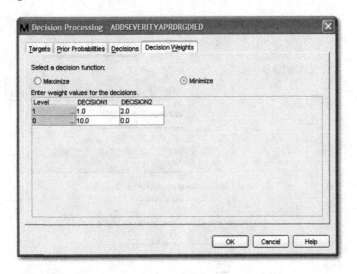

```
proc sort data=nis.sample_addseverity;
by aprdrg_severity;
proc kde data=nis.sample_addseverity;
univar los/gridl=0 gridu=10 out=nis.kdeaprseveritylos1 method=os bwm=1.5;
univar totchg/gridl=0 gridu=30000 out=nis.kdeaprseveritychg1 method=os bwm=1.5;
by aprdrg_severity;
where aprdrg_severity>0 and aprdrg_severity<4;
proc kde data=nis.sample_addseverity;
univar los/gridl=0 gridu=10 out=nis.kdeaprseveritylos2 method=os bwm=.2;
univar totchg/gridl=0 gridu=30000 out=nis.kdeaprseveritychg2 method=os bwm=.2;
by aprdrg_severity;
```

Figure 9. Optimal results with profit/loss

```
Fit Statistics
Model selection based on _TALOSS_

                                Test:       Train:
                                Average     Average
            Selected            Loss for    Squared
            Model   Model Node  DIED        Error

                    AutoNeural14  0.99668    0.16124
                    DmineReg8     4.26132    0.10483
                    MBR14         .          0.16651
                    Neural15      0.89886    0.14321
                    Reg17         0.90256    0.14347
                    Rule9         4.31263    .
            Y       Tree15        0.86770    0.12375
```

Figure 10. Decision tree model using average profit/loss as "best"

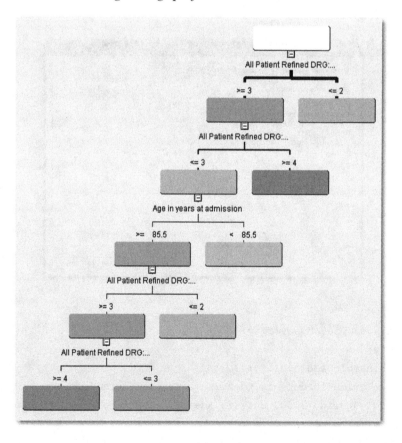

```
where aprdrg_severity=0 or aprdrg_severity=4;
proc sort data=nis.sample_addseverity;
by aprdrg_risk_mortality;
```

```
proc kde data=nis.sample_addseverity;
univar los/gridl=0 gridu=10 out=nis.kdeaprmortalitylos1 method=os bwm=1.5;
univar totchg/gridl=0 gridu=30000 out=nis.kdeaprmortalitychg1 method=os bwm=1.5;
by aprdrg_risk_mortality;
where aprdrg_risk_mortality>0 and aprdrg_risk_mortality<4;
proc kde data=nis.sample_addseverity;
univar los/gridl=0 gridu=10 out=nis.kdeaprmortalitylos2 method=os bwm=.2;
univar totchg/gridl=0 gridu=30000 out=nis.kdeaprmortalitychg2 method=os bwm=.2;
by aprdrg_risk_mortality;
where aprdrg_risk_mortality=0 or aprdrg_risk_mortality=4;
run;
```

Figure 11 gives the length of stay by the APRDRG severity index. It shows that there are differences in length of stay by index level. Figure 12 gives a similar graph for total charges.

As the severity index increases, the likelihood of a longer length of stay increases, with a crossover point at 5 days. Patients in class 4 have considerable variability, so that there is no discernable pattern in the outcomes. That occurs because there are so few patients in that class. Similarly, class 0 is highly variable, which is reasonable since the patients in the category cannot be classified into a severity level.

The graphs in Figure 12 represent a similar result with the higher class having a higher probability of higher total charges. Again, class 4 has considerable variability in its distribution as does class 0. Figures 13 and 14 examine the Mortality Index. The distributions are relatively similar compared to those for total charges.

Figure 11. APRDRG severity index and length of stay

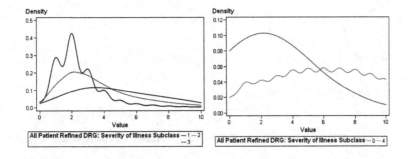

Figure 12. Severity index and total charges

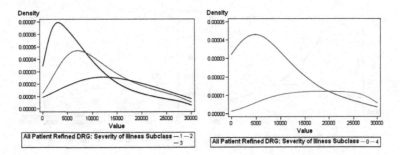

While the distributions are similar compared to Figure 11, it is not until almost day 6 before class 3 has a higher probability compared to class 2. Therefore, for most of the patients, class 2 actually has the higher probability of higher cost compared to class 3. It suggests that providers are successfully shifting patients from class 2 into class 3.

The shifting of patients from class 2 to class 3 is even more pronounced in the mortality index, with class 2 having higher total charges until the $30,000 mark is reached.

COMPARISON TO THE CHARLSON INDEX

We first want to make a comparison between the Charlson Index of the previous chapter and the APRDRG index. There are two indices to consider; one for mortality and the other for patient severity. Table 5 compares the Charlson Index to the APRDRG mortality index.

The value of 0 for APRDRG indicates that an index value cannot be defined given the data, either because the data are missing or because the values given are incorrect. Notice that for none of the Charlson levels does the majority of observations go into the most severe of the APRDRG levels. Charlson levels of 0 and 1 correspond roughly to APRDRG level 1. Charlson levels of 2-5 mostly correspond to APRDRG level 2 with the remaining Charlson levels corresponding largely to APRDRG level 3. However, if we try to predict one index from the other in a linear regression, the r^2 value is only 27%. We also compare the Charlson Index to the APRDRG patient severity index (Table 6).

In Table 6, only the Charlson Index value 1 corresponds to the APRDRG index of 1. Charlson values 1-3 correspond to APRDRG index 2; APRDRG index 3 corresponds to Charlson values 4-12. Only the

Figure 13. Mortality index and length of stay

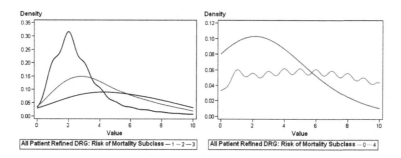

Figure 14. Mortality index and total charges

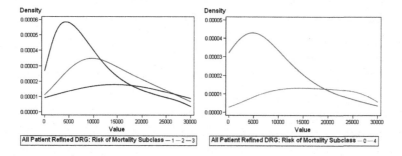

Table 5. Charlson index versus APRDRG mortality index

Table of charlson by APRDRG_Risk_Mortality

charlson Frequency Row Pct Col Pct	\multicolumn{5}{c}{APRDRG_Risk_Mortality(All Patient Refined DRG: Risk of Mortality Subclass)}					Total
	0	**1**	**2**	**3**	**4**	
0	3642 0.08 88.51	3947541 86.96 75.75	414664 9.13 22.63	121476 2.68 17.17	52039 1.15 21.68	4539362
1	286 0.02 6.95	920563 53.86 17.67	549443 32.15 29.99	174866 10.23 24.71	64030 3.75 26.67	1709188
2	115 0.01 2.79	257517 27.77 4.94	453625 48.93 24.76	161738 17.44 22.86	54179 5.84 22.57	927174
3	32 0.01 0.78	57228 12.06 1.10	260272 54.83 14.20	121867 25.67 17.22	35296 7.44 14.70	474695
4	24 0.01 0.58	12248 6.23 0.24	93819 47.72 5.12	70857 36.04 10.01	19635 9.99 8.18	196583
5	11 0.01 0.27	4570 5.45 0.09	37739 45.03 2.06	33454 39.92 4.73	8035 9.59 3.35	83809
6	3 0.01 0.07	8270 19.40 0.16	14923 35.01 0.81	15193 35.64 2.15	4235 9.94 1.76	42624
7	1 0.01 0.02	2520 19.10 0.05	4457 33.78 0.24	4692 35.56 0.66	1526 11.56 0.64	13196
8	1 0.02 0.02	541 9.51 0.01	2399 42.19 0.13	2101 36.95 0.30	644 11.33 0.27	5686
9	0 0.00 0.00	58 3.27 0.00	689 38.80 0.04	776 43.69 0.11	253 14.25 0.11	1776
10	0 0.00 0.00	7 1.07 0.00	187 28.55 0.01	336 51.30 0.05	125 19.08 0.05	655
11	0 0.00 0.00	1 0.46 0.00	63 29.03 0.00	124 57.14 0.02	29 13.36 0.01	217
12	0 0.00 0.00	0 0.00 0.00	9 12.68 0.00	44 61.97 0.01	18 25.35 0.01	71
13	0 0.00 0.00	0 0.00 0.00	2 16.67 0.00	7 58.33 0.00	3 25.00 0.00	12
Total	4115	5211064	1832291	707531	240047	7995048

Table 6. Charlson index versus APRDRG severity index

Table of charlson by APRDRG_Severity						
charlson	APRDRG_Severity(All Patient Refined DRG: Severity of Illness Subclass)					Total
Frequency R o w P c t Col Pct	0	1	2	3	4	
0	3642 0.08 88.51	2667366 58.76 81.20	1414903 31.17 47.71	370066 8.15 26.55	83385 1.84 24.06	4539362
1	286 0.02 6.95	454429 26.59 13.83	816146 47.75 27.52	349367 20.44 25.06	88960 5.20 25.67	1709188
2	115 0.01 2.79	117334 12.66 3.57	426395 45.99 14.38	305035 32.90 21.88	78295 8.44 22.59	927174
3	32 0.01 0.78	30779 6.48 0.94	195968 41.28 6.61	198865 41.89 14.27	49051 10.33 14.15	474695
4	24 0.01 0.58	6000 3.05 0.18	66520 33.84 2.24	98051 49.88 7.03	25988 13.22 7.50	196583
5	11 0.01 0.27	6508 7.77 0.20	25382 30.29 0.86	41284 49.26 2.96	10624 12.68 3.07	83809
6	3 0.01 0.07	2098 4.92 0.06	14302 33.55 0.48	20068 47.08 1.44	6153 14.44 1.78	42624
7	1 0.01 0.02	328 2.49 0.01	3995 30.27 0.13	6715 50.89 0.48	2157 16.35 0.62	13196
8	1 0.02 0.02	142 2.50 0.00	1450 25.50 0.05	2972 52.27 0.21	1121 19.72 0.32	5686
9	0 0.00 0.00	10 0.56 0.00	283 15.93 0.01	1030 58.00 0.07	453 25.51 0.13	1776
10	0 0.00 0.00	1 0.15 0.00	50 7.63 0.00	361 55.11 0.03	243 37.10 0.07	655
11	0 0.00 0.00	1 0.46 0.00	18 8.29 0.00	134 61.75 0.01	64 29.49 0.02	217
12	0 0.00 0.00	0 0.00 0.00	3 4.23 0.00	38 53.52 0.00	30 42.25 0.01	71
13	0 0.00 0.00	0 0.00 0.00	2 16.67 0.00	3 25.00 0.00	7 58.33 0.00	12

Charlson value of 13 corresponds to the APRDRG value of 4. However, there is a small percentage of Charlson value zero patients that have an APRDRG index value of 4; this shows that there can be considerable disagreement in defining the most severe patients.

We next look at the patient diagnoses that are used to define the Charlson Index (Figures 15, 16, and 17). For acute myocardial infarction (AMI) and congestive heart failure (CHF), there is a considerable percentage of patients in the most severe category. Almost half of the CHF cases are in severity class 4. No CHF patients are in class 1. Given the APRDRG distribution for CHF, it is very similar to that for severe liver disease. It should probably have a higher weight in the Charlson Index.

Peripheral vascular disease (PVD) has a much lower proportion contained within APRDRG class #4, as does a cerebral vascular accident (CVA) in spite of the fact that they have identical weights in the Charlson Index, indicating a similar impact on patient outcomes. Almost half are in class 2 with a small proportion in Class 1. The next two diagnoses of connective tissue disorder and peptic ulcer look very similar. It indicates that these four probably should have similar weights in the Charlson Index or that the Charlson Index should be re-evaluated. While diabetes also looks similar, liver disease has a much higher proportion of patients in APRDRG index 4 with half of the patients in APRDRG index 3, and no patients in index 1.

In fact, liver disease results look very similar to those in the pie charts for diabetic complications and paraplegia. It should probably be given the same weight of 2 in the Charlson Index instead of the current weight of 1. At the same time, there is little difference in the APRDRG index for liver disease and severe liver disease. Perhaps they should be combined and receive a Charlson Index weight of 3 rather than 2. Metastatic cancer and HIV have similar distributions of the APRDRG index. However, both appear to be less severe than liver disease. The surprise is that in the distribution for cancer, the risk appears similar to that of AMI (acute myocardial infarction) and diabetes.

We next want to see if the APRDRG index, either alone or in combination with the Charlson Index, can better predict patient outcomes compared to just the Charlson Index. We also want to see if the Charlson Index can predict the APRDRG levels for this specific condition. In addition to the Charlson index, we use patient demographic information to determine whether we can predict the APRDRG mortality index. We use a predictive model on a 10% sample of the NIS dataset.

Figure 18 shows the variable roles for the predictive model. Since the outcome variable is ordinal rather than binary, not all of the predictive models are compatible. Figure 19 shows the predictive model used. Figure 20 gives the misclassification rate, indicating that regression is the optimal model choice. Figure 21 gives the lift function.

In this model, we use age, race, and gender as well as income quartile. We also include length of stay and total charges. ASOURCE, ATYPE, and AWEEKEND indicate the type of hospital admission. We also use the Charlson Index to predict the APRDRG mortality index. ASOURCE indicates whether the patient was admitted from the emergency department. ATYPE indicates whether the admission was elective or not. AWEEKEND indicates whether the admission occurred on the weekend. Generally, elective admissions do not occur on the weekend.

Note that there is little difference in the misclassification rates for 4 of the 5 models used. It indicates that the model is approximately 70% accurate when classifying patients into the APRDRG mortality index. However, the lift function indicates that it is primarily the top decile that can be predicted accurately; starting in the second decile, the lift function is equal to one, indicating that the model does no better than random chance. We also want to know the direction of the misclassification. Therefore, except for these first two deciles, there is no real relationship in the assignment of severity between the

Figure 15. Pie chart of patient diagnoses and APRDRG severity index

Acute Myocardial Infarction

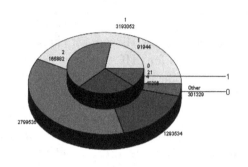

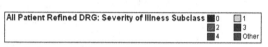

Congestive Heart Failure

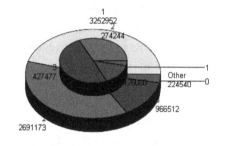

Peripheral Vascular Disease

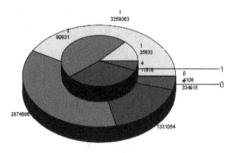

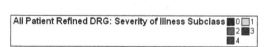

Cerebral Vascular Accident

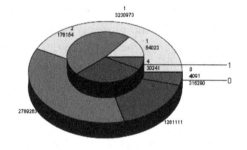

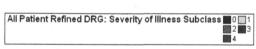

Dementia

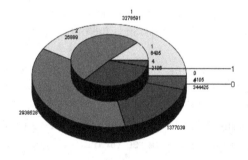

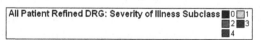

Pulmonary Disease

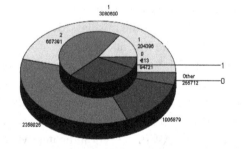

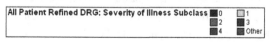

Figure 16. Pie chart of patient diagnoses and APRDRG severity index (continued)

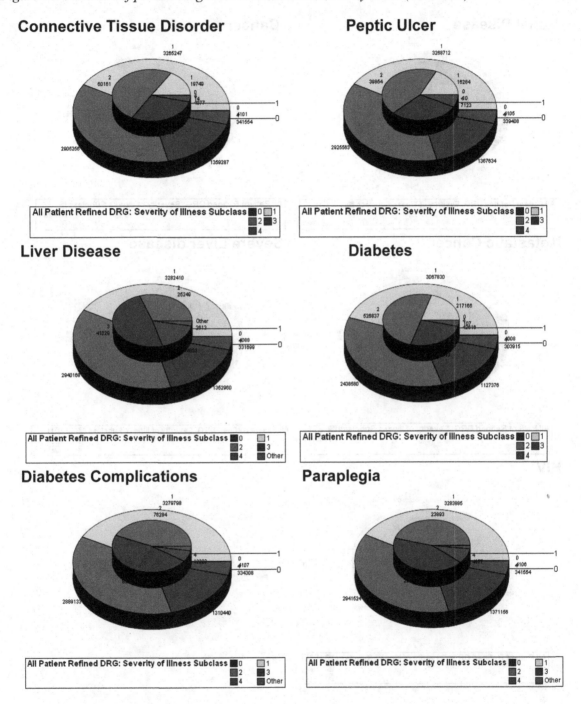

Figure 17. Pie chart of patient diagnoses and APRDRG severity index (continued)

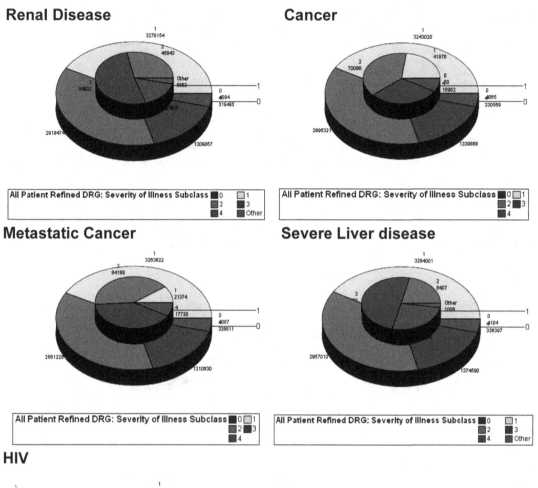

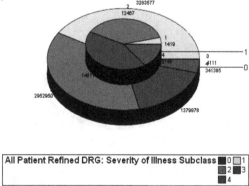

Figure 18. Variable definitions

Name	Role	Level
AGE	Input	Interval
APRDRG_Risk_Mortality	Target	Ordinal
APRDRG_Severity	Rejected	Ordinal
ASOURCE	Input	Nominal
ATYPE	Input	Nominal
AWEEKEND	Input	Nominal
DIED	Input	Binary
DS_LOS_Level	Rejected	Interval
DS_Mrt_Level	Rejected	Interval
DS_RD_Level	Rejected	Interval
FEMALE	Input	Nominal
KEY	ID	Nominal
LOS	Input	Interval
RACE	Input	Nominal
TOTCHG	Input	Interval
ZIPInc_Qrtl	Input	Ordinal
charlson	Input	Nominal

Figure 19. Predictive model to predict the APRDRG

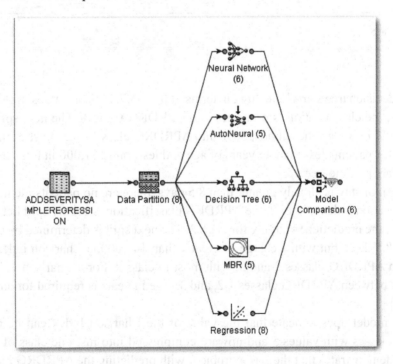

APRDRG severity index and the Charlson Index. This analysis shows that there is a lack of consistency in assigning levels of severity.

Figure 22 gives one branch of the corresponding decision tree. Age, charges, and length of stay are used as classifiers before the introduction of the Charlson Index in branch 3.

Figure 20. Misclassification results

```
Fit Statistics
Model selection based on _TMISC_


                                  Test:
Selected                    Misclassification
  Model        MODEL               Rate

             AutoNeural5          0.43759
             MBR5                 0.29184
             Neural6              0.28494
    Y        Reg8                 0.28229
             Tree6                0.29138
```

Figure 21. Lift function

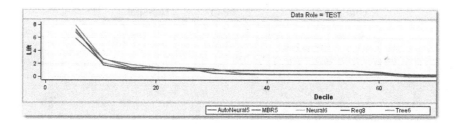

Note that the decision tree starts branching in terms of pairs of Charlson values. If the Charlson Index is equal to 0 or 1, the classification is primarily into APRDRG value 1. The next split shows that the Charlson Index of 2 or 3 classifies almost 50% into APRDRG class 1 with most of the rest in class 2. This branch was for patients less than 45 years of age and less than $51,000 in total charges. Figure 23 shows another branch of the tree.

Since the length of stay is already greater than 8.5 days, there are no patients identified as Charlson Index 0. For a Charlson Index of 1 or 2, the APRDRG classification is evenly split between class 1 and class 2; otherwise, the prediction is largely for class 2. The next split is determined by cost. For a length of stay less than 8.5 days, but with a charge of greater than $45,000, a Charlson index of greater than 1 is split between APRDRG classes 2 and 3, with most in class 2. For a Charlson value of 0 or 1, the prediction is split between APRDRG classes 1,2, and 3. Age in years is required for another split in the prediction.

This decision model does indicate that the value of the Charlson Index can be compressed into approximately 5 classes with values 5 and upward compressed into just one class of patient severity. However, it also demonstrates that there is a problem with predicting the APRDRG index.

Figure 22. Partial diagram starting at branch 3

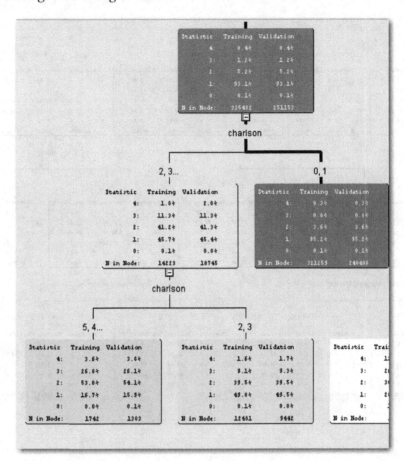

PREDICTION OF APRDRG USING PATIENT DIAGNOSES

We want to consider the relationship between primary and secondary diagnoses, and levels of severity. We consider the condition with the primary diagnosis of congestive heart failure. We next consider the co-morbidities that patients with the disease will also have. Then we take the most frequent co-morbidities to see if the severity and mortality levels can be predicted based upon these co-morbidities. In order to do this, we also look to the primary procedure to divide it into medical and surgical categories.

To investigate this issue, we filter down to all patients with a primary diagnosis of congestive heart failure, code 428. Then we find the most frequently occurring secondary codes using the following SAS code:

```
data nis.chf;
set nis.addseverity;
where rxmatch('428',dx1)>0;
run;
data nis.dx2;
set nis.chf;
```

Figure 23. Tree branch for patients for more than 8.5 days stay

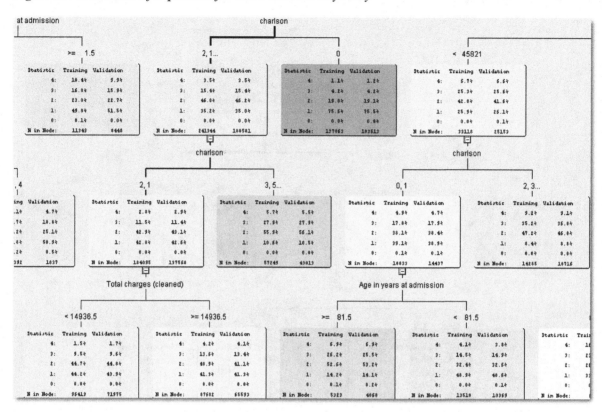

```
dx=dx2;
run;
data nis.dx3;
set nis.chf;
dx=dx3;
run;
data nis.dx4;
set nis.chf;
dx=dx4;
run;
data nis.dx5;
set nis.chf;
dx=dx5;
run;
data nis.dx6;
set nis.chf;
dx=dx6;
run;
data nis.dx7;
set nis.chf;
```

```
dx=dx7;
run;
data nis.dx8;
set nis.chf;
dx=dx8;
run;
data nis.dx9;
set nis.chf;
dx=dx9;
run;
data nis.dx10;
set nis.chf;
dx=dx10;
run;
data nis.dx11;
set nis.chf;
dx=dx11;
run;
data nis.dx12;
set nis.chf;
dx=dx12;
run;
data nis.dx13;
set nis.chf;
dx=dx13;
run;
data nis.dx14;
set nis.chf;
dx=dx14;
run;
data nis.dx15;
set nis.chf;
dx=dx15;
run;
data nis.dxforchf;
set nis.dx2 nis.dx3 nis.dx4 nis.dx5 nis.dx6 nis.dx7 nis.dx8 nis.dx9
nis.dx10 nis.dx11 nis.dx12 nis.dx13 nis.dx14 nis.dx15;
run;
```

The most frequent secondary diagnoses include 428 (congestive heart failure), 401.9 (essential hypertension), 427 (Cardiac dysrhythmias), 496 (Chronic airway obstruction, not elsewhere classified), and 427.31 (Atrial fibrillation). All but the code 496 are directly related to the primary diagnosis of congestive heart failure. According to the documentation, these codes are discarded and not considered in the assignment of severity. Table 7 gives the listed codes that we will use when attempting to predict the APRDRG index value.

We will combine codes 1 and 2 from Table 7. Because the diagnosis code is nominal, '250.00' and '250' are identified as different values. Similarly, we combine 272.4, 272, and 272.0 because of similarity. We will use the diagnoses in Table 7 to see if there is a relationship between the patient diagnoses and the APRDRG index value. We first use a table analysis to compare the APRDRG index to the diagnosis codes (Table 8). The SAS code to define these values is below:

```
Data work.aprdrgcodes;
Set nis.Charlson;
Code=0; code250=0; code272=0; code276=0; code585=0; code491=0 ; code486=0 ;
Code584=0 ; code599=0 ; code5308=0 ; code5939=0 ; code2859=0 ;
Code2449=0 ; code3051=0 ;
If ((rxmatch('250',diagnoses3digits)>0) then code250=1 ;
If ((rxmatch('272',diagnoses3digits)>0) then code272=1 ;
If ((rxmatch('276',diagnoses3digits)>0) then code276=1 ;
If ((rxmatch('585',diagnoses3digits)>0) then code585=1 ;
If ((rxmatch('491',diagnoses3digits)>0) then code491=1 ;
If ((rxmatch('486',diagnoses3digits)>0) then code486=1 ;
If ((rxmatch('584',diagnoses3digits)>0) then code584=1 ;
If ((rxmatch('599',diagnoses3digits)>0) then code599=1 ;
If ((rxmatch('5308',diagnoses4digits)>0) then code5308=1 ;
If ((rxmatch('5939',diagnoses4digits)>0) then code5939=1 ;
```

Table 7. Diagnosis codes used to predict the APRDRG level

Code Number	Code	Frequency	Code Number	Code	Frequency
1	250.00 (Diabetes mellitus without mention of complication of unspecified type)	59,354	11	585 (Chronic kidney disease)	17,197
2	250 (Diabetes mellitus)	46,498	12	491 (Chronic bronchitis)	17,122
3	272.4 (Other and unspecified hyperlipidemia)	35,068	13	584.9 (Acute renal failure, unspecified)	15,977
4	276 (Disorders of fluid, electrolyte, and acid-base balance)	32,577	14	530.81 (Esophageal reflux)	15,617
5	486 (Pneumonia, organism unspecified)	31,253	15	272 (Hyperlipidemia)	14,674
6	593.9 (Unspecified disorder of kidney and ureter)	23,561	16	491.21 (Acute exacerbation of chronic obstructive pulmonary disease)	14,377
7	285.9 (Anemia, unspecified)	22,485	17	276.8 (Hypopotassemia)	13,866
8	244.9 (Unspecified hypothyroidism)	22,402	18	584 (Acute renal failure)	13,346
9	599.0 (Urinary tract infection, site not specified)	18,896	19	305.1 (Tobacco use disorder)	13,043
10	599 (Urinary tract infection)	17,505	20	272.0 (Pure hypercholesterolemia)	12,683

Table 8. APRDRG mortality index compared to patient diagnoses

ICD9 Code	APRDRG 0	APRDRG 1	APRDRG 2	APRDRG 3	APRDRG 4
250	11.34	24.62	37.67	30.96	19.16
272	7.62	29.53	25.90	14.85	6.64
276	45.65	17.94	31.44	46.04	56.21
585	1.76	0.43	3.96	9.22	9.67
491	1.17	4.35	7.19	9.05	8.03
486	4.99	5.45	9.64	21.06	22.95
599	8.02	7.19	16.42	21.39	23.09
584	3.62	0.05	4.03	16.60	48.62
5308	13.29	18.27	12.93	7.68	3.20
5939	1.66	2.65	7.08	5.83	2.80
2859	6.26	8.48	13.88	12.99	6.95
2449	6.16	11.01	12.44	8.53	4.13
3051	29.72	23.54	8.85	5.50	3.03

```
If ((rxmatch('2859',diagnoses4digits)>0) then code2859=1 ;
If ((rxmatch('2449',diagnoses4digits)>0) then code2449=1 ;
If ((rxmatch('3051',diagnoses4digits)>0) then code3051=1 ;
If (code250=1 or code272=1 or code276=1 or code585=1
Or code491=1 or code486=1 or code584=1 or code599=1 or code5939=1
Or code2859 or code2449=1 or code3051=1) then code=1;
Data nis.aprdrgbycodes;
Set work.aprdrgcodes;
Where code=1;
Run;
```

It is clear from Table 8 that some of the codes are used to discriminate in APRDRG indices while others are not. Since 46% of patients with APRDRG code 0 have condition 272, it is not a good classifier; in contrast, code 3051 has decreasing probability of appearing as the class level increases; it is a much better classifier and is likely used to define APRDRG levels. If we substitute the severity index in the place of the mortality index, the proportions of patients with the diagnosis codes is the exact same as those for the mortality index.

PREDICTIVE MODELING OF PROVIDER QUALITY

We again consider the relationship of predicted and actual mortality, with the predicted mortality defined by the APRDRG mortality index. We first look at the example of COPD patients discussed previously in Chapters 3 and 5. Table 8 gives the relationship of APRDRG mortality index by hospital; Table 9 gives the relationship of the APRDRG severity index. Recall that hospital #8 has no patients diagnosed with COPD.

Table 9. APRDRG mortality index and hospital for patients with COPD

Table of DSHOSPID by APRDRG_Risk_Mortality					
Hospital	**APRDRG_Risk_Mortality(All Patient Refined DRG: Risk of Mortality Subclass)**				**Total**
Frequency Row Pct Col Pct	**1**	**2**	**3**	**4**	
1	39 30.71 8.57	63 49.61 12.43	21 16.54 12.50	4 3.15 13.33	127
2	14 22.22 3.08	34 53.97 6.71	12 19.05 7.14	3 4.76 10.00	63
3	13 27.66 2.86	25 53.19 4.93	9 19.15 5.36	0 0.00 0.00	47
4	104 45.22 22.86	94 40.87 18.54	28 12.17 16.67	4 1.74 13.33	230
5	35 40.70 7.69	36 41.86 7.10	14 16.28 8.33	1 1.16 3.33	86
6	60 27.52 13.19	89 40.83 17.55	57 26.15 33.93	12 5.50 40.00	218
7	13 25.00 2.86	36 69.23 7.10	2 3.85 1.19	1 1.92 3.33	52
9	63 28.77 13.85	126 57.53 24.85	25 11.42 14.88	5 2.28 16.67	219
10	114 96.61 25.05	4 3.39 0.79	0 0.00 0.00	0 0.00 0.00	118
Total	455	507	168	30	1160

Very few of the hospitals have patients in APRDRG category 4. Hospital #6 has the highest percentage of patients in category 3; hospital #7 has the lowest, and the differential between the two hospitals is considerable. Note that hospital #10 has no patients in category 3 at all, and almost 97% of its patients are in category 1. We have filtered out all of the APRDRG code values of 0 (Table 10).

The probability of class 4 in the severity index is higher than in the mortality index. However, it is still hospital #6 that has a higher proportion in the higher classes compared to the other hospitals, and hospital #10 has the lowest. It suggests that hospital #6 is very good at shifting its patients into a higher severity level OR it tends to treat sicker patients.

We next look at the APRDRG index restricted to the one procedure, 36.1. Table 6 shows the relationship between the APRDRG mortality index and procedure; Table 7 shows the relationship with the APRDRG severity index. Using both APRDRG indices, the optimal model is the rule induction with 28% misclassification (Figure 24).

The decision tree (Figure 25) has but one branch based upon the mortality index, with a dividing

Table 10. APRDRG severity index and hospital for patients with COPD

Table of DSHOSPID by APRDRG_Severity					
Hospital	**APRDRG_Severity(All Patient Refined DRG: Severity of Illness Subclass)**				**Total**
Frequency Row Pct Col Pct	**1**	**2**	**3**	**4**	
1	9 7.09 4.64	69 54.33 12.13	45 35.43 12.75	4 3.15 9.09	127
2	6 9.52 3.09	30 47.62 5.27	24 38.10 6.80	3 4.76 6.82	63
3	7 14.89 3.61	21 44.68 3.69	16 34.04 4.53	3 6.38 6.82	47
4	32 13.91 16.49	117 50.87 20.56	74 32.17 20.96	7 3.04 15.91	230
5	25 29.07 12.89	40 46.51 7.03	19 22.09 5.38	2 2.33 4.55	86
6	12 5.50 6.19	89 40.83 15.64	97 44.50 27.48	20 9.17 45.45	218
7	7 13.46 3.61	34 65.38 5.98	11 21.15 3.12	0 0.00 0.00	52
9	32 14.61 16.49	120 54.79 21.09	63 28.77 17.85	4 1.83 9.09	219
10	64 54.24 32.99	49 41.53 8.61	4 3.39 1.13	1 0.85 2.27	118
Total	194	569	353	44	1160

level of 3. Greater than a level of three indicates a prediction of mortality. It indicates that 3 is used as the threshold value, and the predicted mortality will be quite high.

By scoring the data, we can define the difference between the actual and predicted value (Table 11). Note that with a threshold value of 3 rather than 4, the predicted values shown in Table 8 are quite high. The trend continues here; a hospital with mortality zero has the lowest ranking and the hospital with the highest mortality level of 4.78 ranks seventh. Table 12 examines the mortality index in relationship to the procedures 36.1x.

Table 12 shows that approximately one third of the patients are in APRDRG category 1 and another third are in category 2 with the remaining split between categories 2 and 3. It does appear that 3616 is somewhat less severe compared to some of the other procedures, having the highest proportion in category 1. Procedures 3613 and 3614 have the highest proportion in category 4. Procedure 3612 is next with almost 8% in category 4. In contrast, almost half (occasionally more) of the patients are in severity category 2 as shown in Table 13, with almost another third in category 3. Procedures 3612, 3613, and

Figure 24. Results of predictive model for mortality

```
Fit Statistics
Model selection based on _TMISC_


                                   Test:
        Selected              Misclassification
        Model      Model Node       Rate

                   AutoNeural    0.39286
                   DMNeural      0.35714
                   DmineReg      0.32143
                   MBR           0.28571
                   Neural        0.35714
                   Reg           0.42857
           Y       Rule          0.28571
                   Tree          0.28571
```

Figure 25. Decision tree for mortality prediction for patients with COPD

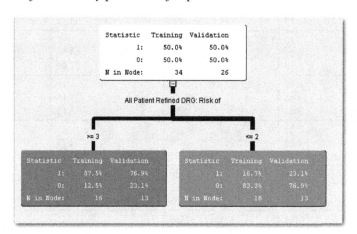

Table 11. Predicted versus actual mortality for COPD patients

Hospital	Actual	Predicted	Difference	Rank
1	3.94	19.69	15.75	4
2	7.94	23.81	15.87	3
3	2.13	19.15	17.02	2
4	4.78	13.91	9.13	7
5	4.65	17.44	12.79	5
6	3.21	31.65	28.44	1
7	3.85	5.77	1.92	8
9	4.11	13.70	9.59	6
10	0	0	0	9

Table 12. APRDRG mortality index and procedure

Table of APRDRG_Risk_Mortality by PR1										
APRDRG_Risk_Mortality	PR1(Principal procedure)									Total
Frequency Row Pct Col Pct	3610	3611	3612	3613	3614	3615	3616	3617	3619	
1	3	1935	4334	3965	2141	2316	213	0	11	14918
	0.02	12.97	29.05	26.58	14.35	15.52	1.43	0.00	0.07	
	37.50	37.85	32.23	30.09	29.70	36.08	41.93	0.00	45.83	
2	5	1921	5285	5207	2917	2561	194	3	9	18102
	0.03	10.61	29.20	28.76	16.11	14.15	1.07	0.02	0.05	
	62.50	37.58	39.30	39.52	40.47	39.90	38.19	100.00	37.50	
3	0	904	2767	2865	1557	1169	80	0	2	9344
	0.00	9.67	29.61	30.66	16.66	12.51	0.86	0.00	0.02	
	0.00	17.68	20.57	21.74	21.60	18.21	15.75	0.00	8.33	
4	0	352	1063	1139	593	373	21	0	2	3543
	0.00	9.94	30.00	32.15	16.74	10.53	0.59	0.00	0.06	
	0.00	6.89	7.90	8.64	8.23	5.81	4.13	0.00	8.33	
Total	8	5112	13449	13176	7208	6419	508	3	24	45907

Table 13. APRDRG severity index and procedure

Table of APRDRG_Severity by PR1										
APRDRG_Severity	PR1(Principal procedure)									Total
Frequency Row Pct Col Pct	3610	3611	3612	3613	3614	3615	3616	3617	3619	
1	1	760	1557	1370	3	786	90	0	3	4570
	0.02	16.63	34.07	29.98	0.07	17.20	1.97	0.00	0.07	
	12.50	14.87	11.58	10.40	0.04	12.24	17.72	0.00	12.50	
2	6	2462	6357	6236	4136	3347	258	1	15	22818
	0.03	10.79	27.86	27.33	18.13	14.67	1.13	0.00	0.07	
	75.00	48.16	47.27	47.33	57.38	52.14	50.79	33.33	62.50	
3	1	1421	4138	4087	2301	1822	125	2	4	13901
	0.01	10.22	29.77	29.40	16.55	13.11	0.90	0.01	0.03	
	12.50	27.80	30.77	31.02	31.92	28.38	24.61	66.67	16.67	
4	0	469	1397	1483	768	464	35	0	2	4618
	0.00	10.16	30.25	32.11	16.63	10.05	0.76	0.00	0.04	
	0.00	9.17	10.39	11.26	10.65	7.23	6.89	0.00	8.33	
Total	8	5112	13449	13176	7208	6419	508	3	24	45907

3614 have the highest proportions in severity category 4.

Similarly, Tables 14 and 15 examine the APRDRG index with the ten hospitals performing cardio-vascular procedures. We want to examine the relationship between hospitals and the index. Table 16 gives the relationship of hospital to procedure. Hospital #7 has the highest proportion of patients in the most severe category.

Note that hospital #1 with 50% of its procedures labeled 3615, which is a milder type of surgery as

Table 14. APRDRG mortality index and hospital

Table of DSHOSPID by APRDRG_Risk_Mortality					
DSHOSPID	**APRDRG_Risk_Mortality(All Patient Refined DRG: Risk of Mortality Subclass)**				**Total**
Frequency Row Pct Col Pct	**1**	**2**	**3**	**4**	
1	122 37.54 27.79	125 38.46 22.08	54 16.62 16.22	24 7.38 18.75	325
2	6 54.55 1.37	5 45.45 0.88	0 0.00 0.00	0 0.00 0.00	11
3	24 21.43 5.47	47 41.96 8.30	25 22.32 7.51	16 14.29 12.50	112
4	81 32.02 18.45	109 43.08 19.26	49 19.37 14.71	14 5.53 10.94	253
5	15 17.05 3.42	27 30.68 4.77	37 42.05 11.11	9 10.23 7.03	88
6	47 26.86 10.71	55 31.43 9.72	57 32.57 17.12	16 9.14 12.50	175
7	78 27.56 17.77	98 34.63 17.31	73 25.80 21.92	34 12.01 26.56	283
8	13 28.89 2.96	23 51.11 4.06	7 15.56 2.10	2 4.44 1.56	45
9	26 33.33 5.92	34 43.59 6.01	11 14.10 3.30	7 8.97 5.47	78
10	27 28.13 6.15	43 44.79 7.60	20 20.83 6.01	6 6.25 4.69	96
Total	439	566	333	128	1466

opposed to 3612-3614, still has the second highest proportion of patients in the highest mortality index; in contrast, hospital #10 with a much higher proportion of more difficult surgeries, has a small percentage of under 5% in the highest mortality category. Hospital #7 has most of its patients in the more difficult surgeries and has the highest proportion in the most severe mortality category. For severity, hospitals #1 and #7 again have the highest proportions in the most severe categories in spite of performing very different types of surgery. There appears to be some definite shifting of patients into more severe categories, especially by hospital #1.

Figure 26 shows the results of the predictive model we used to predict mortality. It shows that the optimal model is rule induction; however, the decision tree is very similar (Figure 27)

For the decision tree, congestive heart failure is first followed by the APRDRG mortality index.

Table 15. APRDRG severity by hospital

Table of DSHOSPID by APRDRG_Severity					
HOSPID	**APRDRG_Severity(All Patient Refined DRG: Severity of Illness Subclass)**				**Total**
Frequency Row Pct Col Pct	**1**	**2**	**3**	**4**	
1	41 12.62 32.54	166 51.08 24.74	91 28.00 17.70	27 8.31 17.42	325
2	2 18.18 1.59	6 54.55 0.89	3 27.27 0.58	0 0.00 0.00	11
3	9 8.04 7.14	44 39.29 6.56	42 37.50 8.17	17 15.18 10.97	112
4	23 9.09 18.25	136 53.75 20.27	78 30.83 15.18	16 6.32 10.32	253
5	3 3.41 2.38	30 34.09 4.47	44 50.00 8.56	11 12.50 7.10	88
6	9 5.14 7.14	65 37.14 9.69	83 47.43 16.15	18 10.29 11.61	175
7	14 4.95 11.11	116 40.99 17.29	109 38.52 21.21	44 15.55 28.39	283
8	2 4.44 1.59	24 53.33 3.58	15 33.33 2.92	4 8.89 2.58	45
9	11 14.10 8.73	40 51.28 5.96	18 23.08 3.50	9 11.54 5.81	78
10	12 12.50 9.52	44 45.83 6.56	31 32.29 6.03	9 9.38 5.81	96
Total	126	671	514	155	1466

The APRDRG severity index was not used at all in the decision tree prediction. In this model, we did not use the Charlson Index in combination with the APRDRG indices, although we did use the specific diagnosis codes related to the Charlson Index. We will also want to determine whether the addition of the Charlson Index will improve the model.

Table 17 shows the actual and predicted values by hospital. Note that this model (in contrast to the Charlson Index in the previous section) has predictive models that are relatively reasonable compared to the actual mortality levels, which is surprising given the proportion of patients in the highest mortality and severity levels. Clearly, the first split based upon the condition of congestive heart failure modifies the threshold value with respect to the APRDRG index. Hospital #3 with the highest actual mortality has the highest rank defining quality. Hospital #2 with zero actual mortality ranks the lowest. We then wanted to see how the results are modified if we include the Charlson Index with the APRDRG indices.

Table 16. Hospital by procedure code

Table of DSHOSPID by PR1								
Hospital	**PR1(Principal procedure)**							**Total**
Frequency Row Pct Col Pct	**3611**	**3612**	**3613**	**3614**	**3615**	**3616**	**3619**	
1	16 4.92 14.81	37 11.38 12.85	47 14.46 11.69	24 7.38 9.09	193 59.38 51.47	8 2.46 28.57	0 0.00 0.00	325
2	3 27.27 2.78	4 36.36 1.39	1 9.09 0.25	0 0.00 0.00	2 18.18 0.53	1 9.09 3.57	0 0.00 0.00	11
3	5 4.46 4.63	10 8.93 3.47	19 16.96 4.73	7 6.25 2.65	69 61.61 18.40	2 1.79 7.14	0 0.00 0.00	112
4	22 8.70 20.37	59 23.32 20.49	82 32.41 20.40	75 29.64 28.41	15 5.93 4.00	0 0.00 0.00	0 0.00 0.00	253
5	2 2.27 1.85	14 15.91 4.86	34 38.64 8.46	29 32.95 10.98	9 10.23 2.40	0 0.00 0.00	0 0.00 0.00	88
6	5 2.86 4.63	23 13.14 7.99	51 29.14 12.69	36 20.57 13.64	58 33.14 15.47	2 1.14 7.14	0 0.00 0.00	175
7	21 7.42 19.44	79 27.92 27.43	95 33.57 23.63	60 21.20 22.73	15 5.30 4.00	12 4.24 42.86	1 0.35 100.00	283
8	7 15.56 6.48	11 24.44 3.82	17 37.78 4.23	9 20.00 3.41	1 2.22 0.27	0 0.00 0.00	0 0.00 0.00	45
9	15 19.23 13.89	23 29.49 7.99	23 29.49 5.72	7 8.97 2.65	9 11.54 2.40	1 1.28 3.57	0 0.00 0.00	78
10	12 12.50 11.11	28 29.17 9.72	33 34.38 8.21	17 17.71 6.44	4 4.17 1.07	2 2.08 7.14	0 0.00 0.00	96
Total	108	288	402	264	375	28	1	1466

In fact, the results are the same. We also examine the length of stay in relationship to the APRDRG index using kernel density estimation. Figure 28 shows the results.

With the average stay of almost 10 days, this error is less than that compared to the Charlson Index alone. The optimal model is Dmine regression, shown in Figure 29.

The results show that both the APRDRG indices and the Charlson Index are both used in the model along with patient demographics.

Figure 26. Predictive model results for mortality using APRDRG index

```
Fit Statistics
Model selection based on _TMISC_


                               Test:
Selected                 Misclassification
Model        Model Node        Rate

             AutoNeural5      0.36842
             DMNeural5        0.26316
             DmineReg5        0.31579
             MBR5             0.47368
             Neural5          0.31579
    Y        Rule2            0.15789
             Tree5            0.15789
```

Figure 27. Decision tree model

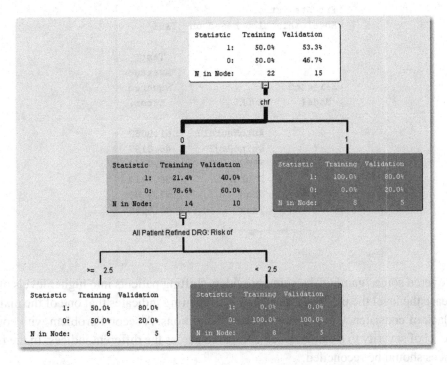

FUTURE TRENDS

As these severity indices will continue to be used to define provider reimbursements, they will come under more scrutiny. It is important to find some means of validating the index. With the APRDRG, patient outcomes are not used to define the index; instead relying on physician panels to reach a consensus. Therefore, we can validate the index using outcomes. In this chapter, we have done exactly that, and

Table 17. Ranking of hospital quality using Charlson index

Hospital	Actual Mortality	Predictive Mortality	Difference	Rank
1	1.23	7.38	6.15	6
2	0	0	0	10
3	4.46	14.29	9.83	1
4	0.79	5.53	4.74	7
5	1.14	10.23	9.09	2
6	0.57	9.14	8.57	3
7	3.53	12.01	8.48	4
8	2.22	4.44	2.22	9
9	1.28	8.97	7.69	5
10	3.13	6.25	3.12	8

Figure 28. Predictive modeling for length of stay with APRDRG indices

```
Fit Statistics
Model selection based on _TASE_

                              Test:
                            Average
      Selected              Squared
        Model     MODEL      Error.

                  AutoNeural7  61.0082
          Y       DmineReg7    46.8197
                  MBR7         50.9164
                  Neural7      56.7914
                  Reg6         57.9200
                  Tree7        47.0236
```

we have discovered some "gaming" by some providers shifting patients into higher levels of severity in order to increase the level the predicted mortality. This gaming indicates that one of the main problems remains the lack of consistency in assigning patient conditions. A second problem with consistency is assigning a level of severity to a patient when compared across the different indices. In the future, these different indices should be reconciled.

DISCUSSION

There appears to be just a few similarities between the severity level as defined by the Charlson Index compared to the APRDRG indices of mortality and severity. Primarily, the Charlson Index restricts itself to a few of the ICD9 codes while omitting all others. In contrast, the APRDRG uses a separate

Figure 29. Dmine regression results

```
The DMINE Procedure

        R-Squares for Target Variable: LOS

Effect                              DF      R-Square

AOV16: APRDRG_Severity               3      0.266862
AOV16: APRDRG_Risk_Mortality         3      0.246181
Var:   APRDRG_Risk_Mortality         1      0.230817
Var:   APRDRG_Severity               1      0.229513
AOV16: charlson                      7      0.049918
AOV16: AGE                          15      0.044500
Var:   charlson                      1      0.030796
Var:   AGE                           1      0.030685
Class: DSHOSPID                      9      0.023798
Group: DSHOSPID                      4      0.023586
Class: FEMALE                        1      0.023507
Class: RACE                          6      0.011729
Group: RACE                          2      0.011553
Class: ZIPInc_Qrtl                   4      0.006520
Group: ZIPInc_Qrtl                   3      0.006469
Class: DIED                          1      0.000534    R2 < MINR2
```

classification of 1-4 that has been identified for each primary patient diagnosis, although with this process, some patients cannot be classified. The proportion of patients that cannot be classified is small, approximately 0.05%.

These classifications were defined using expert panels. For this reason, there will remain a percentage of patients who are assigned a code of 0 because they cannot be placed in any of the levels 1-4. Those who cannot be assigned are not then used to determine the quality of providers.

In this chapter, also, the Charlson Index was compared directly to the APRDRG index values. It shows that there are a number of patient conditions used to define the Charlson Index that are related to high severity levels in the APRDRG classification. However, the comparison also shows that patients can be in the least severe Charlson level while also in the most severe APRDRG. These different results need to be examined carefully to find an explanation as to why a patient can be simultaneously very severe and not at all severe.

REFERENCES

Anonymous-3M. (2008). *3M™ APR-DRG Expert Software*.

Antioch, K. M., & Ellis, R. P. (2007). Risk adjustment policy options for casemix funding: international lessons in financing reform. *The European Journal of Health Economics, 8*(3), 195–212.

Barbash, G., & Safran, C. (1987). Need for better severity indixes of acute myocardial infarction under diagnosis-related groups. *The American Journal of Cardiology, 59*(12), 1052–1056.

Cerrito, P. (2007). Text Mining Coded Information. In H. A. D. Prado & E. Ferneda (Eds.), *Emerging Technologies of Text Mining: Techniques and Applications.* New York: IGI Global.

Ciccone, G., & Bertero, D. (1999). Quality of data or quality of care? Comparisons of diverse standardization methods by clinical severity, based on the discharge form, in the analysis of hospital mortality. *Epidemiologia e Prevenzione, 23*(4), 286–293.

Ciccone, G., & Lorenzoni, L. (1999). Social class, mode of admission, severity of illness and hospital mortality: an analysis with "All patient refined DRG" of discharges from the Molinette hospital in Turin. *Epidemiologia e Prevenzione, 23*(3), 188–196.

Gross, P., & Beyt, B. E. Jr. (1988). Description of case-mix adjusters by the severity of illness working group of the Society of Hospital Epidemiologists of American (SHEA). *Infection Control and Hospital Epidemiology, 9*(7), 309–316.

Horn, S., & Bulkley, G. (1985). Interhospital differences in severity of illness. Problems for prospective payment based on diagnosis-related groups (DRGs). *The New England Journal of Medicine, 313*(1), 20–24.

Lagman, R. L., & Walsh, D. (2007). All patient refined-diagnostic related group and case mix index in acute care palliative medicine. *The Journal of Supportive Oncology, 5*(3), 145–149.

Leary, R., & Leary, R. (1993). Research review: refined diagnosis-related groups-A new perspective on patient classification. *Topics in Health Information Management, 14*(2), 77–87.

Maurici, M., & Rosati, E. (2007). Development of classification and payment system of in patient hospital admissions in the United States: Introduction of Medicare Severity Diagnosis-Related Groups (MS-DRGs) and the present on admission (POA) indicator. *Igiene e Sanita Pubblica, 63*(6), 691–701.

McNeil, B., & Kominski, G. (1988). Modified DRGs as evidence for variability in patient severity. *Medical Care, 26*(1), 53–61.

Naessens, J., & Huschka, T. (2004). Distinguishing hospital complications of care from pre-existing conditions. *International Journal for Quality in Health Care, 16*(Suppl 1), i27–i35.

Pilotto, A., & Scarcelli, C. (2005). All patient refined diagnosis related groups: a new administrative tool for identifying elderly patients at risk of high resource consumption. *Journal of the American Geriatrics Society, 53*(1), 167–168.

Rosen, A., & Loveland, S. (2001). Evaluating diagnosis-based case-mix measures: how well do they apply to the VA population? *Medical Care, 39*(7), 692–704.

Shen, Y. (2003). Applying the 3M all patient refined diagnosis related groups grouper to measure inpatient severity in the VA. *Medical Care, 41*(6Suppl), II103–II110.

Young, J., & Macioce, D. (1990). Identifying inuries and trauma severity in large databases. *The Journal of Trauma Injury Infection and Critical Care, 30*(10), 1220–1230.

Chapter 7
Risk Adjustment Based Upon Resource Utilization

INTRODUCTION

Resource utilization is based upon the assumption that patients with more severe problems will utilize more resources, and the most severe patients will require the most resources. This type of index assumes that no unnecessary resources are utilized and that treatments, medications, and laboratory diagnostics are required because of the severity of the patient condition. However, if the provider is extravagant in the use of resources, the patient will look severe. Then, too, some of the resources used will depend upon the admitting condition.

Suppose, for example, that a patient complains of chest pain. This could be a cold, asthma, acid reflux, or a heart attack. Without expending some resources for diagnostics, it would be impossible to find the actual patient condition. Again, a patient's level of severity is defined using outcomes. Therefore, there will be some problem with validation. We can examine the issue of validation by comparing the index discussed here to the Charlson Index and the APRDRG.

There are three different resource demand indices provided with the National Inpatient Sample: for mortality, for length of stay, and for disease staging. We will examine all three to see how they are similar, and how they are different. This index is also proprietary and was developed by Thomson Medstat.

DOI: 10.4018/978-1-60566-752-2.ch007

Therefore, the exact methodology used to compute the indices is proprietary and unavailable for direct examination.

BACKGROUND

Studies that describe the relationship between healthcare utilization and patient condition and outcome are scarce. The Kessner Adequacy of Prenatal Care Index was developed to examine the relationship between prenatal care and birth outcomes.(Kotelchuck, 1994) It was regarded as flawed because of a heavy reliance on the timing of prenatal care. A second index was developed to overcome these problems. However, the timing of prenatal care was also used to develop this second index, although its importance was reduced.

Another study examined the relationship between compliance with medications and the need for additional resources such as emergency room visits.(Tu et al., 2005) This study suggested that patient compliance is an important factor in resource utilization, indicating that there may be problems with a reliance on such utilization to determine the difference in quality between providers. Patients with diabetes who routinely take their medication and test their blood sugar levels are compliant; patients who do not take their medication regularly enough are not. These patients who are not compliant may have more episodes of uncontrolled blood sugar that require emergency treatment.

A second study examined the relationship between patient body mass index (BMI) and resource utilization, with the result that patients with a BMI of 30 or greater had higher wound infection rates. (Thomas et al., 1997) This study used the following diseases as indicator variables in the regression model: degenerative joint disease, hypertension, cancer, coronary artery disease, peripheral vascular disease, diabetes, emphysema/asthma, congestive heart failure, stroke, liver disease, and renal failure. Note that while this list has some commonalities with the Charlson Index, there are differences. In particular, all of the co-morbidities are given equal weight, and there is no discussion of the validity of this list of co-morbid diseases, or justification as to why the BMI would be the ultimate marker for resource utilization.

Another study, for example, showed that two providers that treated patients with COPD had patients with very different characteristics.(Mapel et al., 2000) One provider has an average age that was approximately 7 years younger compared to the second provider and the patients had fewer co-morbidities. However, the resource utilization was very similar between the two groups, suggesting that the first provider was over-utilizing resources given its patient population.

RESOURCES IN THE MEPS DATA

The MEPS dataset contains very detailed information about reimbursements from payers, including payments by patients, insurers, and government agencies. Therefore, we can look at the relationship between actual reimbursements to patient condition. Moreover, the patient conditions are very detailed and include any ICD9 code that was used to diagnose a patient in the course of a one-year period. Therefore, we can examine actual resource utilization in relationship to patient diagnoses, to the other indices, and to primary and secondary procedures. We can also examine the resource utilization by state and federal governments, by private insurers, and by the patient.

As a special case of resource utilization, we can also examine the relationship between the cost to the patient and the overall costs of the procedures. To investigate the relationship of costs to procedures, we can restrict our attention to a primary procedure. However, because of privacy issues, the specific procedure is not fully identified in the MEPS dataset. Therefore, we will have to approximate the relationship of diagnoses and procedures to costs. We will use the procedure of 36, or Operations on vessels of heart. This procedure of 36 includes all of the procedures of 36.1 that we have used previously. Therefore, we first look to the distribution of costs for inpatient procedures to see if there is a difference in the group of procedures in code 36 that can be deduced from the costs. In addition, since the MEPS datafile follows a cohort of individuals and households, there will be few occurrences of any one condition in any given year. For 2005, there are 9 occurrences of procedure 36 in the inpatient datafile and 45 occurrences in the outpatient datafile. While heart procedures are relatively common, the small number of procedures indicates that in a given cohort of patients in a one year period, the likelihood of requiring such surgery is relatively small. To find a lifetime risk for requiring such surgery, a cohort would need to be followed for a prolonged period of time.

Therefore, in order to get a good indication of resource utilization, we will need to use multiple years. Since it is a good indication that outpatients will use fewer resources compared to inpatients, and that only inpatients have bypass surgery, we will follow the inpatient datafile for multiple years. For the years 1996-2005 combined, there were 148 instances of procedure 36. The SAS code needed to create this dataset is given below:

```
data meps.inpatient_2005;
set meps.h94d;
self_pay=ipfsf05x;
self_pay_physician=ipdsf05x;
private=ipfpv05x+ipfor05x;
private_physician=ipdpv05x+ipdor05x;
public=ipfmr05x+ipfmd05x+ipfva05x+ipftr05x+ipfof05x+ipfsl05x+ipfwc05x+ipfou05x;
public_physician=ipdmr05x+ipdmd05x+ipdva05x+ipdtr05x+ipdof05x+ipdsl05x+ipdwc05x+ipdou05
x;
totalfacilities=ipfxp05x;
totaldoctor=ipdxp05x;
facilitycharge=iptc05x;
physiciancharge=ipdtc05x;
totalreimbursement=ipxp05x;
run;
```

The above code is used to define the outcome measures for the 2005 inpatient data. Similar code must be generated for every other year, changing the '05' in the variables to the correct year for the datafile. Then we need to merge the datasets together.

```
PROC SQL;
CREATE TABLE Meps.APPEND_MEPSTABLE AS
SELECT * FROM Meps.INPATIENT_2005
 OUTER UNION CORR
```

```
SELECT * FROM Meps.INPATIENT_1996
 OUTER UNION CORR
SELECT * FROM Meps.INPATIENT_1997
 OUTER UNION CORR
SELECT * FROM Meps.INPATIENT_1998
 OUTER UNION CORR
SELECT * FROM Meps.INPATIENT_1999
 OUTER UNION CORR
SELECT * FROM Meps.INPATIENT_2000
 OUTER UNION CORR
SELECT * FROM Meps.INPATIENT_2001
 OUTER UNION CORR
SELECT * FROM Meps.INPATIENT_2002
 OUTER UNION CORR
SELECT * FROM Meps.INPATIENT_2003
 OUTER UNION CORR
SELECT * FROM Meps.INPATIENT_2004
;
Quit;
```

The above code appends the inpatient datasets together for the years 1996-2005.

```
PROC SQL;
CREATE TABLE Meps.Bypasspatients AS SELECT MEPS.APPEND_MEPSTABLE.DUID,
    MEPS.APPEND_MEPSTABLE.PID,
    MEPS.APPEND_MEPSTABLE.DUPERSID,
    MEPS.APPEND_MEPSTABLE.EVNTIDX,
    MEPS.APPEND_MEPSTABLE.EVENTRN,
    MEPS.APPEND_MEPSTABLE.ERHEVIDX,
    MEPS.APPEND_MEPSTABLE.FFEEIDX,
    MEPS.APPEND_MEPSTABLE.PANEL,
    MEPS.APPEND_MEPSTABLE.MPCDATA,
    MEPS.APPEND_MEPSTABLE.IPBEGYR,
    MEPS.APPEND_MEPSTABLE.IPBEGMM,
    MEPS.APPEND_MEPSTABLE.IPBEGDD,
    MEPS.APPEND_MEPSTABLE.IPENDYR,
    MEPS.APPEND_MEPSTABLE.IPENDMM,
    MEPS.APPEND_MEPSTABLE.IPENDDD,
    MEPS.APPEND_MEPSTABLE.NUMNIGHX,
    MEPS.APPEND_MEPSTABLE.NUMNIGHT,
    MEPS.APPEND_MEPSTABLE.EMERROOM,
    MEPS.APPEND_MEPSTABLE.SPECCOND,
    MEPS.APPEND_MEPSTABLE.RSNINHOS,
    MEPS.APPEND_MEPSTABLE.ANYOPER,
```

```
      MEPS.APPEND_MEPSTABLE.VAPLACE,
      MEPS.APPEND_MEPSTABLE.IPICD1X,
      MEPS.APPEND_MEPSTABLE.IPICD2X,
      MEPS.APPEND_MEPSTABLE.IPICD3X,
      MEPS.APPEND_MEPSTABLE.IPICD4X,
      MEPS.APPEND_MEPSTABLE.IPPRO1X,
      MEPS.APPEND_MEPSTABLE.IPPRO2X,
      MEPS.APPEND_MEPSTABLE.IPCCC1X,
      MEPS.APPEND_MEPSTABLE.IPCCC2X,
      MEPS.APPEND_MEPSTABLE.IPCCC3X,
      MEPS.APPEND_MEPSTABLE.IPCCC4X,
      MEPS.APPEND_MEPSTABLE.DSCHPMED,
      MEPS.APPEND_MEPSTABLE.FFIPTYPE,
      MEPS.APPEND_MEPSTABLE.IMPFLAG,
      MEPS.APPEND_MEPSTABLE.PERWT05F,
      MEPS.APPEND_MEPSTABLE.VARSTR,
      MEPS.APPEND_MEPSTABLE.VARPSU,
      MEPS.APPEND_MEPSTABLE.self_pay,
      MEPS.APPEND_MEPSTABLE.self_pay_physician,
      MEPS.APPEND_MEPSTABLE.private,
      MEPS.APPEND_MEPSTABLE.private_physician,
      MEPS.APPEND_MEPSTABLE.public,
      MEPS.APPEND_MEPSTABLE.public_physician,
      MEPS.APPEND_MEPSTABLE.totalfacilities,
      MEPS.APPEND_MEPSTABLE.totaldoctor,
      MEPS.APPEND_MEPSTABLE.facilitycharge,
      MEPS.APPEND_MEPSTABLE.physiciancharge,
      MEPS.APPEND_MEPSTABLE.totalreimbursement
FROM MEPS.APPEND_MEPSTABLE AS MEPS.APPEND_MEPSTABLE;
WHERE meps.append_mepstable.IPPRO1X = "36";
QUIT;
```

The remaining code filters the appended data to those observations with a primary procedure of "36". Table 1 gives the summary statistics by year for the payment variables. It gives the number of procedures by year.

There is no question that there is an increase in costs by year, so that resource utilization as estimated by payments must include some variable related to inflation. The best way to do this is to normalize the costs for each year. Then we can identify the patients by order of costs, and examine their diagnoses. The code to normalize is below:

```
Proc sort data= Meps.Bypasspatients;
By IPBEGYR;
DATA WORK.keepvariablenames;
   SET meps.bypasspatients;
```

Table 1. Summary statistics for payment variables by year

EVENT START DATE - YEAR	N Obs	Variable	Mean	Std Dev	Minimum	Maximum
1996	8	self_pay	140.8275000	376.7019637	0	1072.62
		self_pay_physician	2.7000000	7.6367532	0	21.6000000
		private	4998.14	8504.87	0	22308.03
		private_physician	1555.29	1726.83	28.1100000	4710.40
		public	.	.	.	.
		public_physician	.	.	.	.
		totalfacilities	17351.35	10334.00	1122.00	29376.54
		totaldoctor	3603.06	3638.14	140.5400000	11430.51
		facilitycharge	.	.	.	.
		physiciancharge	6778.15	5379.27	444.4400000	15255.00
1997	11	self_pay	114.8181818	298.0761038	0	985.0000000
		self_pay_physician	14.5600000	43.8755296	0	146.2500000
		private	3508.68	6450.33	0	20641.81
		private_physician	213.6145455	330.1217615	0	794.2900000
		public	.	.	.	.
		public_physician	.	.	.	.
		totalfacilities	15381.87	10197.91	229.0000000	29228.16
		totaldoctor	547.1354545	957.7178278	0	3274.78
		facilitycharge	18834.53	9893.12	229.0000000	30335.25
		physiciancharge	1248.73	2678.13	0	9176.00
1998	10	self_pay	10.0000000	31.6227766	0	100.0000000
		self_pay_physician	57.5330000	122.8719621	0	370.0000000
		private	5622.41	9214.22	0	27715.82
		private_physician	1772.56	3371.06	0	8833.00
		public	.	.	.	.
		public_physician	.	.	.	.
		totalfacilities	12824.10	7249.03	124.1700000	27715.82
		totaldoctor	2479.78	3249.68	0	9203.00
		facilitycharge	29881.65	21434.11	5625.54	78453.29
		physiciancharge	4940.55	5195.36	0	14428.00
1999	10	self_pay	343.8810000	985.6739665	0	3144.81
		self_pay_physician	63.3160000	187.3211523	0	595.6600000
		private	3955.28	10484.64	0	33662.74
		private_physician	242.1490000	347.9493636	0	845.8800000
		public	83352.00	.	83352.00	83352.00
		public_physician	0	.	0	0
		totalfacilities	21287.54	24602.18	800.0000000	83352.00
		totaldoctor	1574.42	1724.50	0	4310.97
		facilitycharge	39900.32	31433.79	3968.00	83352.00
		physiciancharge	5052.48	5938.77	0	16839.32
2000	13	self_pay	2.3076923	8.3205029	0	30.0000000
		self_pay_physician	123.2815385	371.9524621	0	1354.05
		private	5799.69	14090.40	0	46493.68
		private_physician	1022.23	1513.50	0	5046.95
		public	12195.25	11743.07	0	32801.74
		public_physician	1811.04	2604.40	0	9306.57
		totalfacilities	17997.26	13937.00	219.1200000	46493.68
		totaldoctor	2956.56	2598.67	0	9306.57
		facilitycharge	42012.33	29833.54	939.0600000	95680.95
		physiciancharge	6054.26	5021.79	0	14591.00

Table 1. continued

EVENT START DATE - YEAR	N Obs	Variable	Mean	Std Dev	Minimum	Maximum
2001	13	self_pay	69.7100000	116.5962158	0	318.8400000
		self_pay_physician	161.8184615	400.5448184	0	1403.07
		private	7436.04	11265.53	0	33000.01
		private_physician	2219.23	2131.56	34.9800000	5497.89
		public	8130.85	14757.64	0	53323.83
		public_physician	468.0761538	818.5731194	0	2842.73
		totalfacilities	15636.60	16158.90	226.6100000	58306.83
		totaldoctor	2849.13	2112.22	625.8600000	6632.72
		facilitycharge	39538.36	21795.16	3772.49	72903.30
		physiciancharge	6340.50	4636.07	1057.83	11744.00
2002	26	self_pay	299.4015385	841.4442546	0	4097.30
		self_pay_physician	143.6203846	434.8967158	0	2072.67
		private	7627.84	11804.42	0	40925.86
		private_physician	1983.44	3486.43	0	13753.27
		public	7422.46	12192.26	0	43327.41
		public_physician	999.5469231	1731.28	0	5127.71
		totalfacilities	15372.22	13360.34	585.5200000	45023.16
		totaldoctor	3126.61	3378.89	0	13753.27
		facilitycharge	50075.85	55169.16	1350.50	188272.36
		physiciancharge	7943.20	8782.72	0	32545.86
2003	18	self_pay	17.2672222	70.6066281	0	300.0000000
		self_pay_physician	62.0844444	185.2119540	0	780.1900000
		private	12492.57	22540.83	0	61482.71
		private_physician	1726.38	3353.71	0	9833.06
		public	11419.55	11399.28	0	37964.36
		public_physician	1302.89	1733.11	0	4843.79
		totalfacilities	23929.39	19271.37	943.5100000	61482.71
		totaldoctor	3091.36	3216.34	0	9859.72
		facilitycharge	57975.92	40939.44	943.5200000	139495.50
		physiciancharge	8081.84	7670.10	0	22579.00
2004	30	self_pay	43.9463333	134.2028882	0	655.5600000
		self_pay_physician	38.4930000	130.4942161	0	658.2200000
		private	4093.98	9857.20	0	44007.29
		private_physician	894.7710000	1846.82	0	6955.95
		public	14019.17	20841.47	0	116093.69
		public_physician	1610.60	1840.06	0	6210.20
		totalfacilities	18157.10	21405.31	2804.36	121044.49
		totaldoctor	2543.87	2450.05	0	7762.75
		facilitycharge	54475.65	60829.34	6110.65	256269.96
		physiciancharge	7186.77	6500.98	0	25575.81
2005	9	self_pay	866.2766667	2283.73	0	6945.53
		self_pay_physician	21.5844444	21.5710936	0	46.9800000
		private	6260.31	13779.88	0	40944.77
		private_physician	669.9700000	964.6273653	0	2645.70
		public	11578.62	13191.90	0	37056.71
		public_physician	927.7111111	843.8795768	0	2095.46
		totalfacilities	18705.21	13500.46	740.0000000	40944.77
		totaldoctor	1619.27	874.6678531	0	2688.90
		facilitycharge	54868.57	23610.97	11563.87	87400.63
		physiciancharge	7268.86	3566.49	2833.00	12125.00

```
    stnd_self_pay = self_pay;
    LABEL stnd_self_pay="Standardized self_pay: mean = 0 standard deviation = 1";
    stnd_self_pay_physician = self_pay_physician;
    LABEL stnd_self_pay_physician="Standardized self_pay_physician: mean = 0 standard
deviation = 1";
    stnd_private = private;
    LABEL stnd_private="Standardized private: mean = 0 standard deviation = 1";
    stnd_private_physician = private_physician;
    LABEL stnd_private_physician="Standardized private_physician: mean = 0 standard de-
viation = 1";
    stnd_public = public;
    LABEL stnd_public="Standardized public: mean = 0 standard deviation = 1";
    stnd_public_physician = public_physician;
    LABEL stnd_public_physician="Standardized public_physician: mean = 0 standard devia-
tion = 1";
    stnd_totalfacilities = totalfacilities;
    LABEL stnd_totalfacilities="Standardized totalfacilities: mean = 0 standard devia-
tion = 1";
    stnd_totaldoctor = totaldoctor;
    LABEL stnd_totaldoctor="Standardized totaldoctor: mean = 0 standard deviation = 1";
    stnd_facilitycharge = facilitycharge;
    LABEL stnd_facilitycharge="Standardized facilitycharge: mean = 0 standard deviation
= 1";
    stnd_physiciancharge = physiciancharge;
    LABEL stnd_physiciancharge="Standardized physiciancharge: mean = 0 standard devia-
tion = 1";
    stnd_totalreimbursement = totalreimbursement;
    LABEL stnd_totalreimbursement="Standardized totalreimbursement: mean = 0 standard
deviation = 1";
RUN;
PROC STANDARD;
DATA= WORK.keepvariablenames
OUT=meps.standardizedbypass
    MEAN=0
    STD=1
    ;
    VAR stnd_self_pay stnd_self_pay_physician stnd_private stnd_private_physician stnd_
public stnd_public_physician stnd_totalfacilities stnd_totaldoctor stnd_facilitycharge
stnd_physiciancharge stnd_totalreimbursement;
    BY IPBEGYR;
RUN;
```

Once we have standardized the variables, we can investigate the patient conditions. Table 2 lists the ten patients with the least cost and the ten patients with the greatest costs along with their diagnoses listed.

Table 2. Contrast patients with greatest and least costs

Row number	3-DIGIT ICD-9-CM CONDITION CODE	3-DIGIT ICD-9-CM CONDITION CODE	3-DIGIT ICD-9-CM CONDITION CODE	3-DIGIT ICD-9-CM CONDITION CODE	Standardized totalreimbursement: mean = 0 standard deviation = 1
1	-1	-1	-1	-1	-1.78629
2	-8	-1	-1	-1	-1.41160
3	429	-1	-1	-1	-1.31158
4	414	-1	-1	-1	-1.28103
5	-1	-1	-1	-1	-1.19145
6	414	410	-1	-1	-1.13326
7	414	410	-1	-1	-1.08304
8	-1	-1	-1	-1	-1.04587
9	444	429	786	786	-1.03820
10	410	-1	-1	-1	-1.02175
139	794	-1	-1	-1	1.53877
140	-1	-1	-1	-1	1.63953
141	410	-1	-1	-1	1.74980
142	429	786	-1	-1	1.88893
143	-8	-1	-1	-1	1.90818
144	-1	-1	-1	-1	1.99283
145	-1	-1	-1	-1	2.02380
146	-8	-1	-1	-1	2.45501
147	429	-1	-1	-1	2.55625
148	-1	-1	-1	-1	4.68343

Only one patient has three diagnosis codes; the diagnosis codes do not seem to be different. Therefore, the patient's severity does not appear to explain the difference in costs and resource utilization; that is, there is no apparent relationship between the reported diagnosis codes and the total costs for treating each patient. Patient 148 with a standardized reimbursement of 4.68 has no diagnosis codes listed. Therefore, we need to look at the patient conditions dataset (which is a separate data file in the MEPS collection) that contains all diagnoses given to each patient in the course of the year. We can look at these most crucial patients. Table 3 gives the reimbursements for the patients with procedure '36' for the year 2005. As there are just nine patients, we can look at each individually.

The total reimbursement ranges from a low of $2750 to a high of $41,000. Because the '36' is incomplete, it is not known if these patients have similar procedures, or if the difference is enough to account for the difference in payments. We can first look to see if they have different secondary procedures. Table 4 gives the patient conditions for these nine patients as identified in the conditions dataset. In contrast to the inpatients file, which lists just a handful of diagnoses, there are a total of 72 diagnoses for these nine patients.

There is no obvious reason that patient #37357013 should cost more compared to patient #55776017 just by comparing the patient conditions.

Table 3. Reimbursements for 2005 patients

Row number	PERSON ID (DUID + PID)	self_pay	self_pay_physician	private	private_physician	public
1	56299025	100.00	0.00	640.00	2008.65	0.00
2	57185015	6945.53	0.00	0.00	179.82	0.00
3	34035011	0.00	46.98	0.00	187.91	12870.03
4	55776017	0.00	46.98	0.00	187.91	12870.03
5	32614023	309.75	43.20	13937.25	2645.70	0.00
6	31252015	350.00	27.00	0.00	0.00	16410.83
7	38475011	0.00	0.00	0.00	337.62	25000.00
8	34054027	91.21	30.10	820.79	482.12	37056.71
9	37357013	0.00	0.00	40944.77	0.00	0.00

Row number	public_physician	totalfacilities	totaldoctor	facilitycharge
1	0.00	740.00	2008.65	39928.60
2	719.26	6945.53	899.08	11563.87
3	939.58	12870.03	1174.47	42624.75
4	939.58	12870.03	1174.47	42624.75
5	0.00	14247.00	2688.90	62913.86
6	2037.01	16760.83	2064.01	61578.30
7	1618.51	25000.00	1956.13	84107.20
8	2095.46	37968.71	2607.68	87400.63
9	0.00	40944.77	0.00	61075.16

Row number	PERSON ID (DUID + PID)	physiciancharge	totalreimbursement
1	56299025	12125.00	2748.65
2	57185015	4175.00	7844.61
3	34035011	2833.00	14044.50
4	55776017	2833.00	14044.50
5	32614023	9519.00	16935.90
6	31252015	11329.00	18824.84
7	38475011	7252.00	26956.13
8	34054027	9596.50	40576.39
9	37357013	5757.27	40944.77

Table 4. Secondary procedure codes for 2005 patients

PERSON ID (DUID + PID)	Diagnosis Codes	Translation
56299025	272, 429, 723, 401, 477	Disorders of lipoid metabolism, Ill-defined descriptions and complications of heart disease, Other disorders of cervical region, Essential hypertension, Allergic rhinitis
57185015	716, 424, 724, V76, 366, 722, 473, 477, 536, 429, 272, 401	Other and unspecified arthropathies, Other diseases of endocardium, Other and unspecified disorders of back, Special screening for malignant neoplasms, Cataract, Intervertebral disc disorders, Chronic sinusitis, Allergic rhinitis, Disorders of function of stomach, Ill-defined descriptions and complications of heart disease, Disorders of lipoid metabolism, Essential hypertension
34035011	780, 724, 311, 401, 274, 250, 716, 354, 185, 429	General symptoms, Other and unspecified disorders of back, Depressive disorder, not elsewhere classified, Essential hypertension, Gout, Diabetes Mellitus, Other and unspecified arthropathies, Mononeuritis of upper limb and mononeuritis multiplex, Malignant neoplasm of prostate, Ill-defined descriptions and complications of heart disease
55776017	V70, V72, V58, 996, 490, 401, 173, 602, 530, 272	General medical examination, Special investigations and examinations, Encounter for other and unspecified procedures and aftercare, Complications peculiar to certain specified procedures, Bronchitis, not specified as acute or chronic, Essential hypertension, Other malignant neoplasm of skin, Other disorders of prostate, Diseases of esophagus, Disorders of lipoid metabolism
32614023	300, 414, 487	Anxiety, dissociative and somatoform disorders, Other forms of chronic ischemic heart disease, Influenza
31252015	362, 444, 401, 592, V77, 355	Other retinal disorders, Arterial embolism and thrombosis, Essential hypertension, Calculus of kidney and ureter, Special screening for endocrine, nutritional, metabolic, and immunity disorders, Mononeuritis of lower limb
38475011	274, V77, 246, 427, 486, 401, 493, 250	Gout, Special screening for endocrine, nutritional, metabolic, and immunity disorders, Other disorders of thyroid, Cardiac dysrhythmias, Pneumonia, organism unspecified, Essential hypertension, Asthma, Diabetes mellitus
34054027	V72, 959, 780, V81, 366, 429, 782, 530	Special investigations and examinations, Injury, other and unspecified, General symptoms, Special screening for cardiovascular, respiratory, and genitourinary diseases, Cataract, Ill-defined descriptions and complications of heart disease, Symptoms involving skin and other integumentary tissue, Diseases of esophagus
37357013	311, 780, 276, 794, 355, 272, 401, 250	Depressive disorder, not elsewhere classified, General symptoms, Disorders of fluid, electrolyte, and acid-base balance, Nonspecific abnormal results of function studies, Mononeuritis of lower limb, Disorders of lipoid metabolism, Essential hypertension, Diabetes Mellitus

COMPARISONS OF THE RESOURCE DEMAND LEVEL TO PATIENT OUTCOMES

There are a number of proprietary indices that are based upon resource utilization. The NIS dataset contains such an index developed by Medstat. There are four different scales: length of stay, mortality, resource demand level, and the stage of principal disease category. We will focus on the first three levels in this chapter. We will first look at the relationship of the resource demand level to patient outcomes.

Comparisons in the NIS Data

We will compare this index to the Charlson and APRDRG indices that were defined in Chapters 5 and 6. Since the NIS data has all three indices, we can make direct comparisons. Again, we want to see if there is any consistency in the definition of severity, or if patients can be identified as severe depending upon the choice of the index.

Comparison to the Charlson Index

We first look at the relationship of the Charlson Index to the disease staging: length of stay (Table 5).

Note that the Charlson code of 0 is divided between the first three disease staging levels with a Charlson code of 1 divided between 50% in the disease staging level 3 and 25% in level 4. By Charlson index 4, the majority of patients are contained within disease staging level 4. There is only a slight shift to index 5 at Charlson index level 11 and above.

Figures 1,2, and 3 compares the Disease Staging: Resource Level (DS) to the individual conditions that define the Charlson Index using a series of pie charts. Virtually every condition is defined using DS levels 3, 4, and 5. What does change is the proportion of levels 3 and 4. For both acute myocardial infarction and congestive heart failure, half of the patients have staging level 3 with a small proportion in the most severe category of 5. There is a larger proportion of level 3 for diabetes and liver disease with a higher proportion of level 4 for metastatiic cancer and paraplegia. From this spread, it is clear that there is no one disease that is considered in the most severe category in and of itself.

Since every one of these conditions is high on the disease staging level, this result explains why only a value of zero for the Charlson Index is in the first three disease staging levels. It shows that the Charlson Index is focused on very severe patients compared to the resource demand index, which appears to focus on more mild conditions and has a much higher proportion of patients in the more severe categories.

Similarly to the predictive model using the Charlson Index to predict the APRDRG index, we can use a predictive model to determine whether the Charlson Index can compare to the disease staging level. Figure 4 gives the variable definitions and identified roles in the predictive model; Figure 5 gives the predictive model. The misclassification rate is given in Figure 6, and the Lift is given in Figure 7.

Note that the misclassification rate is much higher compared to the predictive model for the APRDRG in the previous chapter. The decision tree remains the best model as it was in Chapter 5.

However, the lift results indicate that the model is effective only to the second decile, indicating that the Charlson Index can make very few predictions accurately of the disease staging: resource demand level. Figure 8 has part of the decision tree; only a small portion of this tree is dependent upon the Charlson Index after total charges and age at admission. Therefore, the relationship between the Charlson Index and the disease staging model is very slight.

If the Charlson Index is 0, the next measures are for total charges and admission type. If the Charlson Index is greater than one but less than or equal to 3, then admission type is next in the tree with a slight division for resource level 4. Otherwise, the admission type then splits the patients into resource level 4 versus resource level 3.

It seems quite reasonable that the resource demand level would depend more upon charges and length of stay than patient condition. Therefore, we will also consider the disease staging: mortality level as well. We perform a similar analysis, changing only the target variable. Figure 9 gives the misclassification rate; Figure 8 gives the Lift function.

Figure 10 indicates that the optimal model is a decision tree. However, the misclassification rate is extremely high at 42%. The relationship between the Charlson Index and the disease staging indices is extremely poor.

The prediction decile is now at 3 so that 30% of the patients can be classified more accurately using the model compared to random chance. Therefore, for the most critical patients, the model has reasonable predictability.

Figure 11 shows a part of the decision tree, starting with the third branch and the Charlson Index. Interestingly enough, the Charlson Index is somewhat scattered throughout the tree, and the other vari-

Table 5. Charlson index and disease staging: length of stay

charlson	Disease Staging: Length of Stay Level					Total
Frequency Row Pct Col Pct	1	2	3	4	5	
0	234037 5.16 77.51	1226126 27.03 86.76	2381418 52.50 57.56	539219 11.89 31.70	155472 3.43 35.51	4536272
1	51830 3.03 17.16	133132 7.79 9.42	961228 56.25 23.23	449931 26.33 26.45	112811 6.60 25.77	1708932
2	13227 1.43 4.38	38714 4.18 2.74	461011 49.73 11.14	331913 35.80 19.51	82206 8.87 18.78	927071
3	1801 0.38 0.60	9631 2.03 0.68	207722 43.76 5.02	208733 43.98 12.27	46759 9.85 10.68	474646
4	268 0.14 0.09	2092 1.06 0.15	73819 37.56 1.78	98419 50.07 5.79	21964 11.17 5.02	196562
5	586 0.70 0.19	2622 3.13 0.19	31391 37.46 0.76	40335 48.13 2.37	8868 10.58 2.03	83802
6	165 0.39 0.05	685 1.61 0.05	14575 34.20 0.35	21326 50.04 1.25	5866 13.76 1.34	42617
7	28 0.21 0.01	151 1.14 0.01	4152 31.47 0.10	6777 51.36 0.40	2086 15.81 0.48	13194
8	10 0.18 0.00	48 0.84 0.00	1600 28.14 0.04	2897 50.96 0.17	1130 19.88 0.26	5685
9	0 0.00 0.00	10 0.56 0.00	475 26.75 0.01	889 50.06 0.05	402 22.64 0.09	1776
10	0 0.00 0.00	3 0.46 0.00	167 25.50 0.00	324 49.47 0.02	161 24.58 0.04	655
11	0 0.00 0.00	0 0.00 0.00	35 16.13 0.00	126 58.06 0.01	56 25.81 0.01	217
12	0 0.00 0.00	0 0.00 0.00	16 22.54 0.00	39 54.93 0.00	16 22.54 0.00	71
13	0 0.00 0.00	0 0.00 0.00	0 0.00 0.00	8 66.67 0.00	4 33.33 0.00	12
Total	301952	1413214	4137609	1700936	437801	7991512

Figure 1. Disease staging compared to Charlson index diagnoses

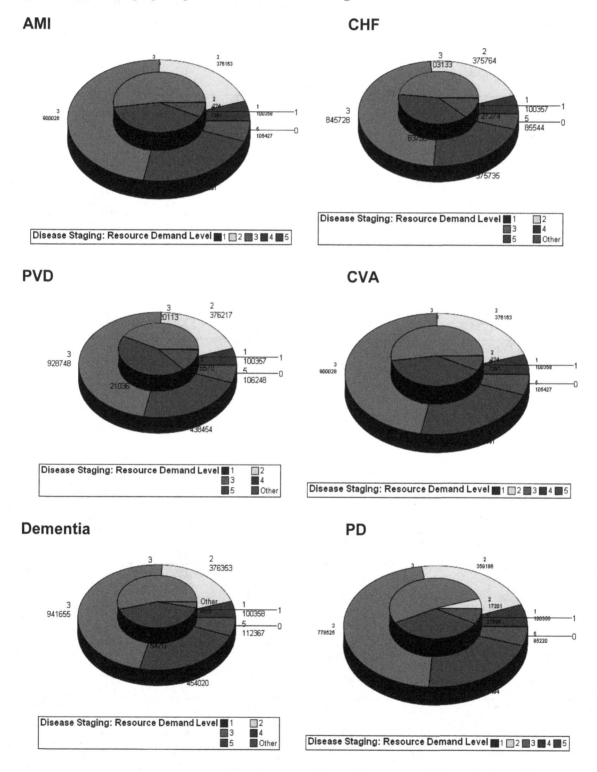

Figure 2. Disease staging compared to Charlson index diagnoses (continued)

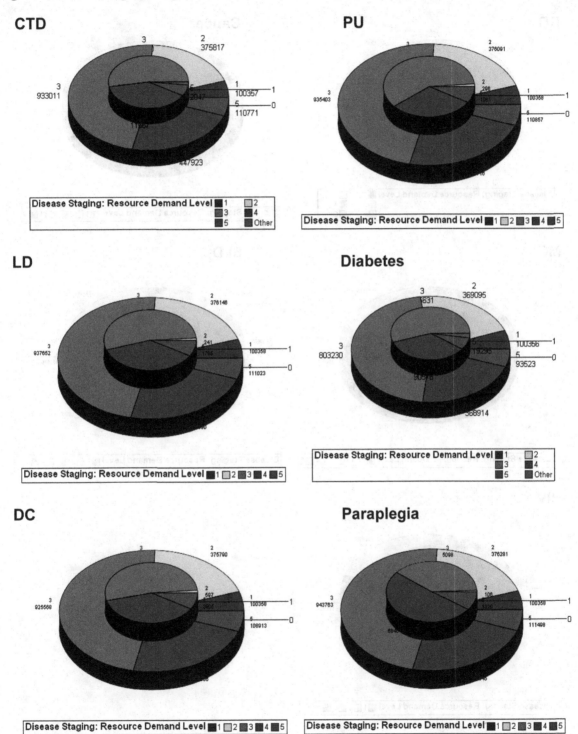

Figure 3. Disease staging compared to Charlson index diagnoses (continued)

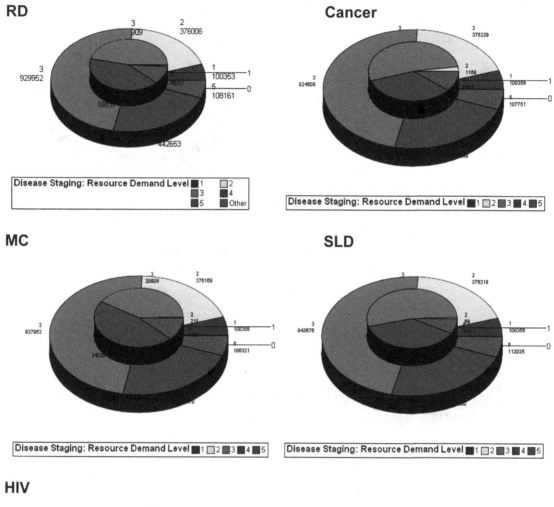

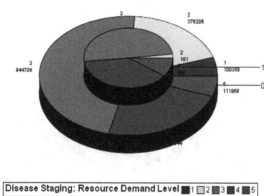

Figure 4. Variable definitions

Name	Role	Level
AGE	Input	Interval
APRDRG_Risk_Mortality	Rejected	Ordinal
APRDRG_Severity	Rejected	Ordinal
ASOURCE	Input	Nominal
ATYPE	Input	Nominal
AWEEKEND	Input	Nominal
DIED	Input	Binary
DS_LOS_Level	Rejected	Interval
DS_Mrt_Level	Rejected	Interval
DS_RD_Level	Target	Ordinal
FEMALE	Input	Nominal
KEY	ID	Nominal
LOS	Input	Interval
RACE	Input	Nominal
TOTCHG	Input	Interval
ZIPInc_Qrtl	Input	Ordinal
charlson	Input	Nominal

Figure 5. Predictive model

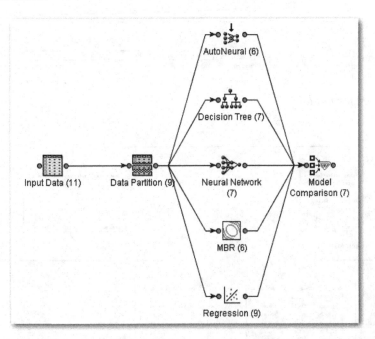

ables are given more importance in the model. This indicates yet again that disease staging still has a somewhat limited relationship to the Charlson Index.

There is no question that these two indices will give wildly divergent results for a substantial portion of the patient population. For this reason, we need to be very concerned about the use of the results for reimbursements to providers, and to drill down into details to discover the reasons for this divergence.

Figure 6. Misclassification rates

```
Fit Statistics
Model selection based on _TMISC_


                                     Test:
         Selected                  Misclassification
         Model        MODEL            Rate.


                      AutoNeural6     0.52022
                      MBR6            0.37965
                      Neural7         0.44446
                      Reg9            0.44682
             Y        Tree7           0.36792
```

Figure 7. Lift results

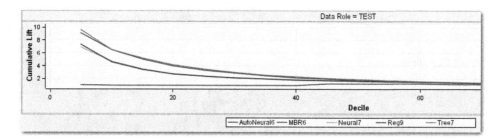

Figure 8. Partial tree for model

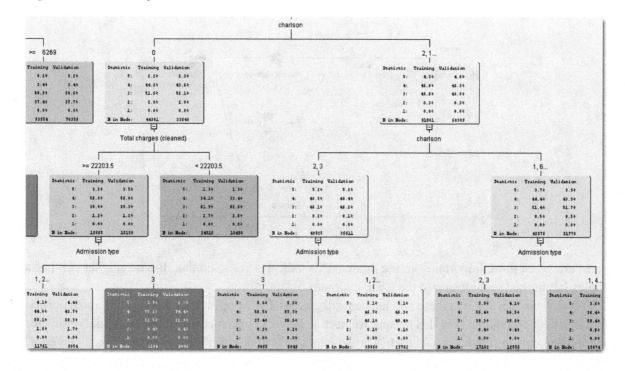

Figure 9. Misclassification rate for model

```
Fit Statistics
Model selection based on _TMISC_


                                      Test:
        Selected                Misclassification
          Model      MODEL           Rate.

                     AutoNeural6     0.57789
                     MBR6            0.44046
                     Neural7         0.51276
                     Reg9            0.51086
            Y        Tree7           0.42321
```

Figure 10. Lift function for model

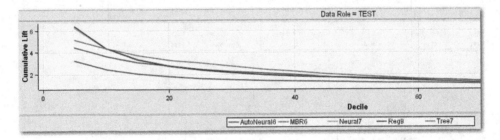

Comparison to the APRDRG

Unlike the APRDRG coding, all patients can be classified using the patient utilization indices. Tables 6,7 give the relationship between the different indices.

In Table 6, note that almost 95% of patients from disease staging length of stay classes 1-2 are in APRDRG class 1; 71% from class 3 are also in APRDRG class 1. Most of the patients are in class 1 because most of the patients are in APRDRG class 1. Patients in the most severe disease staging LOS are in APRDRG class two 30% of the time, and in class 4 only 17% of the time. In fact, there are almost twice as many patients in DS LOS class 5 compared to APRDRG class 4.

Table 7 gives the comparison of APRDRG mortality to disease staging mortality level. A similar result occurs here, with slight shifts in classes. Over 95% of the patients in the first three disease staging levels are in APRDRG class 1; 32% of the patients in disease staging level 5 are in APRDRG class 4. This table indicates that far more patients are identified as least severe in the APRDRG index compared to the disease staging indices.

We add the APRDRG mortality and severity indices to the predictive model to determine whether multiple indices can predict the disease staging levels. Figure 12 gives the variable roles; Figure 13 gives the misclassification rate, and Figure 14 gives the Lift function. The clear conclusion is that there is still little ability for one index to predict another.

Figure 11. Decision tree branch including Charlson

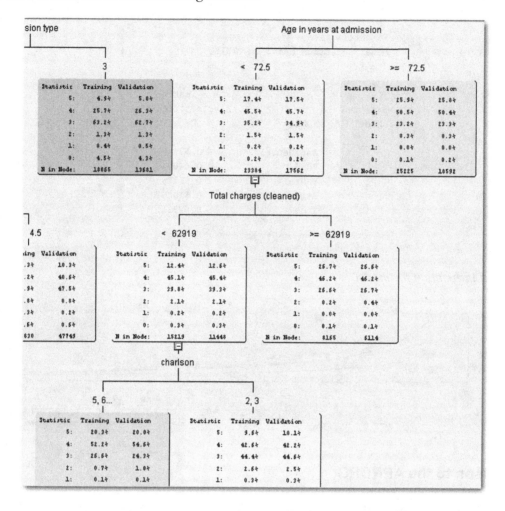

The misclassification rate appears to be little changed from that defined with only the Charlson Index and not the APRDRG. However, as shown in Figure 12, the lift function has moved to the fourth decile. Therefore, the model can give fairly accurate predictions for approximately 40% of the patients in the data set.

The APRDRG index is used in the first branch of the tree, with patients in classes 0 (unknown) or 1 following the path in Figure 15. The Charlson Index is little used in the predictive model.

The entire tree is given in Figure 16. It shows that for the APRDRG of 2 or larger in the first branch, there is a further split between class 2 and classes 3-4. Note that the Charlson Index still does not appear in the model. We can conclude from this that the APRDRG is more closely related to the disease staging indices than is the Charlson Index.

Table 6. Table of DS_LOS_Level by APRDRG_Risk_Mortality

DS_LOS_Level	APRDRG_Risk_Mortality					Total
Frequency Row Pct Col Pct	0	1	2	3	4	
1	86 0.03 4.60	285507 94.55 5.48	14542 4.82 0.79	1375 0.46 0.19	442 0.15 0.18	301952
2	272 0.02 14.54	1347185 95.33 25.86	57593 4.08 3.14	5880 0.42 0.83	2284 0.16 0.95	1413214
3	944 0.02 50.45	2936176 70.96 56.35	946599 22.88 51.67	212867 5.14 30.09	41023 0.99 17.10	4137609
4	314 0.02 16.78	530921 31.21 10.19	680532 40.01 37.14	368619 21.67 52.11	120550 7.09 50.26	1700936
5	255 0.06 13.63	110532 25.25 2.12	132830 30.34 7.25	118623 27.10 16.77	75561 17.26 31.50	437801
Total	1871	5210321	1832096	707364	239860	7991512

Table 7. APRDRG mortality compared to DIS: mortality level

DS_Mrt_Level	APRDRG_Risk_Mortality					Total
Frequency Row Pct Col Pct	0	1	2	3	4	
0	194 0.01 10.21	1321899 98.79 25.37	14704 1.10 0.80	1017 0.08 0.14	260 0.02 0.11	1338074
1	188 0.07 9.89	272775 96.51 5.23	8714 3.08 0.48	798 0.28 0.11	161 0.06 0.07	282636
2	272 0.02 14.31	1091830 96.67 20.95	32539 2.88 1.78	3671 0.33 0.52	1162 0.10 0.48	1129474
3	764 0.02 40.19	2206633 65.47 42.35	966978 28.69 52.78	173451 5.15 24.52	22396 0.66 9.34	3370222
4	381 0.03 20.04	302412 20.48 5.80	708109 47.97 38.65	377066 25.54 53.30	88305 5.98 36.81	1476273
5	102 0.03 5.37	15204 3.85 0.29	101065 25.56 5.52	151374 38.29 21.40	127582 32.27 53.19	395327
Total	1901	5210753	1832109	707377	239866	7992006

Figure 12. Variable definitions adding APRDRG mortality and severity as inputs

Name	Role	Level
AGE	Input	Interval
APRDRG_Risk_Mortality	Input	Ordinal
APRDRG_Severity	Input	Ordinal
ASOURCE	Input	Nominal
ATYPE	Input	Nominal
AWEEKEND	Input	Nominal
DIED	Input	Binary
DS_LOS_Level	Rejected	Nominal
DS_Mrt_Level	Target	Ordinal
DS_RD_Level	Rejected	Interval
FEMALE	Input	Nominal
KEY	ID	Nominal
LOS	Input	Interval
RACE	Input	Nominal
TOTCHG	Input	Interval
ZIPInc_Qrtl	Input	Ordinal
charlson	Input	Nominal

Figure 13. Misclassification rate with APRDRG indices as inputs

```
Fit Statistics
Model selection based on _TMISC_


                                        Test:
Selected                        Misclassification
Model        MODEL                      Rate


             AutoNeural6               0.57821
             MBR6                      0.44046
             Neural7                   0.57315
             Reg9                      0.50031
   Y         Tree7                     0.39505
```

Figure 14. Lift function with APRDRG indices as inputs

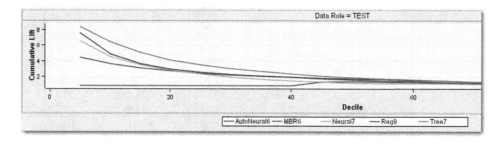

Figure 15. Tree path for patients in APRDRG class 0,1

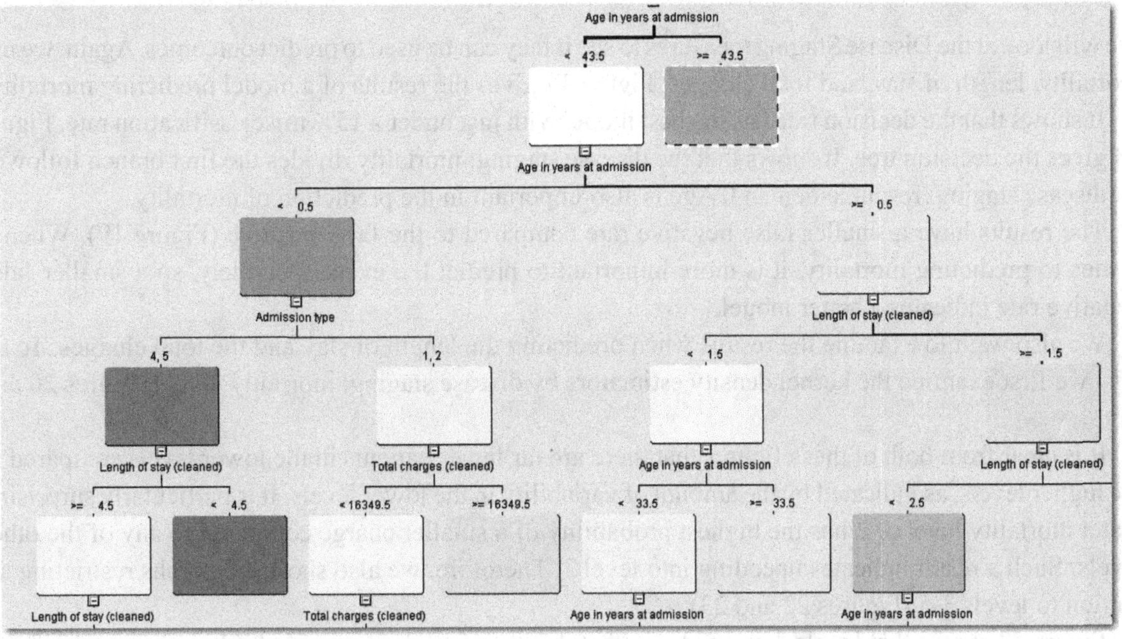

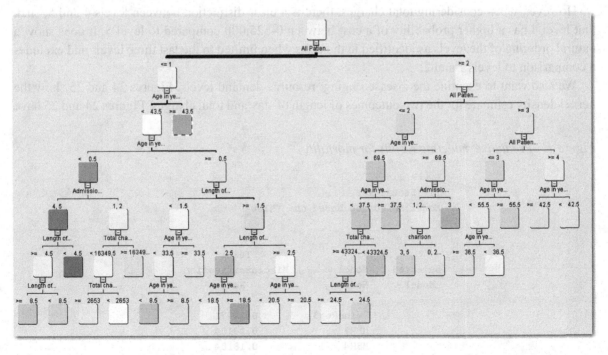

Figure 16. Decision tree for model

DISEASE STAGING COMPARED TO OUTCOMES

We will look at the Disease Staging measures to see if they can be used to predict outcomes. Again, we use mortality, length of stay, and total charges. Figure 17 gives the results of a model predicting mortality.

It shows that the decision tree has the best model with just under a 15% misclassification rate. Figure 18 gives the decision tree. It shows that the disease staging: mortality divides the first branch followed by disease staging: resource demand. Age is also important in the prediction of mortality.

The results have a smaller false negative rate compared to the false positive (Figure 19). When it comes to predicting mortality, it is more important to predict the event accurately, so a smaller false negative rate indicates a better model.

We also want to examine the results when predicting the length of stay and the total charges. To do this, we first examine the kernel density estimators by disease staging: mortality level (Figures 20 and 21).

It is clear from both of these figures that there are far fewer patients in the lower levels compared to the higher levels, as indicated by the amount of variability in the lower levels. It is particularly surprising that a mortality level of 2 has the highest probability of a smaller charge compared to any of the other levels. Such a result indicates upcoding into level 2. Therefore, we also show the graphs restricting attention to levels 3-5 (Figures 22 and 23).

Figure 22 shows that levels 4 and 5 do, in fact, have a much higher probabililty of a length of stay greater than 4 days, and have virtually the same probability of a stay of greater than 7 days. This shows that the distinction in patient severity between levels 4 and 5 is not demonstrated in the patient outcomes.

However, when considering total charges, there is a clear distinction between levels 4 and 5, such that level 4 has a higher probability of a cost between 0-$25,000 compared to level 5. It does show a natural ordering of the levels as identified in the costs when limited to the last three levels and excludes a comparison to levels 1 and 2.

We also want to examine the disease staging: resource demand levels. Figures 24 and 25 show the kernel density estimate for the two outcomes of length of stay and total charges. Figures 24 and 25 have

Figure 17. Predictive modeling results for mortality

```
Fit Statistics
Model selection based on _TMISC_


                                    Test:
    Selected    Model       Misclassification
    Model       Node              Rate


                DmineReg3         0.14971
                MBR3              0.18104
                MBR4              0.18104
                Neural3           0.29050
                Reg3              0.29057
                Rule3             0.14840
        Y       Tree3             0.14745
```

Figure 18. Decision tree to predict mortality

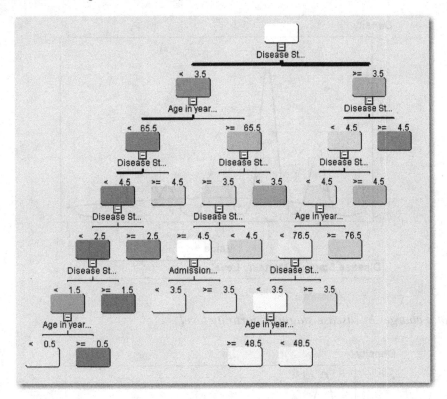

Figure 19. Results of predictive model

```
Event Classification Table
Model selection based on _TMISC_
```

MODEL	Data Role	Target	False Negative	True Negative	False Positive	True Positive
Reg3	TRAIN	DIED	930	7946	8847	15863
Reg3	VALIDATE	DIED	779	5956	6639	11816
Rule3	TRAIN	DIED	1360	13230	3563	15433
Rule3	VALIDATE	DIED	1125	9994	2601	11470
Neural3	TRAIN	DIED	789	7840	8953	16004
Neural3	VALIDATE	DIED	677	5887	6708	11918
Tree3	TRAIN	DIED	1393	13276	3517	15400
Tree3	VALIDATE	DIED	1158	10028	2567	11437
DmineReg3	TRAIN	DIED	1291	13086	3707	15502
DmineReg3	VALIDATE	DIED	1080	9887	2708	11515
MBR3	TRAIN	DIED	2750	13834	2959	14043
MBR3	VALIDATE	DIED	2301	10331	2264	10294
MBR4	TRAIN	DIED	2750	13834	2959	14043
MBR4	VALIDATE	DIED	2301	10331	2264	10294

the graphs for length of stay and total charges; figures 26 and 27 have the graphs restricted to level 3 and above.

Note that in the above two figures, there is a considerable difference in levels 1 and 2, with the probability of low cost and a length of stay of 3.5 days or less that is greater for level 1 compared to the other

Figure 20. Length of stay by disease staging: mortality level

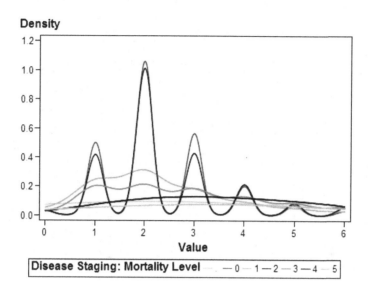

Figure 21. Total charges by disease staging: mortality level

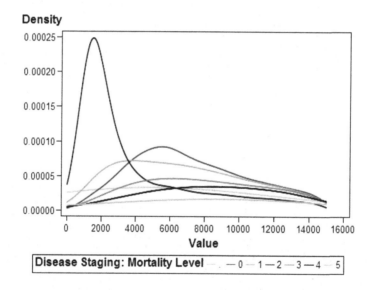

levels. This is in direct contrast to the results using the mortality index that show that level two has the highest probability of a low cost. It indicates that it is easier to "game" the mortality index than it is to "game" the resource demand level. The next two graphs are restricted to levels 3 and higher.

Figure 26 shows that as the level increases, the probability of a stay of greater than ten days increases while the probability of a stay of less than four days decreases as the level increases. However, the probability of a stay of between four and eight days is greater for level 4 than it is for level 5.

Figure 27 shows that the probability of costs less than $30,000 are generally less for level 5 than for level 4; at some point beyond 30,000, the two curves will intersect. Of interest, however, is that the

Figure 22. Length of stay by disease staging: mortality level for levels 3-5

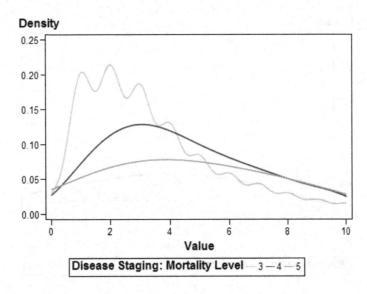

Figure 23. Total charges by disease staging: mortality level for levels 3-5

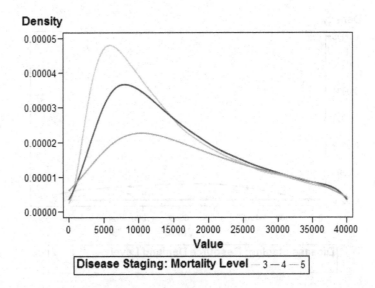

probability of a stay costing between $20,000 and $30,000 is greater for level 3 compared to level 5 as well. The results are similar to those using the resource mortality level.

However, compared to both the Charlson Index and the APRDRG Index, the overall probability for a stay of greater than 10 days is less for patients overall, indicating that this disease staging index is good for patients with generally less severity while the other two measures will better account for patients with much higher levels of severity. In other words, the disease staging indices do not help to predict the outcomes for the outlier patients.

Figure 24. Kernel density for length of stay by resource demand level

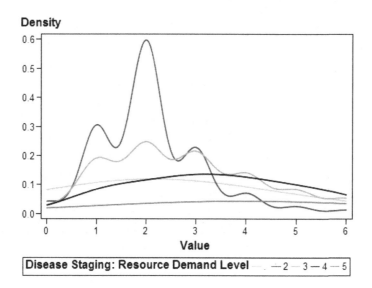

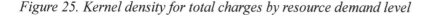

Figure 25. Kernel density for total charges by resource demand level

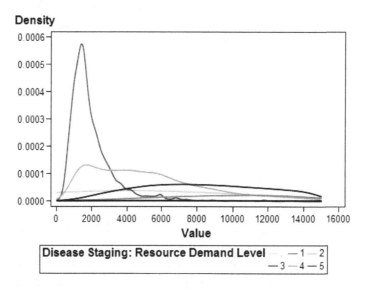

If we perform predictive modeling for length of stay, the optimal model is a decision tree. The tree is extensive with many different branches. Figure 28 shows the left-hand part of the tree; Figure 29 shows the center, and Figure 30 shows the right hand side. The left side predicts a shorter length of stay; the right side predicts a much higher length of stay. All three disease staging measures were used in the model.

Because of its extensiveness, we give some of the English Rules below:

```
IF Admission type < 3.5
AND 1.5 <= Disease Staging: Length of Stay Level < 2.5
```

Figure 26. Kernel density of length of stay for resource demand levels 3 and higher

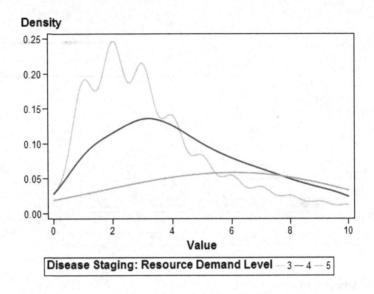

Figure 27. Kernel density of total charges for resource demand levels 3 and higher

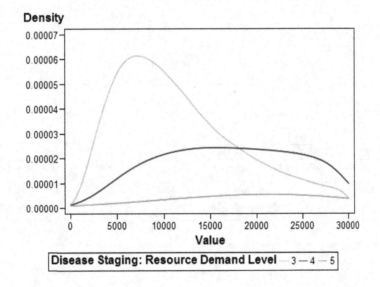

```
THEN
  NODE: 16
  N: 106547
  AVE: 1.96887
  SD: 2.90575
```

This first split gives the extremes in terms of the length of stay, splitting between an average of 1.5 days versus an average of 4.5 days.

Figure 28. Left side of decision tree

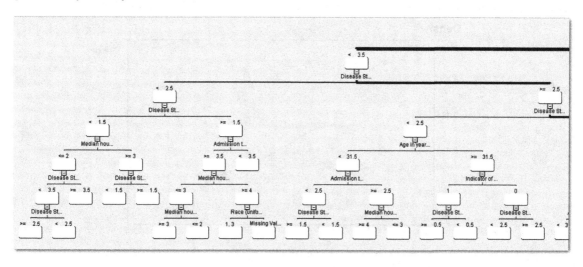

Figure 29. Center of decision tree

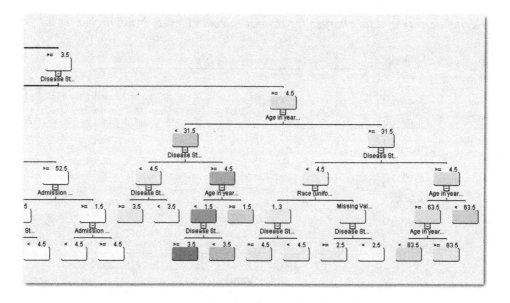

```
IF 1.5 <= Age in years at admission < 31.5
AND 4.5 <= Disease Staging: Resource Demand Level
AND 4.5 <= Disease Staging: Length of Stay Level
   THEN
   NODE: 41
   N: 1566
   AVE: 21.6903
   SD: 23.9904
IF 31.5 <= Age in years at admission < 63.5
AND 4.5 <= Disease Staging: Mortality Level
```

Figure 30. Right side of decision tree

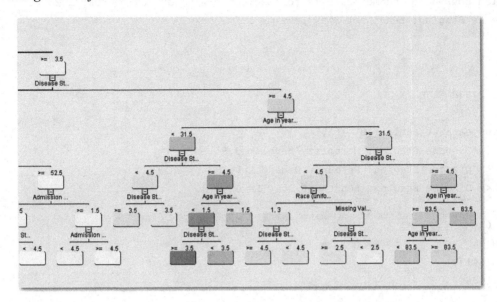

```
AND 4.5 <= Disease Staging: Length of Stay Level
THEN
  NODE: 44
  N: 2651
  AVE: 22.3093
  SD: 23.3815
IF Disease Staging: Resource Demand Level < 3.5
AND Age in years at admission < 31.5
AND 4.5 <= Disease Staging: Length of Stay Level
THEN
  NODE: 52
  N: 947
  AVE: 12.434
  SD: 18.2126
```

The next split is between an average of 12 days and an average of 22 days.

```
IF 3.5 <= Disease Staging: Resource Demand Level < 4.5
AND Age in years at admission < 31.5
AND 4.5 <= Disease Staging: Length of Stay Level
THEN
  NODE: 53
  N: 1581
  AVE: 15.0006
  SD: 15.3814
IF 3.5 <= Disease Staging: Resource Demand Level
```

```
AND Median household income quartile for patient's ZIP Code IS ONE OF: 1 2
AND Disease Staging: Length of Stay Level < 1.5
THEN
   NODE: 55
   N: 2670
   AVE: 1.27978
   SD: 0.74301
IF Age in years at admission < 65.5
AND 0.5 <= Disease Staging: Mortality Level < 3.5
AND 2.5 <= Disease Staging: Resource Demand Level
AND 2.5 <= Disease Staging: Length of Stay Level < 3.5
THEN
   NODE: 60
   N: 139408
   AVE: 3.54198
   SD: 3.18064
```

The last split shown separates an average stay of 1.2 days and 3.5 days. There is a strong possibility that this tree is too extensive and should be pruned. Such pruning is beyond the scope of this text, and we refer the reader to more detailed information on decision trees. (Ville, 2006) We also consider the outcome of total charges. The decision tree is again the best model. Since it is equally as complicated as the one for length of stay, we provide the beginning English rules. This tree does differ in that income quartile and race are prominently featured in the tree, although the disease staging levels form the first branches.

```
IF Disease Staging: Length of Stay Level < 4.5
AND Admission type < 1.5
AND 4.5 <= Disease Staging: Mortality Level
AND 4.5 <= Disease Staging: Resource Demand Level
THEN
   NODE: 42
   N: 1522
   AVE: 74756.2
   SD: 68010.7
```

This first level depends upon the disease staging, separating level 5 from the remaining levels.

```
IF Admission type IS MISSING
AND 4.5 <= Disease Staging: Mortality Level
AND 4.5 <= Disease Staging: Resource Demand Level
THEN
   NODE: 45
   N: 1437
   AVE: 208045
```

```
SD: 186099
```

Starting with the next level, race and income quartile are used to make the splits in the tree.

```
IF Race (uniform) IS ONE OF: 1 2 5
AND Median household income quartile for patient's ZIP Code IS ONE OF: 3 4
AND Admission type < 1.5
AND 2.5 <= Disease Staging: Resource Demand Level < 3.5
THEN
   NODE: 62
   N: 71128
   AVE: 18367.9
   SD: 19320.2
IF Race (uniform) IS ONE OF: 3 4 6
AND Median household income quartile for patient's ZIP Code IS ONE OF: 3 4
AND Admission type < 1.5
AND 2.5 <= Disease Staging: Resource Demand Level < 3.5
THEN
   NODE: 63
   N: 13072
   AVE: 21539.1
   SD: 24382
IF Median household income quartile for patient's ZIP Code IS ONE OF: 1 2
3
AND Race (uniform) EQUALS 1
AND Admission type < 2.5
AND 3.5 <= Disease Staging: Resource Demand Level < 4.5
THEN
   NODE: 64
   N: 43987
   AVE: 29756.9
   SD: 29730.3
IF Median household income quartile for patient's ZIP Code EQUALS 4
AND Race (uniform) EQUALS 1
AND Admission type < 2.5
AND 3.5 <= Disease Staging: Resource Demand Level < 4.5
THEN
   NODE: 65
   N: 15506
   AVE: 33577.4
   SD: 33142.4
IF Race (uniform) IS ONE OF: 1 5
AND 3.5 <= Admission source (uniform)
AND 2.5 <= Admission type
```

```
AND 3.5 <= Disease Staging: Resource Demand Level < 4.5
THEN
  NODE: 66
  N: 34346
   AVE: 38300.6
   SD: 32272.1
IF Race (uniform) IS ONE OF: 3 4 2 6
AND 3.5 <= Admission source (uniform)
AND 2.5 <= Admission type
AND 3.5 <= Disease Staging: Resource Demand Level < 4.5
THEN
  NODE: 67
  N: 7576
```

Table 8. Hospital by resource demand level: mortality

Table of DSHOSPID by DS_Mrt_Level					
Hospital	DS_Mrt_Level(Disease Staging: Mortality Level)				Total
Frequency Row Pct Col Pct	0	3	4	5	
1	0 0.00 0.00	35 27.56 8.93	75 59.06 10.98	17 13.39 20.48	127
2	1 1.59 50.00	17 26.98 4.34	43 68.25 6.30	2 3.17 2.41	63
3	0 0.00 0.00	12 25.53 3.06	33 70.21 4.83	2 4.26 2.41	47
4	1 0.43 50.00	75 32.61 19.13	140 60.87 20.50	14 6.09 16.87	230
5	0 0.00 0.00	42 48.84 10.71	38 44.19 5.56	6 6.98 7.23	86
6	0 0.00 0.00	45 20.64 11.48	148 67.89 21.67	25 11.47 30.12	218
7	0 0.00 0.00	11 21.15 2.81	39 75.00 5.71	2 3.85 2.41	52
9	0 0.00 0.00	38 17.35 9.69	166 75.80 24.30	15 6.85 18.07	219
10	0 0.00 0.00	117 99.15 29.85	1 0.85 0.15	0 0.00 0.00	118
Total	2	392	683	83	1160

AVE: 43274.3
SD: 41720

PREDICTIVE MODELING FOR QUALITY RANKING

We first look at our example of patients with COPD amongst the 9 hospitals to examine the relationship to the resource demand level measures. Tables 8, 9, and 10 give the proportion of patients in each level.

While hospital #6 has the highest proportion in level 4, hospitals #7 and 9 have a high proportion in the combined categories of 3 and 4. In contrast, hospital #10, with no actual mortality, has virtually all of its patients in mortality level 3. At level 3, we need to consider what the predicted mortality would be, and to consider that to be a valid measure, the predicted mortality should be less than it is for levels 1 and 2.

Table 9. Hospital by resource demand level: length of stay

Table of DSHOSPID by DS_LOS_Level				
Hospital	DS_LOS_Level(Disease Staging: Length of Stay Level)			Total
Frequency Row Pct Col Pct	3	4	5	
1	62 48.82 10.37	57 44.88 10.75	8 6.30 25.00	127
2	24 38.10 4.01	38 60.32 7.17	1 1.59 3.13	63
3	19 40.43 3.18	28 59.57 5.28	0 0.00 0.00	47
4	115 50.00 19.23	107 46.52 20.19	8 3.48 25.00	230
5	69 80.23 11.54	17 19.77 3.21	0 0.00 0.00	86
6	40 18.35 6.69	173 79.36 32.64	5 2.29 15.63	218
7	36 69.23 6.02	16 30.77 3.02	0 0.00 0.00	52
9	122 55.71 20.40	89 40.64 16.79	8 3.65 25.00	219
10	111 94.07 18.56	5 4.24 0.94	2 1.69 6.25	118
Total	598	530	32	1160

Table 10. Hospital by resource demand level: disease staging

Table of DSHOSPID by DS_RD_Level					
Hospital	**DS_RD_Level(Disease Staging: Resource Demand Level)**				**Total**
Frequency Row Pct Col Pct	**2**	**3**	**4**	**5**	
1	0 0.00 0.00	78 61.42 11.56	42 33.07 10.82	7 5.51 29.17	127
2	3 4.76 4.11	35 55.56 5.19	23 36.51 5.93	2 3.17 8.33	63
3	0 0.00 0.00	30 63.83 4.44	17 36.17 4.38	0 0.00 0.00	47
4	14 6.09 19.18	130 56.52 19.26	83 36.09 21.39	3 1.30 12.50	230
5	9 10.47 12.33	66 76.74 9.78	11 12.79 2.84	0 0.00 0.00	86
6	4 1.83 5.48	77 35.32 11.41	135 61.93 34.79	2 0.92 8.33	218
7	0 0.00 0.00	46 88.46 6.81	6 11.54 1.55	0 0.00 0.00	52
9	0 0.00 0.00	143 65.30 21.19	68 31.05 17.53	8 3.65 33.33	219
10	43 36.44 58.90	70 59.32 10.37	3 2.54 0.77	2 1.69 8.33	118
Total	73	675	388	24	1160

For patients with COPD, the levels of 1 and 2 are not assigned. Hospital #6 again has the highest proportion of patients in category 4; very few of the patients are in category #5. Hospital #10, again with no mortality has 94% of its patients in level 3; hospital #5 has 80% of its patients in that level.

Figure 31 shows the results of the predictive model to predict mortality rates. It shows that the memory based reasoning node is the most accurate with 28% misclassification. Figure 32 gives the decision tree for the results.

Note that the tree uses the patient's age only and none of the disease staging levels. This tree indicates that the results are highly questionable since the severity level is not used to predict the patient outcome of mortality. The ability of the model to predict mortality is extremely poor (Table 11).

Even though the predictive ability is extremely poor, we can still define a ranking, regardless of the accuracy of that ranking. In this case, because the demand resource levels skew toward the higher levels in comparison to the APRDRG levels, the threshold will have a high proportion of predicted mortality.

Figure 31. Results of predictive modeling

```
Fit Statistics
Model selection based on _TMISC_


                                        Test:
      Selected                    Misclassification
      Model         Model Node           Rate


                    AutoNeural2         0.46429
                    DMNeural2           0.28571
                    DmineReg2           0.53571
      Y             MBR2                0.28571
                    Neural2             0.39286
                    Reg2                0.46429
                    Rule2               0.35714
                    Tree2               0.32143
```

Figure 32. Decision tree model for predicting mortality

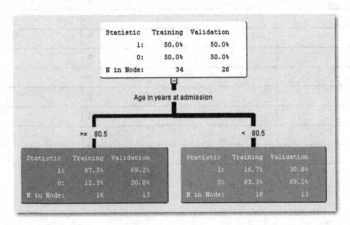

It is clear that predicted mortality of 55% and 85% is much too high to be useful. Table 12 compares the rankings of the APRDRG indices to the disease staging levels defined in this chapter.

Note that the rankings are very different between the two sets of index measures. For the APRDRG index, hospital #6 has the highest ranking; for the disease staging indices, hospital #3 has the highest ranking. In addition, the demand staging has difficulty in separating providers, giving two of the providers the same ranking. Table 12 again shows the lack of consistency across measures of patient severity.

We look to see how the disease staging measures compare with cardiovascular procedure 36.1. Tables 13, 14, and 15 compare the severity measures to the procedure. Note that all of the patients are in categories 3,4, and 5 for length of stay, indicating that this measure does recognize the more severe level of these patients.

Approximately ¾ of these patients are in category 4, with procedures 3612-3614 having the highest proportion in category 5. In Table 5, which focuses on mortality, the majority of patients are in category 3 rather than 4.

Table 11. Predicted versus actual mortality for COPD patients

Hospital	Actual	Predicted	Difference	Rank
1	3.94	62.20	58.26	5
2	7.94	61.90	53.96	6
3	2.13	85.11	82.98	1
4	4.78	54.78	50	7
5	4.65	54.65	50	7
6	3.21	61.93	58.72	4
7	3.85	78.85	75	2
9	4.11	77.63	73.52	3
10	0	0	0	9

Table 12. Comparison of APRDRG to demand resource level rankings

Hospital	APRDRG Ranking	Demand Staging Ranking
1	4	5
2	3	6
3	2	1
4	7	7
5	5	7
6	1	4
7	8	2
9	6	3
10	9	9

Table 13. Length of stay by procedure for disease staging

Table of DS_LOS_Level by PR1

DS_LOS_Level	PR1(Principal procedure)									Total
Frequency Row Pct Col Pct	3610	3611	3612	3613	3614	3615	3616	3617	3619	
3	3 / 0.05 / 37.50	800 / 13.01 / 15.65	1761 / 28.64 / 13.10	1608 / 26.15 / 12.20	857 / 13.94 / 11.89	1013 / 16.47 / 15.78	100 / 1.63 / 19.69	0 / 0.00 / 0.00	7 / 0.11 / 29.17	6149
4	5 / 0.01 / 62.50	3896 / 10.80 / 76.21	10566 / 29.30 / 78.58	10496 / 29.10 / 79.67	5757 / 15.96 / 79.87	4948 / 13.72 / 77.08	382 / 1.06 / 75.20	3 / 0.01 / 100.00	13 / 0.04 / 54.17	36066
5	0 / 0.00 / 0.00	416 / 11.28 / 8.14	1120 / 30.36 / 8.33	1071 / 29.03 / 8.13	594 / 16.10 / 8.24	458 / 12.42 / 7.14	26 / 0.70 / 5.12	0 / 0.00 / 0.00	4 / 0.11 / 16.67	3689
Total	8	5112	13447	13175	7208	6419	508	3	24	45904

Table 14. Mortality level by procedure

Table of DS_Mrt_Level by PR1										
DS_Mrt_Level	**PR1(Principal procedure)**									**Total**
Frequency Row Pct Col Pct	**3610**	**3611**	**3612**	**3613**	**3614**	**3615**	**3616**	**3617**	**3619**	
0	0	20	42	22	16	20	1	0	0	121
	0.00	16.53	34.71	18.18	13.22	16.53	0.83	0.00	0.00	
	0.00	0.39	0.31	0.17	0.22	0.31	0.20	0.00	0.00	
1	0	47	100	78	51	60	5	0	0	341
	0.00	13.78	29.33	22.87	14.96	17.60	1.47	0.00	0.00	
	0.00	0.92	0.74	0.59	0.71	0.93	0.98	0.00	0.00	
2	0	93	192	181	116	106	19	0	2	709
	0.00	13.12	27.08	25.53	16.36	14.95	2.68	0.00	0.28	
	0.00	1.82	1.43	1.37	1.61	1.65	3.74	0.00	8.33	
3	7	3406	9041	8893	4875	4412	365	2	15	31016
	0.02	10.98	29.15	28.67	15.72	14.22	1.18	0.01	0.05	
	87.50	66.63	67.23	67.50	67.63	68.73	71.85	66.67	62.50	
4	1	1244	3170	3103	1654	1465	96	1	6	10740
	0.01	11.58	29.52	28.89	15.40	13.64	0.89	0.01	0.06	
	12.50	24.33	23.57	23.55	22.95	22.82	18.90	33.33	25.00	
5	0	302	902	898	496	356	22	0	1	2977
	0.00	10.14	30.30	30.16	16.66	11.96	0.74	0.00	0.03	
	0.00	5.91	6.71	6.82	6.88	5.55	4.33	0.00	4.17	
Total	8	5112	13447	13175	7208	6419	508	3	24	45904
Frequency Missing = 3										

Table 15. Resource demand by procedure

Table of DS_RD_Level by PR1										
DS_RD_Level	**PR1(Principal procedure)**									**Total**
Frequency Row Pct Col Pct	**3610**	**3611**	**3612**	**3613**	**3614**	**3615**	**3616**	**3617**	**3619**	
3	0	0	1	1	0	0	0	0	0	2
	0.00	0.00	50.00	50.00	0.00	0.00	0.00	0.00	0.00	
	0.00	0.00	0.01	0.01	0.00	0.00	0.00	0.00	0.00	
4	3	404	926	747	415	518	50	0	2	3065
	0.10	13.18	30.21	24.37	13.54	16.90	1.63	0.00	0.07	
	37.50	7.90	6.89	5.67	5.76	8.07	9.84	0.00	8.33	
5	5	4708	12520	12427	6793	5901	458	3	22	42837
	0.01	10.99	29.23	29.01	15.86	13.78	1.07	0.01	0.05	
	62.50	92.10	93.11	94.32	94.24	91.93	90.16	100.00	91.67	
Total	8	5112	13447	13175	7208	6419	508	3	24	45904
Frequency Missing = 3										

In Table 15, the overwhelming majority (90% or above) of patients are in the highest resource demand category. It indicates that this one index recognizes that the patients undergoing bypass procedures are

Table 16. Length of stay by hospital for cardiovascular surgery

Table of DSHOSPID by DS_LOS_Level				
DSHOSPID	**DS_LOS_Level(Disease Staging: Length of Stay Level)**			**Total**
Frequency Row Pct Col Pct	**3**	**4**	**5**	
1	25 7.69 15.53	284 87.38 24.03	16 4.92 13.01	325
2	2 18.18 1.24	8 72.73 0.68	1 9.09 0.81	11
3	11 9.82 6.83	89 79.46 7.53	12 10.71 9.76	112
4	24 9.49 14.91	211 83.40 17.85	18 7.11 14.63	253
5	5 5.68 3.11	72 81.82 6.09	11 12.50 8.94	88
6	20 11.43 12.42	140 80.00 11.84	15 8.57 12.20	175
7	42 14.84 26.09	217 76.68 18.36	24 8.48 19.51	283
8	4 8.89 2.48	37 82.22 3.13	4 8.89 3.25	45
9	19 24.36 11.80	54 69.23 4.57	5 6.41 4.07	78
10	9 9.38 5.59	70 72.92 5.92	17 17.71 13.82	96
Total	161	1182	123	1466

in very serious condition, and will require considerable resources to treat. However, with so many of the patients in the same index level, it will be extremely difficult to use this measure to predict patient outcomes, and to distinguish between providers in terms of quality.

We compare these same three indices to the ten hospitals that perform cardiovascular surgery (Table 16). Hospital #7 has the highest proportion in the most severe category. This reconfirms the results from the APRDRG indices showing that #7 has the most severe patients while performing the most difficult surgeries compared to the other hospitals. However, hospital #1 also has a high proportion in category 4 in spite of having less severe surgeries. Table 17 shows the mortality index. Note that 36% of the patients in hospital #7 are in the highest mortality category; this is far higher than for any other hospital.

Table 18 shows the resource demand level. Note again that for the cardiovascular patients, there are

Table 17. Mortality disease staging by hospital

Table of DSHOSPID by DS_Mrt_Level							
DSHOSPID	**DS_Mrt_Level(Disease Staging: Mortality Level)**						**Total**
Frequency Row Pct Col Pct	**0**	**1**	**2**	**3**	**4**	**5**	
1	0 0.00 0.00	2 0.62 33.33	4 1.23 19.05	223 68.62 24.11	83 25.54 20.85	13 4.00 11.30	325
2	0 0.00 0.00	0 0.00 0.00	0 0.00 0.00	7 63.64 0.76	4 36.36 1.01	0 0.00 0.00	11
3	0 0.00 0.00	0 0.00 0.00	4 3.57 19.05	66 58.93 7.14	34 30.36 8.54	8 7.14 6.96	112
4	0 0.00 0.00	1 0.40 16.67	0 0.00 0.00	171 67.59 18.49	66 26.09 16.58	15 5.93 13.04	253
5	0 0.00 0.00	0 0.00 0.00	0 0.00 0.00	57 64.77 6.16	24 27.27 6.03	7 7.95 6.09	88
6	0 0.00 0.00	0 0.00 0.00	4 2.29 19.05	126 72.00 13.62	34 19.43 8.54	11 6.29 9.57	175
7	0 0.00 0.00	0 0.00 0.00	5 1.77 23.81	150 53.00 16.22	86 30.39 21.61	42 14.84 36.52	283
8	1 2.22 100.00	0 0.00 0.00	2 4.44 9.52	25 55.56 2.70	13 28.89 3.27	4 8.89 3.48	45
9	0 0.00 0.00	2 2.56 33.33	2 2.56 9.52	50 64.10 5.41	15 19.23 3.77	9 11.54 7.83	78
10	0 0.00 0.00	1 1.04 16.67	0 0.00 0.00	50 52.08 5.41	39 40.63 9.80	6 6.25 5.22	96
Total	1	6	21	925	398	115	1466

only two categories where patients are classified. Almost every hospital has 95% or higher in category 5. The lone exception is hospital #7, with the most crucial patients, the patients with the highest risk of mortality and severity, but with the lowest proportion of high resource demand. It appears that not only is hospital #1 "gaming" the system by shifting patients into higher categories, hospital #7 is "anti-gaming" by having its patients look less severe than they really are since hospital #7 has the highest level of mortality.

Figure 33 shows the results of the predictive model using just the resource demand level indices. Both the tree and rule induction models give a 26% misclassification level; all of the other models have much higher misclassification rates, indicating that these indices generally are poor predictors.

Figure 34 gives the decision tree for the model. Note that the model is based entirely upon the disease staging: mortality level.

Table 18. Resource demand level by hospital

Table of HOSPID by DS_RD_Level			
HOSPID	**DS_RD_Level(Disease Staging: Resource Demand Level)**		**Total**
Frequency Row Pct Col Pct	**4**	**5**	
1	2 0.62 2.90	323 99.38 23.12	325
2	0 0.00 0.00	11 100.00 0.79	11
3	2 1.79 2.90	110 98.21 7.87	112
4	14 5.53 20.29	239 94.47 17.11	253
5	1 1.14 1.45	87 98.86 6.23	88
6	10 5.71 14.49	165 94.29 11.81	175
7	26 9.19 37.68	257 90.81 18.40	283
8	1 2.22 1.45	44 97.78 3.15	45
9	9 11.54 13.04	69 88.46 4.94	78
10	4 4.17 5.80	92 95.83 6.59	96
Total	69	1397	1466

Because of the simplicity of the model, it is clear that level 5 mortality is the threshold to predict mortality. However, because of the severity of the patients, a high proportion of them already exist in level 5; this indicates that those patients in level 5 will be predicted for mortality. The predicted mortality is given in Table 19, compared to the actual mortality by hospital. We can compare these results to those from previous chapters.

Table 20 shows the relationship of the predicted mortality as given in Table 19 above to the actual proportion of patients in mortality index level 5 by hospital as listed in Table 17. The two columns are identical. Shifting patients into this level will increase the predicted mortality and improve the ranking of the provider.

These rankings are considerably different from those defined using the APRDRG indices (Table 21). Rank #1 from APRDRG becomes rank #9 for Resource Demand Level. Therefore, there is still the

Figure 33. Results of prediction of mortaility

```
Fit Statistics
Model selection based on _TMISC_


                                         Test:
  Selected                         Misclassification
   Model        Model Node               Rate


                AutoNeural8             0.57895
                DMNeural7               0.42105
                DmineReg8               0.42105
                MBR8                    0.47368
                Neural8                 0.57895
                Reg7                    0.47368
       Y        Rule4                   0.26316
                Tree8                   0.26316
```

Figure 34. Decision tree to predict mortality

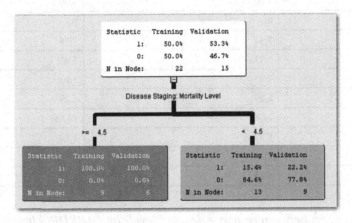

problem of robustness since providers can appear better or worse depending upon the measure used.

We now include the values of the Charlson Index and the APRDRG indices to the resource demand levels to see if we can improve the predictions. As shown in Figure 35, Dmine regression provides the best result with a very similar misclassification rate (21% versus 26%). The Dmine regression results are in Figure 36.

The resource demand level for mortality has the most importance followed by the APRDRG indices. The Charlson Index has lower importance compared to the hospitals. The results are in Tables 22 and 23. Again, note the similarity between the values in Table 17 for mortality level 5 and the predicted values as listed in Table 22.

Notice that while the rank using all indices is similar to the one using just the resource demand levels, there are still differences. We also examine the length of stay using all of the indices. The decision tree is the optimal model, with average error as given in Figure 37. This average error is 46, or less than the value of the mean. The decision tree is given in Figure 38.

Table 19. Predicted mortality versus actual mortality by hospital

Hospital	Actual Mortality	Predictive Mortality	Difference	Rank
1	1.23	4.00	2.77	8
2	0	0	0	10
3	4.46	7.14	2.68	9
4	0.79	5.93	5.14	6
5	1.14	7.95	6.81	3
6	0.57	6.29	5.72	5
7	3.53	14.84	11.31	1
8	2.22	8.89	6.67	4
9	1.28	11.54	10.26	2
10	3.13	6.25	3.12	7

Table 20. Predicted mortality versus mortality level 5

Hospital	Predicted Mortality	Mortality Level 5
1	4.00	4.00
2	0	0
3	7.14	7.14
4	5.93	5.93
5	7.95	7.95
6	6.29	6.29
7	14.84	14.84
9	8.89	8.89
10	11.54	11.54
	6.25	6.25

Table 21. Rank comparisons between resource demand levels and APRDRG indices

Hospital	APRDRG Rank	Resource Demand Rank
1	6	8
2	10	10
3	1	9
4	7	6
5	2	3
6	3	5
7	4	1
8	9	4
9	5	2
10	8	7

Figure 35. Predictive model results using all three indices

```
Fit Statistics
Model selection based on _TMISC_


                                        Test:
        Selected              Misclassification
        Model     Model Node        Rate


                  AutoNeural9       0.36842
                  DMNeural8         0.26316
          Y       DmineReg9         0.21053
                  MBR9              0.47368
                  Neural9           0.42105
                  Reg8              0.21053
                  Rule5             0.26316
                  Tree9             0.26316
```

Figure 36. Dmine regression results

```
The DMINE Procedure

                R-Squares for Target Variable: DIED

Effect                        DF      R-Square

AOV16: DS_Mrt_Level            2      0.781818
Var:   DS_Mrt_Level            1      0.774799
AOV16: APRDRG_Severity         2      0.688312
Var:   APRDRG_Severity         1      0.683891
AOV16: APRDRG_Risk_Mortality   3      0.630303
Var:   APRDRG_Risk_Mortality   1      0.582734
AOV16: AGE                    10      0.575758
Class: DSHOSPID                8      0.418182
Group: DSHOSPID                3      0.418182
AOV16: charlson                4      0.318903
AOV16: DS_LOS_Level            2      0.318182
Var:   DS_LOS_Level            1      0.310345
Var:   charlson                1      0.288889
Class: FEMALE                  1      0.142857
Class: ZIPInc_Qrtl             3      0.133838
Class: RACE                    3      0.068687
Group: RACE                    2      0.067769
Var:   AGE                     1      0.047311
Var:   DS_RD_Level             1             0   R2 < MINR2
AOV16: DS_RD_Level             0             0   R2 < MINR2
```

The APRDRG indices are used for the first branch; disease staging starts at the second. This shows that the indices are not redundant, but provide different information, and provide different answers for the problem of severity indices.

Table 22. Predicted mortality versus actual mortality by hospital using all indices

Hospital	Actual Mortality	Predictive Mortality	Difference	Rank
1	1.23	4.00	2.77	8
2	0	0	0	10
3	4.46	7.14	2.68	9
4	0.79	5.93	5.14	6
5	1.14	7.95	6.81	4
6	0.57	6.29	5.72	5
7	3.53	14.84	11.31	1
8	2.22	8.89	6.67	3
9	1.28	11.54	10.26	2
10	3.13	6.25	3.12	7

Table 23. Rank comparisons between resource demand levels and APRDRG indices, and all three indices combined

Hospital	APRDRG Rank	Resource Demand Rank	All Indices Combined
1	6	8	8
2	10	10	10
3	1	9	9
4	7	6	6
5	2	3	4
6	3	5	5
7	4	1	1
8	9	4	3
9	5	2	2
10	8	7	7

FUTURE TRENDS

While resource utilization should be a valid measure of patient severity since it seems safe to assume that patients with many co-morbidites will require more resources, there seems to be a problem since the use of these measures consistently under-value the conditions of the most severe patients. Moreover, the predicted models indicate that the mortality resource level is used primarily for prediction, and the threshold value for the logistic regression is defined as level 5 of the mortality index. Perhaps this index can be modified by adding more categories, and using an index with ten levels rather than 5.

Figure 37. Average error for length of stay using all indices

```
Fit Statistics
Model selection based on _TASE_

                                    Test:
                                    Average
        Selected                    Squared
        Model       MODEL           Error.

                    AutoNeural10     64.4857
                    DMNeural9        48.0283
                    DmineReg10       77.9684
                    MBR10            49.6799
                    Neural10         57.7048
                    Reg9             57.3475
        Y           Tree10           46.9658
```

Figure 38. Decision tree for prediction of length of stay

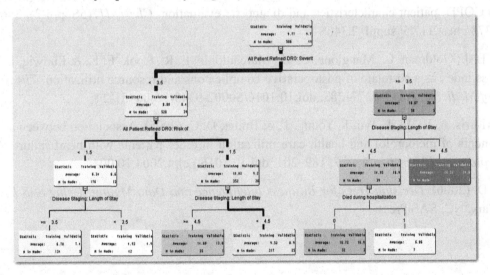

DISCUSSION

The disease staging for mortality, severity, and resource usage still has problems with the misclassification rate. The three types of models studied in this and the previous two chapters: Charlson, APRDRG, and Disease Staging have only a low level of correlation. Therefore, there remains a serious lack of consistency when defining the patient condition. Unfortunately, as we have also shown, the tendency to upcode to improve a provider's standing will remain a serious problem as long as regression-based models remain dominant in the methodology. Since it is clear that the threshold value is defined by the level 5 mortality index for disease staging, it would be a relatively simple matter to shift patients into level 5 to increase the prediction of mortality.

The disease staging indices appear to assume a lesser degree of severity in the patient population compared to the previous Charlson and APRDRG indices. For this reason, a significant portion of the patient population is in the highest level of severity. Moreover, for patients undergoing cardiovascular surgery, none are classified in the lowest two index levels. The main problem here with a substantial portion of the patients in the highest levels is that there is no ability to classify the sickest patients into a higher category of severity, and the sickest patients are combined into the same class level as patients with more moderate conditions. Therefore, predictions for length of stay and total charges will not reach as high as they should given the gamma distributions of the outcome variables. These disease staging models have difficulty with predicting true patient outliers.

REFERENCES

Kotelchuck, M. (1994). An evaluation of the Kessner adequacy of prenatal care index and a proposed adequacy of prenatal care utilization index. *American Journal of Public Health*, *84*(9), 1414–1420. doi:10.2105/AJPH.84.9.1414

Mapel, D. W., Picchi, M. A., Hurley, J. S., Frost, F. J., Petersen, H. V., & Mapel, V. M. (2000). Utilization in COPD: patient characteristics and diagnostic evaluation. *Chest*, *117*(5Suppl 2), 346s–353s. doi:10.1378/chest.117.5_suppl_2.346S

Thomas, E. J., Goldman, L., Mangione, C. M., Marcantonio, E. R., Cook, E. F., & Ludwig, L. (1997). Body mass index as a correlate of postoperative complicatons and resource utilization. *The American Journal of Medicine*, *102*(3), 277–283. doi:10.1016/S0002-9343(96)00451-2

Tu, W., Morris, A. B., Li, J., Wu, J., Young, J., & Brater, D. C. (2005). Association between adherence measurements of metoprolol and health care utilization in older patients with heart failure. *Clinical Pharmacology and Therapeutics*, *77*, 189–201. doi:10.1016/j.clpt.2004.10.004

Ville, B. D. (2006). *Decision Trees for Business Intelligence and Data Mining: Using SAS Enterprise Miner*. Cary, NC: SAS Press.

Chapter 8
Text Mining and Patient Severity Clusters

INTRODUCTION

The problem with using the diagnosis codes is that there are just too many to be able to use them all in a predictive model or regression. The requirements of a predictive model are that categorical data have just a small number of levels; this requirement will lead to the need to compress the number of levels in the variable. Therefore, thus far, there is a predetermined list of codes that count in risk adjustment, leaving many codes not included (as in the case of the Charlson Index). Otherwise, consensus panels are used to determine categories of severity, as in the case of the APRDRG Index. We have shown that in many cases, some of the omitted codes include as much, if not more, risk compared to those codes that are included; patients with the omitted conditions will be identified as less severe compared to patients with included conditions. In this chapter, we will introduce a method that can compress the diagnoses into clusters while still using all of the codes, without relying upon consensus panels. Moreover, outcomes are not used to define the severity index, so they can be used to validate the model; outcomes can then be used to consider the quality of providers.

Perhaps the major reason to use the modeling here is that the methodology described does not require that the diagnosis codes used are independent as is required for regression models; in fact, the modeling

DOI: 10.4018/978-1-60566-752-2.ch008

makes use of the dependency in the codes as defined by co-morbidities. Moreover, the methodology does not require the assumption of the uniformity of data entry. Again, the method described in this chapter has the capacity to ignore the upcoding of some healthcare providers; moreover, it can be used to identify those providers who are upcoding. Since uniformity is a false assumption that is required to use regression models, it is possible to generate a patient severity index using text mining that is superior to those in current use defined by using logistic regression models.

Text mining diagnosis codes takes advantage of the linkage across patient conditions instead of trying to force the assumption of independence. Combinations of diagnoses are used to define groups of patients. For example, patients with diabetes have a high probability of heart disease and kidney failure compared to the general population. Instead of relying on these three conditions and assuming that the general population is just as likely to acquire them in combination, text mining examines the combinations of diabetes, diabetes with kidney failure, diabetes with heart failure, and diabetes with both conditions.

BACKGROUND

Nominal data have always been difficult to use in quantitative analyses. There always has to be some way to compress text into a small number of categories. Under recent development, methods have been devised that can use grammar, syntax, and natural language to quantify information that is locked in text format. The methodologies developed are labeled under the general topic of text mining.

The process of text analysis generally involves the following steps:

1. Transpose the data so that the observational unit is the identifier and all nominal values are defined in the observational unit.
2. Tokenize the nominal data so that each nominal value is defined as one token.
3. Concatenate the nominal tokens into a text string such that there is one text string per identifier. Each text string is a collection of tokens; each token represents a noun.
4. Use text mining to cluster the text strings so that each identifier belongs to one cluster.
5. Use other statistical methods to define a natural ranking in the clusters.
6. Use the clusters defined by text mining in other statistical analyses.

The first step in analyzing text data is to define a term by document matrix. Each document forms a row of the matrix; each term forms a column. The resulting matrix will be extremely large, but very sparse, with most of the cells containing zeros. The matrix can be compressed using the technique of singular value decomposition with the matrix restricted to a maximum of N dimensions. In our example, the document consists of a text string of ICD9 codes, and each of the codes forms a column. Each cell contains a count of the number of times a code appears in a document. In this case, the document is defined as the patient's condition, and each code defines one diagnosis of the condition. Since there are only a handful of diagnoses connected to any one patient, most of the cells will contain the value, '0'. Therefore, the matrix will be very large, but most of the cells will be empty.

Singular value decomposition is based upon an assignment of weights to each term in the dataset. Terms that are common and appear frequently, such as 'of', 'and', 'the' are given low or zero weight while terms that appear in only a handful of documents are given a high weight (entropy). Other weighting schemes take into consideration target or outcome variables (information gain, chi-square). In our example, there are only diagnosis codes, and common terms are in fact common diagnoses. It is the less common diagnoses that are given higher weights compared to more common terms. Therefore, 'flu' will have a low weight while 'metastatic lung cancer' will have a much higher weight. We initially use the standard entropy weighting method, so that the most common ICD9 codes (hypertension, disorder of lipid metabolism or high cholesterol) will be given low weights while less common (uncontrolled Type I diabetes with complications) will be given higher weights.

Clustering was performed using the expectation maximization algorithm. (Cerrito, 2007) It is a relatively new, iterative clustering technique that works well with nominal data in comparison to the K-means and hierarchical methods that are more standard. The clusters are identified by the terms that most clearly represent the text strings contained within the cluster. It does not mean that every patient has the representative combination of terms. It does mean that the linkages within the terms are the ones that have the highest identified weights.

This chapter gives an application of the use of text mining to the development of a patient severity index. It is not intended to give a complete discussion on how text mining is performed, and how natural language processing has enhanced the development of text mining. Instead, we refer the interested reader to several textbooks that provide detailed information on the process of text mining.(Feldman & Sanger, 2006; Kao & Poteet, 2006; Weiss, Indurkhya, Zhang, & Damerau, 2004)

In this chapter, we will develop an artificial language of text strings that are composed of nouns. The nouns in the string represent patient conditions and/or procedures. Then, the methodology that was initially developed to analyze sentences and paragraphs can also be used on these text strings. The natural language methods take advantage of the linkage between codes that are related to any one patient. It is the combinations of codes rather than the individual codes that are used to define clusters of patients.

Consider one such string: 682.7, 250.02, 730.17, 681.10, 401.9, 593.9, and 285.29. The translations are Other cellulitis and abscess of foot except toe, Type II diabetes without complications, Chronic osteomyelitis of the ankle and foot, Cellulitis and abscess, unspecified, Essential hypertension, Unspecified disorder of kidney and ureter, and Anemia of other chronic illness. This patient has diabetes and long-term problems with foot ulcers, cellulitis, and infection in the bone. In addition, this patient has kidney problems with anemia. A second string is 682.7, 041.11, v09.0, and 042. This patient has Other cellulitis and abscess of foot except toe, Staphylococcus aureus, Infection with microorganisms resistant to penicillins, and Human immunodeficiency virus [HIV] disease. This patient has foot ulcers with resistant infection related to HIV rather than to diabetes.

TEXT ANALYSIS OF DIAGNOSIS CODES

We first look at the diagnosis codes for the patients. Using all of the 3 digit codes in one text string, we can use the text analysis to define a total of ten different clusters. Using a 1% sample of the National Inpatient Sample for 2005 because of the computational time involved, we find the clusters given in Table 1. Once the clusters are defined, the scoring mechanism can be used in SAS Enterprise Miner to place all of the patients into the identified text clusters.

It is clear that clusters 2 and 4 are focused primarily upon childbirth. We will first look at the relationship of these text clusters to patient outcomes. Then we can also define clusters after first eliminating all diagnoses related to childbirth, which are very specific and not specifically related to patients with other diagnoses. Table 2 gives the probability of mortality by cluster. At this point, the clusters were not

Table 1. Ten clusters of diagnosis codes using 1% sample

Cluster	ICD9 Codes	Translation	Frequency
1	410, 486, 428, 401, 411, 272, 599, 496, v45, 276	Acute Myocardial Infarction, Pneumonia, Heart Failure, Organism Unspecified, Essential Hypertension, Acute And Subacute Forms Of Ischemic Heart Disease, Disorders Of Lipoid Metabolism, Other Disorders Of Urethra And Urinary Tract, Chronic Airway Obstruction, Other Postprocedural States, Disorders Of Fluid, Electrolyte, And Acid-base Balance	23,213
2	770, v30, v05, 663, 652, 654, 766, 650, v27, 661	Other Respiratory Conditions Of Fetus And Newborn, Single Liveborn, Need For Other Prophylactic Vaccination And Inoculation Against Single Diseases, Umbilical Cord Complications During Labor And Delivery, Malposition And Malpresentation Of Fetus, Abnormality Of Organs And Soft Tissues Of Pelvis, Disorders Relating To Long Gestation And High Birthweight, Normal Delivery, Outcome Of Delivery, Abnormality Of Forces Of Labor	27,095
3	995, 530, 305, 285, 276, 571, 785, 493, 486	Certain Adverse Effects NEC, Diseases Of Esophagus, Nondependent Abuse Of Drugs, Other And Unspecified Anemias, Disorders Of Fluid, Electrolyte, And Acid-base Balance, Chronic Liver Disease And Cirrhosis, Symptoms Involving Cardiovascular System, Asthma	17,657
4	745, 770, 530, v30, 771, 747, 785, 493, 486, 774	Bulbus Cordis Anomalies And Anomalies Of Cardiac Septal Closure, Other Respiratory Conditions Of Fetus And Newborn, Diseases Of Esophagus, Single Liveborn, Infections Specific To The Perinatal Period, Other Congenital Anomalies Of Circulatory System, Symptoms Involving Cardiovascular System, Asthma, Pneumonia, Organism Unspecified, Other Perinatal Jaundice	5665
5	285, 787, 998, 496, 560, 250, 530, 278, v15, 574	Other And Unspecified Anemias, Symptoms Involving Digestive System, Other Complications Of Procedures, NEC, [INSERT FIGURE 001]Chronic Airway Obstruction, NEC, Intestinal Obstruction Without Mention Of Hernia, Diabetes, Diseases Of Esophagus, Overweight, Obesity And Other Hyperalimentation, Other Personal History Presenting Hazards To Health, Cholelithiasis	27,663
6	401, v58, 278, v12, 733, 424, 715, 427, 428, 272	Essential Hypertension, Encounter For Other And Unspecified Procedures And Aftercare, Overweight, Obesity And Other Hyperalimentation, Personal History Of Certain Other Diseases, Other Disorders Of Bone And Cartilage, Other Diseases Of Endocardium, Osteoarthrosis And Allied Disorders, Cardiac Dysrhythmias, Heart Failure, Disorders Of Lipoid Metabolism	14,615
7	300, 311, 309, 296, v15, 295, 722, 304, 278, 493	Anxiety, Dissociative And Somatoform Disorders, Depressive Disorder, NEC, Adjustment Reaction, Episodic Mood Disorders, Other Personal History Presenting Hazards To Health, Schizophrenic Disorders, Intervertebral Disc Disorders, Drug Dependence, Overweight, Obesity And Other Hyperalimentation, Asthma	12,956
8	311, 780, v57, 285, 781, 438, v43, 331, 401, 733	Depressive Disorder, NEC, General Symptoms, Care Involving Use Of Rehabilitation Procedures, Other And Unspecified Anemias, Symptoms Involving Nervous And Musculoskeletal Systems, Late Effects Of Cerebrovascular Disease, Organ Or Tissue Replaced By Other Means, Other Cerebral Degenerations, Essential Hypertension, Other Disorders Of Bone And Cartilage	7850
9	041, 197, 486, 276, 790, 707, v10, 682, 780, v09	Bacterial Infection In Conditions Classified Elsewhere And Of Unspecified Site, Secondary Malignant Neoplasm Of Respiratory And Digestive Systems, Pneumonia, Organism Unspecified, Disorders Of Fluid, Electrolyte, And Acid-base Balance, Nonspecific Findings On Examination Of Blood, Chronic Ulcer Of Skin, Personal History Of Malignant Neoplasm, Other Cellulitis And Abscess, General Symptoms, Infection With Drug-resistant Microorganisms	14,412
10	654, 644, 658, v23, 663, 646, 645, 652, 661, v27	Abnormality Of Organs And Soft Tissues Of Pelvis, Early Or Threatened Labor, Other Problems Associated With Amniotic Cavity And Membranes, Supervision Of High-risk Pregnancy, Umbilical Cord Complications During Labor And Delivery, Other Complications Of Pregnancy, NEC, Late Pregnancy, Malposition And Malpresentation Of Fetus, Abnormality Of Forces Of Labor, Outcome Of Delivery	8775

defined using any of the outcome variables. Therefore, we can examine the clusters in relationship to the outcomes and we can look at mortality, charges, and length of stay with respect to the different clusters.

In terms of mortality, there is a natural ordering in the ten defined clusters, $10<7<2<4<6<5<8<9<1<3$.

Table 2. Mortality by cluster

Table of allclusters by DIED			
allclusters	**DIED**		**Total**
Frequency **Row Pct** **Col Pct**	**0**	**1**	
1	22253 95.90 14.23	952 4.10 27.76	23205
2	27035 99.80 17.29	55 0.20 1.60	27090
3	16572 93.91 10.60	1074 6.09 31.32	17646
4	5625 99.29 3.60	40 0.71 1.17	5665
5	27187 98.32 17.38	464 1.68 13.53	27651
6	14413 98.66 9.22	196 1.34 5.72	14609
7	12936 99.89 8.27	14 0.11 0.41	12950
8	7657 97.63 4.90	186 2.37 5.42	7843
9	13956 96.90 8.92	447 3.10 13.04	14403
10	8772 99.99 5.61	1 0.01 0.03	8773

Consider cluster 3 with anemia, dehydration, liver and heart disease, and asthma. These patients have multiple and severe co-morbidities. Note that anemia and asthma are not contained within the list of Charlson Index conditions, although liver and heart disease are included.

Similarly, the patients in cluster 1 mostly have severe heart disease with no non-heart related co-morbidities. In contrast, cluster 10 is related to complications of pregnancy and delivery that will very seldom result in death. None of the diagnoses in cluster 10 are included in the Charlson Index. Patients in cluster 7 have serious mental disorders; severe depression can result in suicide. Again, none of the conditions are included in the Charlson Index. Cluster 8 also has mental disorders that accompany some difficult physical problems.

Table 3 gives the summary statistics for length of stay and total charges. Note the ordering of the clusters, 2<10<6<7<1<4<9<5<3<8 for length of stay. For total charges, the order is 2<10<7<4<9<8<6<5<1<3. Note that the orders are slightly different for the two outcomes. As means are susceptible to outliers,

Table 3. Summary statistics by cluster

Cluster Number	N Obs	Variable	Mean	Std Dev	Minimum	Maximum
1	23213	LOS	4.9532589	6.2661966	0	160.0000000
		TOTCHG	31049.85	41923.65	75.0000000	878999.00
2	27095	LOS	2.7629083	4.3595463	0	142.0000000
		TOTCHG	6709.54	17419.82	29.0000000	690811.00
3	17657	LOS	5.6405392	8.8703964	0	219.0000000
		TOTCHG	31784.15	60821.73	35.0000000	993107.00
4	5665	LOS	5.1419241	12.6491378	0	265.0000000
		TOTCHG	21622.08	53211.10	35.0000000	838707.00
5	27663	LOS	5.3739426	6.3360912	0	154.0000000
		TOTCHG	27290.85	40271.16	35.0000000	966378.00
6	14615	LOS	4.0107431	4.3202349	0	191.0000000
		TOTCHG	26859.63	31417.12	35.0000000	919723.00
7	12956	LOS	4.5065998	6.2346689	0	149.0000000
		TOTCHG	17698.05	22699.33	35.0000000	755327.00
8	7850	LOS	6.5688623	8.2627672	0	315.0000000
		TOTCHG	23245.37	32148.28	263.0000000	797968.00
9	14412	LOS	5.2954892	7.0770023	0	233.0000000
		TOTCHG	22256.87	34559.13	35.0000000	705743.00
10	8775	LOS	2.8694017	3.3940094	0	122.0000000
		TOTCHG	9835.06	12656.74	494.0000000	740929.00

we can avoid this susceptibility by looking at the kernel density probabilities as well (Figures 1 and 2).

Cluster 2, for treating a newborn, has both the lowest costs and total charges, followed by cluster 10 for labor and delivery. Cluster 7, for patients with severe mental disorders, very likely has low costs because the facilities in the NIS exclude psychiatric institutions so that those patients with severe prob-

Figure 1. Probability density for length of stay

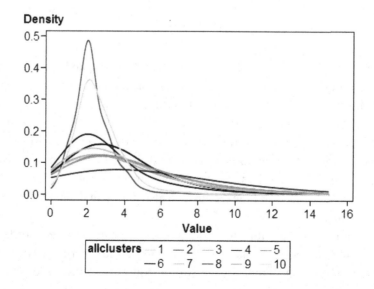

Figure 2. Probability density for total charges

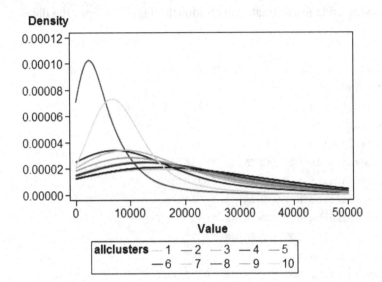

lems are discharged to other providers that are more specific to their diagnoses. Cluster 6, with more mild co-morbidities, is also on the lower end for both length of stay and total charges, but a slightly higher risk of mortality. Figure 1 gives the probability distribution for length of stay; Figure 2 gives the probability for total charges. We want to see if there is a hierarchy embedded within the kernel density distributions that can identify the order of severity.

From the distribution, 2<10<4<7<3<1<5<9<6<8 for length of stay. We define this ordering by the probabilityof having a length of stay between 0 and 4 days. The higher the curve, the greater the probability of having 0-4 days of stay. There is a crossover point where the ordering changes, so that the cluster with the lowest probability of a stay of 4 days or less has the highest probability of a stay of 8 or more days. In Figure 1, there are two cutpoints (or crossover points). The first occurs just beyond the 4-day mark where clusters 2 and 10 crossover, with the lowest probability of a stay beyond 5 days. Cluster 4 also crosses over at that point. The second cutpoint occurs at 6 days where the remaining clusters switch from lower to higher probabilities.

Note that the ordering in Figure 1 is not the same as it is when just using the mean. Since the mean is unduly influenced by the presence of outliers, when the distributions are as highly skewed as they are in Figure 2, it is better to use medians.

For total charges, 2<10<4<7<9<3<5<8<6<1. The distribution for total charges has an ordering that is almost the same as it is for length of stay. There are also three cutpoints in Figure 2. The first occurs at just over $10,000 when cluster 2 moves from the highest probability of a total charge of less than 10,000 to the lowest probability of a charge of greater than 10,000. The second cutpoint occurs for cluster ten at approximately $15,000. The third cutpoint for the remaining clusters is at just over $20,000.

Because of the dominance of childbirth and delivery in two of the clusters, the results are not quite as representative as they should be. Therefore, we want to re-cluster after first eliminating any patient conditions that are related to childbirth. We also want to eliminate all newborn conditions, as they are also related to childbirth. Therefore, we use SAS coding to remove from consideration all patients with ICD9 codes 630-677 (related to labor and delivery), 760-779 (related to newborns), and V20-V39 (pre-existing conditions related to childbirth).

We use the following code to eliminate the childbirth diagnoses from the dataset:

```
PROC SQL
CREATE TABLE Public.reduceddiagnoses AS SELECT Public.textmining
FROM Public.TEXTMINING AS textmining
WHERE textmining.diagnoses3digits NOT CONTAINS "630" and
textmining.diagnoses3digits NOT CONTAINS "631" and
textmining.diagnoses3digits NOT CONTAINS "632" and
textmining.diagnoses3digits NOT CONTAINS "633" and
textmining.diagnoses3digits NOT CONTAINS "634" and
textmining.diagnoses3digits NOT CONTAINS "635" and
textmining.diagnoses3digits NOT CONTAINS "636" and
textmining.diagnoses3digits NOT CONTAINS "637" and
textmining.diagnoses3digits NOT CONTAINS "638" and
textmining.diagnoses3digits NOT CONTAINS "639" and
textmining.diagnoses3digits NOT CONTAINS "640" and
textmining.diagnoses3digits NOT CONTAINS "641" and
textmining.diagnoses3digits NOT CONTAINS "642" and
textmining.diagnoses3digits NOT CONTAINS "643" and
textmining.diagnoses3digits NOT CONTAINS "644" and
textmining.diagnoses3digits NOT CONTAINS "645" and
textmining.diagnoses3digits NOT CONTAINS "646" and
textmining.diagnoses3digits NOT CONTAINS "647" and
textmining.diagnoses3digits NOT CONTAINS "648" and
textmining.diagnoses3digits NOT CONTAINS "649" and
textmining.diagnoses3digits NOT CONTAINS "650" and
textmining.diagnoses3digits NOT CONTAINS "651" and
textmining.diagnoses3digits NOT CONTAINS "652"and
textmining.diagnoses3digits NOT CONTAINS "653" and
textmining.diagnoses3digits NOT CONTAINS "654" and
textmining.diagnoses3digits NOT CONTAINS "655" and
textmining.diagnoses3digits NOT CONTAINS "656" and
textmining.diagnoses3digits NOT CONTAINS "657" and
textmining.diagnoses3digits NOT CONTAINS "658" and
textmining.diagnoses3digits NOT CONTAINS "659" and
textmining.diagnoses3digits NOT CONTAINS "660" and
textmining.diagnoses3digits NOT CONTAINS "661" and
textmining.diagnoses3digits NOT CONTAINS "662" and
textmining.diagnoses3digits NOT CONTAINS "663" and
textmining.diagnoses3digits NOT CONTAINS "664" and
textmining.diagnoses3digits NOT CONTAINS "665" and
textmining.diagnoses3digits NOT CONTAINS "666" and
textmining.diagnoses3digits NOT CONTAINS "667" and
```

```
textmining.diagnoses3digits NOT CONTAINS "668" and
textmining.diagnoses3digits NOT CONTAINS "669" and
textmining.diagnoses3digits NOT CONTAINS "670" and
textmining.diagnoses3digits NOT CONTAINS "671" and
textmining.diagnoses3digits NOT CONTAINS "672" and
textmining.diagnoses3digits NOT CONTAINS "673" and
textmining.diagnoses3digits NOT CONTAINS "674" and
textmining.diagnoses3digits NOT CONTAINS "675" and
textmining.diagnoses3digits NOT CONTAINS "676" and
textmining.diagnoses3digits NOT CONTAINS "677" and
textmining.diagnoses3digits NOT CONTAINS "760" and
textmining.diagnoses3digits NOT CONTAINS "761" and
textmining.diagnoses3digits NOT CONTAINS "762" and
textmining.diagnoses3digits NOT CONTAINS "763" and
textmining.diagnoses3digits NOT CONTAINS "764" and
textmining.diagnoses3digits NOT CONTAINS "765" and
textmining.diagnoses3digits NOT CONTAINS "766" and
textmining.diagnoses3digits NOT CONTAINS "767" and
textmining.diagnoses3digits NOT CONTAINS "768" and
textmining.diagnoses3digits NOT CONTAINS "769" and
textmining.diagnoses3digits NOT CONTAINS "770" and
textmining.diagnoses3digits NOT CONTAINS "771" and
textmining.diagnoses3digits NOT CONTAINS "772" and
textmining.diagnoses3digits NOT CONTAINS "773" and
textmining.diagnoses3digits NOT CONTAINS "774" and
textmining.diagnoses3digits NOT CONTAINS "775" and
textmining.diagnoses3digits NOT CONTAINS "776" and
textmining.diagnoses3digits NOT CONTAINS "777" and
textmining.diagnoses3digits NOT CONTAINS "778" and
textmining.diagnoses3digits NOT CONTAINS "779" and
textmining.diagnoses3digits NOT CONTAINS "v20" and
textmining.diagnoses3digits NOT CONTAINS "v21" and
textmining.diagnoses3digits NOT CONTAINS "v22" and
textmining.diagnoses3digits NOT CONTAINS "v23" and
textmining.diagnoses3digits NOT CONTAINS "v24" and
textmining.diagnoses3digits NOT CONTAINS "v25" and
textmining.diagnoses3digits NOT CONTAINS "v26" and
textmining.diagnoses3digits NOT CONTAINS "v27" and
textmining.diagnoses3digits NOT CONTAINS "v28" and
textmining.diagnoses3digits NOT CONTAINS "v29" and
textmining.diagnoses3digits NOT CONTAINS "v30" and
textmining.diagnoses3digits NOT CONTAINS "v31" and
textmining.diagnoses3digits NOT CONTAINS "v32" and
textmining.diagnoses3digits NOT CONTAINS "v33" and
```

```
textmining.diagnoses3digits NOT CONTAINS "v34" and
textmining.diagnoses3digits NOT CONTAINS "v35" and
textmining.diagnoses3digits NOT CONTAINS "v36" and
textmining.diagnoses3digits NOT CONTAINS "v37" and
textmining.diagnoses3digits NOT CONTAINS "v38" and
textmining.diagnoses3digits NOT CONTAINS "v39"
;
Run;
```

We next examine the ICD9 codes that occur most often in the National Inpatient Sample, omitting all codes related to childbirth (Table 4).

It is not surprising that hypertension and diabetes are more common than any other patient conditions. Because they are so common, they will not be able to distinguish between different groups of patients; therefore, some of the less common conditions will be of more value when used to define the patient clusters (Table 5).

Patients in Cluster 1 have some severe problems largely related to shortness of air and/or pneumonia. Cluster 2 patients have some severe mental disorders, including drug and alcohol abuse. In contrast, patients in cluster 4 have diagnoses that are almost exclusively related to drug abuse with no depression. Those in Cluster 3 have some severe infections, including cellulitis and skin ulcers that are related to diabetes. Patients in cluster 3 can also have an infection of the blood.

In Cluster 5, patients have problems of the head, neck, and spine. This can also include the condition of stroke. Cluster 6 patients have kidney failure plus complications that are largely related to dialysis, including urinary tract infections. In Cluster 7, patients have anxiety plus other chronic problems including arthritis, shortness of air, and artificial devices. These artifical devices can include orthopedic replacement joints as well as pacemakers. These patients have a need for rehabilitation of some type. Cluster 7, if examined, will very likely have older patients compared to some of the other clusters. Cluster 8

Table 4. Most common ICD9 codes

Code	Translation	Frequency	Code	Translation	Frequency
401	Essential hypertension	113,294	285	Other and unspecified anemias	33,153
250	Diabetes	63,615	530	Diseases of esophagus	33,055
276	Disorders of fluid, electrolyte, and acid-base balance	59,845	599	Other disorders of urethra and urinary tract	27,347
414	Other forms of chronic ischemic heart disease	58,221	496	Chronic airway obstruction, not elsewhere classified	24,863
272	Disorders of lipoid metabolism	53,956	244	Acquired hypothyroidism	23,097
427	Cardiac dysrhythmias	46,402	715	Osteoarthrosis and allied disorders	22,257
428	Heart failure	43,391	486	Pneumonia, organism unspecified	21,193
305	Nondependent abuse of drug	38,414	493	Asthma	21,170
780	General symptoms	36,393	V15	Other personal history presenting hazards to health	20,438
V45	Other postprocedural states (renal dialysis, cardiac device in situ)	34,947	518	Other diseases of lung	19,182

classifies patients with problems in the female reproductive system. Patients in Cluster 9 have a serious heart problem, including ischemic heart disease. Cluster 10 generally contains patients with abdominal problems, and problems in the digestive system. These patients appear to have milder conditions compared to some of the other clusters. Note that diseases of the esophagus are fairly common across the

Table 5. Ten clusters of diagnosis codes eliminating childbirth using a 5% sample

Cluster	ICD9 Codes	Translation	Frequency
1	530, 278, 786, 305, 493, 496, 518, 491, 486, 272	Diseases of esophagus, Overweight, obesity and other hyperalimentation, Symptoms involving respiratory system and other chest symptoms, Nondependent abuse of drugs, Asthma, Chronic airway obstruction, not elsewhere classified, Other diseases of lung, Chronic bronchitis, Pneumonia, organism unspecified, Disorders of lipoid metabolism	35,484
2	304, 311, 300, 303, 305, 295, 788, 291, 592, 724	Drug dependence, Depressive disorder, not elsewhere classified, Anxiety, dissociative and somatoform disorders, Alcohol dependence syndrome, Nondependent abuse of drugs, Schizophrenic disorders, Symptoms involving urinary system, Alcohol-induced mental disorders, Calculus of kidney and ureter, Other and unspecified disorders of back	30,608
3	995, 403, 038, 682, 707, 599, 518, 584, 780, 041	Certain adverse effects not elsewhere classified, Hypertensive kidney disease, Septicemia, Other cellulitis and abscess, Chronic ulcer of skin, Other disorders of urethra and urinary tract, Other diseases of lung, Acute renal failure, General symptoms, Bacterial infection in conditions classified elsewhere and of unspecified site	62,321
4	303, 493, 724, 304, 309, v62, v15, 305, 301, 314	Alcohol dependence syndrome, Asthma, Other and unspecified disorders of back, Alcohol dependence syndrome, Adjustment reaction, Other psychosocial circumstances, Other personal history presenting hazards to health, Nondependent abuse of drugs, Personality disorders, Hyperkinetic syndrome of childhood	9838
5	434, 401, v15, 278, 784, 272, 722, 244, v12, v58	Occlusion of cerebral arteries, Essential hypertension, Other personal history presenting hazards to health, Overweight, obesity and other hyperalimentation, Symptoms involving head and neck, Disorders of lipoid metabolism, Intervertebral disc disorders, Acquired hypothyroidism, Personal history of certain other diseases, Encounter for other and unspecified procedures and aftercare	38,634
6	585, 285, 995, 403, 996, 041, v45, 038, 250, 599	Chronic kidney disease (CKD), Other and unspecified anemias, Certain adverse effects not elsewhere classified, Hypertensive kidney disease, Complications peculiar to certain specified procedures, Bacterial infection in conditions classified elsewhere and of unspecified site, Other postprocedural states, Septicemia, Diabetes, Other disorders of urethra and urinary tract	7971
7	300, 244, 530, 272, 294, v43, v57, 496, 331, 715	Anxiety, dissociative and somatoform disorders, Acquired hypothyroidism, Diseases of esophagus, Disorders of lipoid metabolism, Persistent mental disorders due to conditions classified elsewhere, Organ or tissue replaced by other means, Care involving use of rehabilitation procedures, Chronic airway obstruction, not elsewhere classified, Other cerebral degenerations, Osteoarthrosis and allied disorders	33,194
8	618, 614, 625, 577, 617, 620, 621, 616, 574, 278	Genital prolapse, Inflammatory disease of ovary, fallopian tube, pelvic cellular tissue, and peritoneum, Pain and other symptoms associated with female genital organs, Diseases of pancreas, Endometriosis, Noninflammatory disorders of ovary, fallopian tube, and broad ligament, Disorders of uterus, not elsewhere classified, Inflammatory disease of cervix, vagina, and vulva, Cholelithiasis, Overweight, obesity and other hyperalimentation	9340
9	402, 411, 428, 427, v45, 414, 272, 410, 424, 496	Hypertensive heart disease, Other acute and subacute forms of ischemic heart disease, Heart failure, Cardiac dysrhythmias, Other postprocedural states, Other forms of chronic ischemic heart disease, Disorders of lipoid metabolism, Acute myocardial infarction, Other diseases of endocardium, Chronic airway obstruction, not elsewhere classified	55,198
10	276, 280, 562, 553, 560, 535, 787, 530, 564, 998	Disorders of fluid, electrolyte, and acid-base balance, Iron deficiency anemias, Diverticula of intestine, Other hernia of abdominal cavity without mention of obstruction or gangrene, Intestinal obstruction without mention of hernia, Gastritis and duodenitis, Symptoms involving digestive system, Diseases of esophagus, Functional digestive disorders, not elsewhere classified, Other complications of procedures, NEC	32,328

clusters. The mortality is given in Table 6.

In this second example, 4<8<2<5<10<7<1<6<9<3. Since patients in cluster 3 have some serious and high risk infections, it is reasonable to conclude that they also have the highest risk of mortality, followed by the patients in Cluster 9 with severe heart problems. Patients with problems of drug abuse have the least risk of mortality, as do those patients chiefly with problems in the female reproductive system. Roughly in the center, with 4% mortality, are the patients with problems in the abdomen and the digestive system.

Table 7 shows the relationship to length of stay and total charges. For length of stay, the ordering is 8<5<2<1<9<10<7<3<4<6. For total charges, the ordering is 4<8<2<1<5<7<10<3<9<6. Again, note that patients with a higher risk of mortality do not always have the greatest length of stay or the highest

Table 6. Mortality by revised clusters

Table of allclusters by DIED			
allclusters	**DIED**		**Total**
Frequency Row Pct Col Pct	**0**	**1**	
1	34495 97.23 11.63	981 2.77 12.08	35476
2	30432 99.51 10.26	151 0.49 1.86	30583
3	59074 94.84 19.91	3216 5.16 39.61	62290
4	9822 99.92 3.31	8 0.08 0.10	9830
5	28354 99.05 9.56	271 0.95 3.34	28625
6	7723 96.95 2.60	243 3.05 2.99	7966
7	32750 98.75 11.04	415 1.25 5.11	33165
8	9327 99.89 3.14	10 0.11 0.12	9337
9	52697 95.51 17.76	2478 4.49 30.52	55175
10	31971 98.93 10.78	347 1.07 4.27	32318
Total	296645	8120	304765
Frequency Missing = 151			

costs. Patients in Cluster 3 with serious infections may be discharged to home health once the infection is initially treated. Similarly, patients with problems of drug abuse may be discharged to a psychiatric facility or a drug rehabilitation center. Note that these patients have a lower amount of total charges, but a higher length of stay compared to other clusters.

Figure 3 shows the probability density for length of stay; Figure 4 shows the density for total charges. For Figure 3, the ordering is 8<5<2<1<9<10<7<3<4<6. There are some slight differences compared to the ordering for the average values. Again, this occurs because of the outliers in some of the clusters. Clearly, cluster 8 has the highest probability of a length of stay between 0 and 4 days, and the lowest probability of a stay of 8 days or more. Cluster 6 has the lowest probability of a length of stay between 0 and 4 days. Generally, the cutpoint occurs at day number six, with the exception of the cutpoint for cluster 8 that occurs at day number 4. Note that this is the same ordering as it is for the means, suggesting that the outliers are not skewing the averages as much as it did for our first example.

Figure 4, for total charges is not so clean, with the ordering somewhat confused. While the general ordering for the probability of low charges is equal to 4<1<2<10<3<5<7<9<6, it is difficult to place cluster 8 as it is shifted to the right of the other clusters. In addition, cluster 6 has the fewest number of patients, and the bandwidth is too large for an accurate depiction of that probability distribution.

We next want to compare the results using text mining to those of the indices in the previous chapters that specify a list of patient conditions.

Table 7. Length of stay and total charges by revised cluster

Cluster ID	N Obs	Variable	Mean	Std Dev	Minimum	Maximum	N
1	35484	LOS	4.3271708	5.6830914	0	140.0000000	35483
		TOTCHG	21099.41	36398.82	29.0000000	954673.00	35118
2	30608	LOS	4.0709665	5.5011898	0	266.0000000	30606
		TOTCHG	19668.37	27756.17	26.0000000	805168.00	30225
3	62321	LOS	6.3920055	9.1064411	0	361.0000000	62318
		TOTCHG	29854.70	53636.12	29.0000000	998508.00	61549
4	9838	LOS	6.9217321	9.8362611	0	242.0000000	9838
		TOTCHG	13804.80	22434.25	35.0000000	746092.00	9809
5	28634	LOS	3.8345791	5.4602312	0	325.0000000	28630
		TOTCHG	24567.71	29502.42	35.0000000	669559.00	27968
6	7971	LOS	7.9941029	11.4332685	0	270.0000000	7970
		TOTCHG	51977.70	78645.89	52.0000000	998088.00	7849
7	33194	LOS	5.3695502	6.5327041	0	335.0000000	33189
		TOTCHG	24605.86	26415.07	29.0000000	877351.00	32739
8	9340	LOS	2.8922797	6.0833226	0	364.0000000	9339
		TOTCHG	18061.29	17559.88	35.0000000	700591.00	9194
9	55198	LOS	4.9769182	5.7734597	0	285.0000000	55195
		TOTCHG	33038.66	43700.06	45.0000000	985950.00	54481
10	32328	LOS	5.1153525	6.6699273	0	226.0000000	32327
		TOTCHG	25939.36	40362.08	35.0000000	926560.00	31889

Text Mining and Patient Severity Clusters

Figure 3. Probability density for revised clusters 1-10 for length of stay

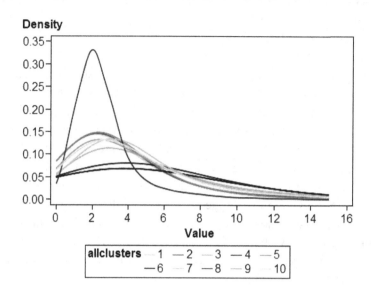

Figure 4. Probability density for revised clusters 1-10 for total charges

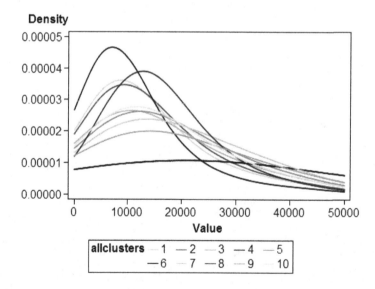

CLUSTERING IN SAS TEXT MINER

In order to use the National Inpatient Sample and SAS Text Miner, we must first concatenate the text strings. In order to do this, we use the following code:

```
Data nis.nistextstrings;
Set nis.nis2005;
Diagnoses=catx (' ',dx1,dx2,dx3,dx4,dx5,dx6,dx7,
```

Figure 5. SAS text miner

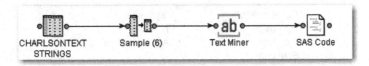

Figure 6. Scoring all data

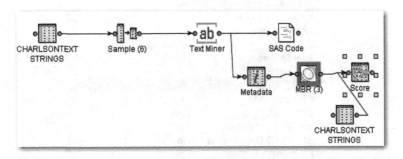

```
dx8,dx9,dx10,dx11,dx12,dx13,dx14,dx15);
Procedures=catx(' ',pr1,pr2,pr3,pr4,pr5,pr6,pr7,
pr8,pr9,pr10,pr11,pr12,pr13,pr14,pr15);
Run;
```

Then, we use the following diagram in SAS Enterprise Miner (Figure 5).

We generally use a sample of the data because of the amount of computer resources required to perform Text Miner. We can then score the remaining data, meaning that we use a small sample to define the clusters and then we use the remaining data as test data (Figure 6). The metadata node is used to change the definition of the cluster value as a target variable; the MBR node is used to define the prediction of the cluster. The score node is used to define the cluster value for the remaining data.

In order to run the process shown in Figure 6, the data role for the scored data must be changed to "score". The Text Miner node has some defaults that need to be changed in order to work with ICD9 codes (Figure 7).

In particular, we must allow Text Miner to cluster using numbers, since numbers are all that are available. Generally, the default is not to use numbers. We also don't want Text Miner to attempt to distinguish between different parts of speech since all of the ICD9 codes are nouns, and we don't want to use noun groups. Once the singular value decomposition is completed, we can go ahead and cluster the patient records. For a patient severity index, we want to define a small number of clusters, so we define the total number of clusters exactly. In this case, we use a total of ten diagnosis clusters.

We can similarly cluster based upon procedures, although we have to make a slight modification in the dataset, or we will overwrite the cluster numbers. We use the created dataset, emws.text_documents and define a new dataset with the code:

```
Data nis.diagnosisclusters (drop=_SVD_1-_SVD_100 prob1-prob100);
Set emws.text_documents;
```

Figure 7. Changing default options in Text Miner

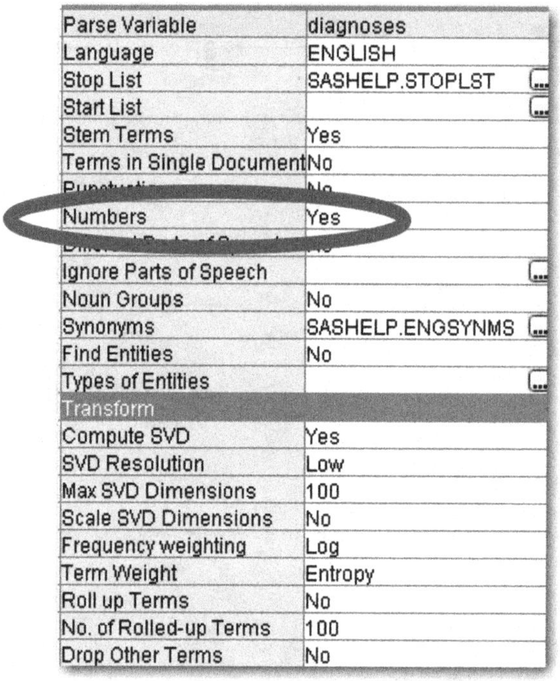

Parse Variable	diagnoses
Language	ENGLISH
Stop List	SASHELP.STOPLST
Start List	
Stem Terms	Yes
Terms in Single Document	No
Punctuati	No
Numbers	Yes
Different Parts of S...	No
Ignore Parts of Speech	
Noun Groups	No
Synonyms	SASHELP.ENGSYNMS
Find Entities	No
Types of Entities	
Transform	
Compute SVD	Yes
SVD Resolution	Low
Max SVD Dimensions	100
Scale SVD Dimensions	No
Frequency weighting	Log
Term Weight	Entropy
Roll up Terms	No
No. of Rolled-up Terms	100
Drop Other Terms	No

```
Diagnosisclusters=_CLUSTER_;
Run;
```

Then we can run Text Miner on the new dataset using the procedure clusters. We can use both diagnosis and procedure clusters to define a severity index.

COMPARISON TO CHARLSON INDEX

We next want to compare these results to those of Chapter 5 with the Charlson Index. As shown in the previous figures, the procedure and diagnosis clusters are not ordered numerically. Therefore, we consider first the comparison of Charlson score to cluster number. To make this comparison, we used a 10% subsample. Figure 8 has the proportion of each Charlson Index by each diagnosis cluster, restricted to the first 5 Index values; Figure 9 has the proportion for the remaining Index values. We will also examine the Charlson Index in relation to the procedure clusters in the same manner.

Note that there seems to be some order to each of the clusters. For example, for cluster 9, Charlson index 0 has fewer than 10% classified. This increases to almost 35% for Index 1 followed by Index values 4 and 5. Index value 2 has a rate that is the same as for index value 4. In contrast, only the Charlson Index value of 0 is present in clusters 1 and 3 with positive probability.

It appears from Figure 8 that clusters 7 and 9 have the highest risk in relationship to the Charlson Index, followed by clusters 3 and 6. That is relatively similar to the ordering defined by using patient

Figure 8. Charlson index by diagnosis cluster for index values 1-5

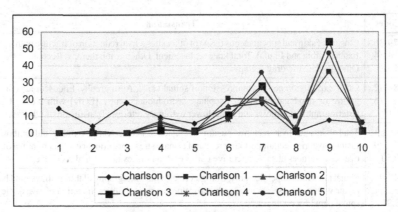

Figure 9. Charlson index by diagnosis cluster for index values 6-10

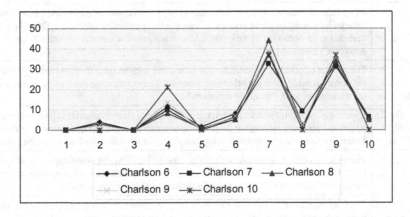

outcomes. However, as we saw in Chapter 5, the Charlson Index itself is not linear in that patients at a higher index can have higher average charges and length of stay compared to a patient at a lower index.

Figure 9 also shows that clusters 7 and 9 have the highest risk compared to the remaining clusters. However, clusters 3 and 6 show a much lower occurrence of these higher Charlson values; cluster 4 appears to have a higher occurrence, but not as high as clusters 7 and 9. This is not unreasonable since the higher Charlson Index values should not have cluster levels that have a lower rate of risk.

Similarly, we consider the relationship of the Charlson Index to the procedure clusters as identified in Table 8 (Figures 10 and 11). Here, it is clearly cluster 6 with the highest proportion for all index levels. The pattern is quite similar for Index levels 6-10 (Figure 11).

Overall, these graphs show that there is a pattern to the diagnosis and procedure clusters, but the pattern differs from the one used to develop the Charlson Index. We use the predictive model to determine whether the inclusion of patient demographic information will allow us to predict the Charlson Index using both the diagnosis and procedure clusters. The best model is a decision tree with a 38% misclassification rate. Figure 12 gives the tree. It shows the importance of both diagnosis and procedure clusters to predict the Charlson level, along with the patient's age and mortality.

Table 8. Clusters of patient procedures with a 1% sample

Cluster	ICD9 Codes	Translation	Frequency
1	86.59, 79.36, 81.54, 94.44, 93.81, 94.25	Closure of skin and subcutaneous tissue of other sites, Open reduction of fracture with internal fixation (tibia and fibula), Total knee replacement, Other group therapy, Recreation therapy, Other psychiatric drug therapy	9933
2	03.09, 88.42, 44.43, 45.16, 88.48, 99.07	Other exploration and decompression of spinal canal, Aortography, Endoscopic control of gastric or duodenal bleeding, Esophagogastroduodenoscopy [EGD] with closed biopsy, Arteriography of femoral and other lower extremity arteries, Transfusion of other serum	9991
3	68.4, 81.63, 81.08, 59.79, 65.61, 70.50	Total abdominal hysterectomy, Fusion or refusion of 4- 8 vertebrae, Lumbar and lumbosacral fusion, posterior technique, Other repair of urinary stress incontinence, Other removal of both ovaries and tubes at same operative episode, Repair of cystocele and rectocele	5347
4	03.31, 47.09, 87.41, 53.61, 38.95, 03.91	Spinal tap, Other appendectomy, Computerized axial tomography of thorax, Incisional hernia repair with prosthesis, Venous catheterization for renal dialysis, Injection of anesthetic into spinal canal for analgesia	18,052
5	94.69, 94.61, 07.61, 86.93, 11.64, 60.69	Combined alcohol and drug rehabilitation and detoxification, Alcohol rehabilitation, Partial excision of pituitary gland, transfrontal approach, Insertion of tissue expander, Other penetrating keratoplasty, Other prostatectomy	77,028
6	75.34, 73.01, 03.90, 66.39, 03.91, 73.6	Other fetal monitoring, Induction of labor by artificial rupture of membranes, Insertion of catheter into spinal canal for infusion of therapeutic or palliative substances, Other bilateral destruction or occlusion of fallopian tubes, Injection of anesthetic into spinal canal for analgesia, Episiotomy	20,840
7	99.05, 79.35, 99.60, 88.72, 96.04, 81.52	Transfusion of platelets, Open reduction of fracture with internal fixation (femur), Cardiopulmonary resuscitation, not otherwise specified, Diagnostic ultrasound of heart, Insertion of endotracheal tube, Partial hip replacement	17275
8	99.20, 37.72, 36.07, 99.21, 93.94, 37.83	Injection or infusion of platelet inhibitor, Initial insertion of transvenous leads [electrodes] into atrium and ventricle, Insertion of drug-eluting coronary artery stent(s), Injection of antibiotic, Respiratory medication administered by nebulizer, Initial insertion of dual-chamber device	17,348
9	86.07, 51.23, 59.8, 99.25, 87.74, 68.51	Insertion of totally implantable vascular access device [VAD], Laparoscopic cholecystectomy, Ureteral catheterization, Injection or infusion of cancer chemotherapeutic substance, Retrograde pyelogram, Laparoscopically assisted vaginal hysterectomy (LAVH)	6643
10	95.41, 33.27, 99.15, 34.91, 43.11, 38.93	Audiometry, Closed endoscopic biopsy of lung, Parenteral infusion of concentrated nutritional substances, Thoracentesis, Percutaneous [endoscopic] gastrostomy [PEG], Venous catheterization, not elsewhere classified	17,419

Figure 10. Charlson index by procedure cluster for index values 1-5

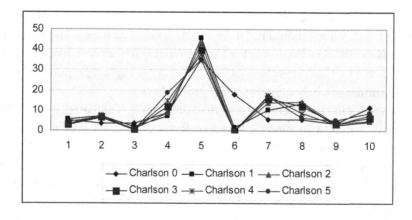

Figure 11. Charlson index by procedure cluster for index values 6-10

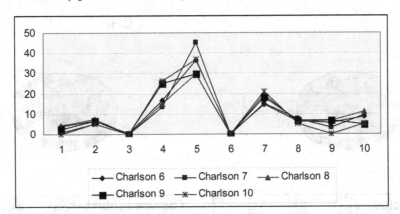

Figure 12. Decision tree to predict Charlson level

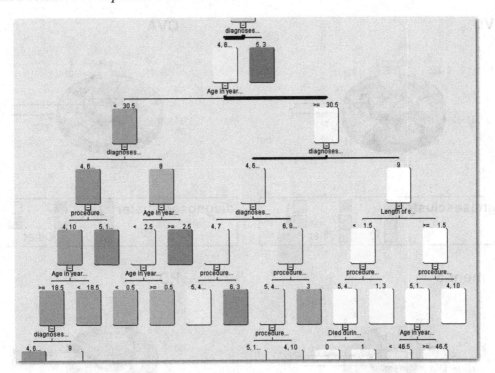

Figure 12 shows the relationship of the diagnosis clusters to each of the codes that define the Charlson Index; Figures 13, 14, and 15 show the procedure clusters.

It is not surprising that a much higher proportion of patients with liver disease are in cluster 4, which is focused on alcohol abuse as such abuse does damage the liver. An even higher proportion of patients with severe liver disease are in cluster 4. In addition, both acute myocardial infarction and congestive heart failure are concentrated in cluster 9, which tends to identify with heart disease. One of the reasons that the Charlson Index conditions are scattered across the clusters is because many are in fact related. Many patients with renal disease also have heart disease, and conversely. Also, a higher proportion of

Figure 13. Diagnosis clusters compared to Charlson index diagnoses

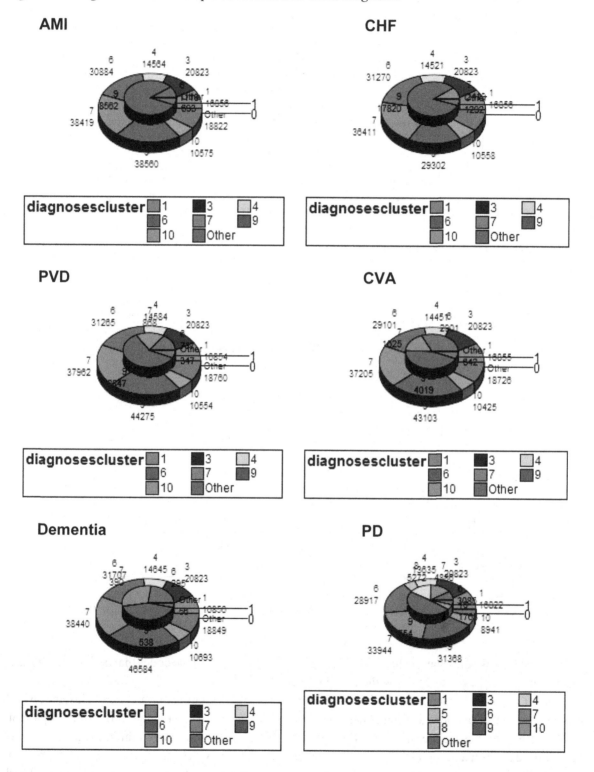

Figure 14. Diagnosis clusters compared to Charlson index diagnoses (continued)

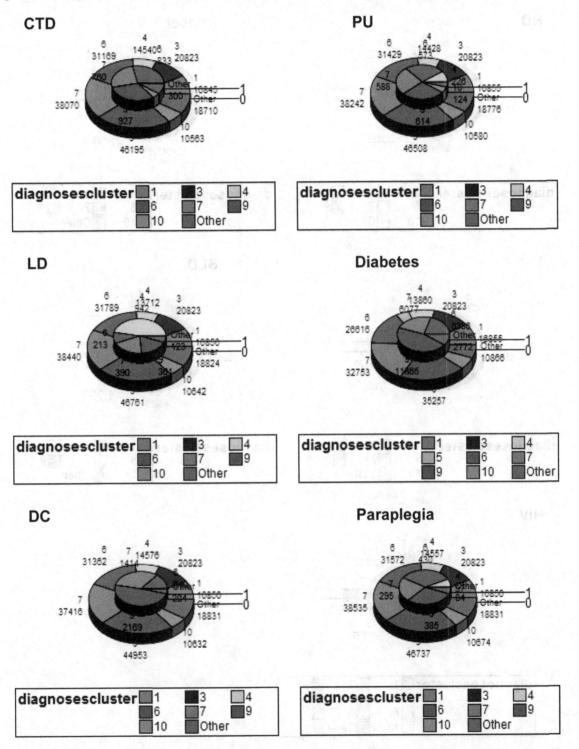

Figure 15. Diagnosis clusters compared to Charlson index diagnoses (continued)

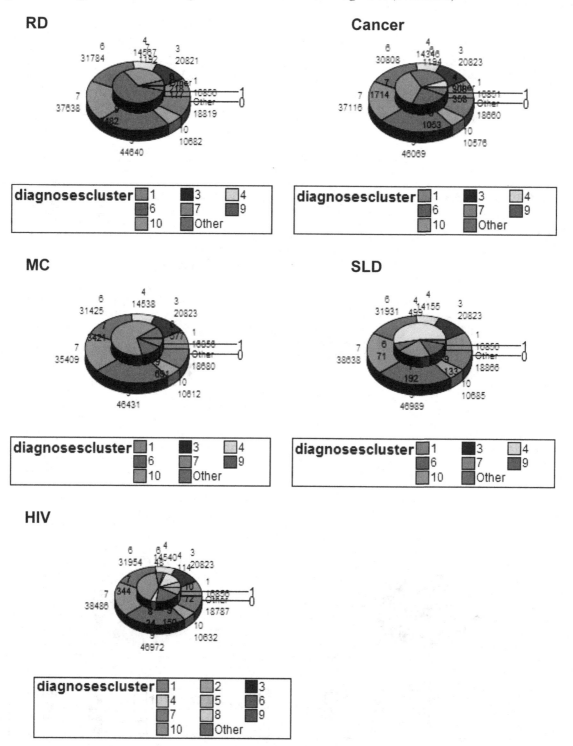

cancer patients are in cluster 7, related to anxiety disorders, which seems inherently reasonable. It is even more prevalent for patients with metastatic cancer, and for patients with HIV. The reason some of these diagnoses that define the Charlson Index are scattered across the diagnosis clusters is that different diagnoses are used to define the clusters. Figures 16, 17, and 18 give the procedure clusters as they are related to these same patient conditions.

Cluster 5 is so prominent and related to so many of the Charlson Index diagnosis, that it is possible that it is into this cluster where some upcoding may occur. Patient with peptic ulcers do not appear to be in this cluster very prominently, or surprisingly, for patients with liver disease. Cancer and metastatic cancer have a significant proportion in cluster 9, which contains procedures related to chemotherapy.

COMPARISON TO APRDRG

In a similar manner, we can compare the text clusters to the APRDRG index. Table 9 shows the proportion of patients in each diagnosis cluster by APRDRG mortality index.

As Table 9 shows, there are some similarities. There are also some benefits to the use of the diagnosis clusters since most of the patients in APRDRG category 0 that cannot be classified, were classified in the clusters. Figure 19 shows where similarities occur. Note that over 90% of the patients in cluster 1 cannot be classified using the APRDRG Index. Over 80% of the patients in cluster 3 are in APRDRG category 2. However, the remaining clusters tend to cross all of the APRDRG levels.

A graph of the APRDRG severity index by diagnosis cluster gives a similar result. We again use a predictive model to determine whether the clusters can predict the APRDRG mortality level. The misclassification rate on the testing set is 25%, indicating that this model predicts slightly better than predicting the Charlson Index levels. The memory based reasoning model is the best, but the decision tree misclassifies at a rate of 28%. It indicates that the first split is on age, but the second split is based on diagnosis codes followed by procedure codes (Figure 20).

Since we define both the APRDRG Index and the clusters as nominal, we can include the entire APRDRG index, including the patients that cannot be classified with the value of 0.

COMPARISON TO RESOURCE UTILIZATION

We do a similar examination in Table 10 using the Disease Staging: Mortality Level.

The clusters have a range of 0 to 10% (in cluster 9) of the patients in the highest severity level. A total of 92% of the values in diagnosis cluster 1 are in the mortality level of 0. Table 11 gives the comparison by procedure levels.

Some of the clusters are scattered across the mortality levels, while others such as cluster 6 are concentrated within one mortality level. We again want to see how well the clusters can predict the resource level. We attempt to predict the disease staging: mortality level. The regression model is optimal, but the error rate is 58%.

Figure 16. Procedure clusters compared to Charlson index diagnoses

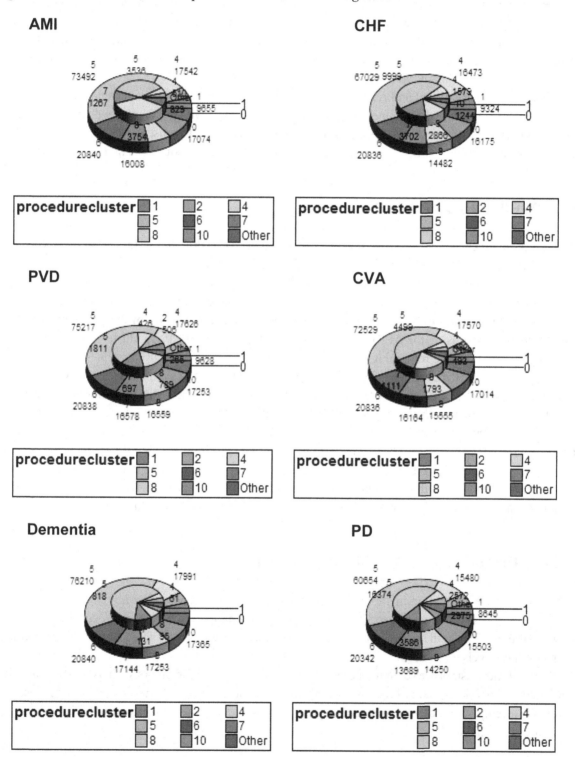

Figure 17. Procedure clusters compared to Charlson index diagnoses (continued)

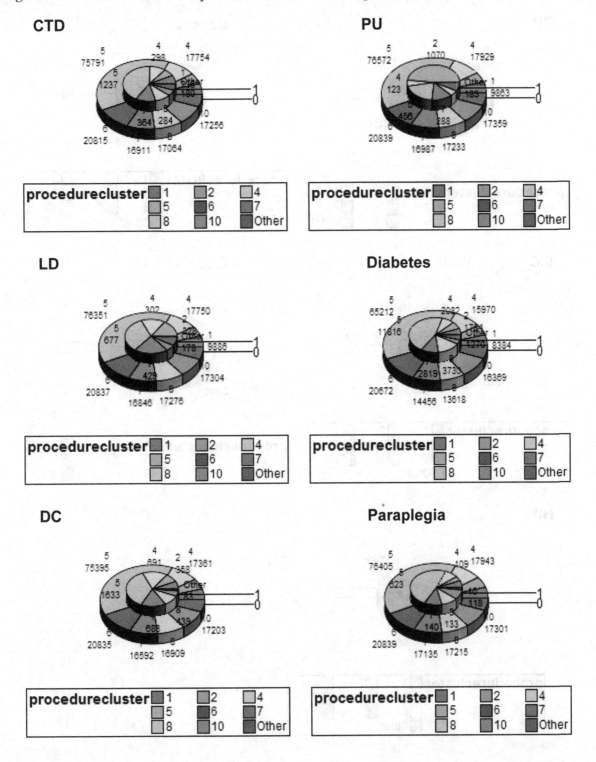

Figure 18. Procedure clusters compared to Charlson index diagnoses (continued)

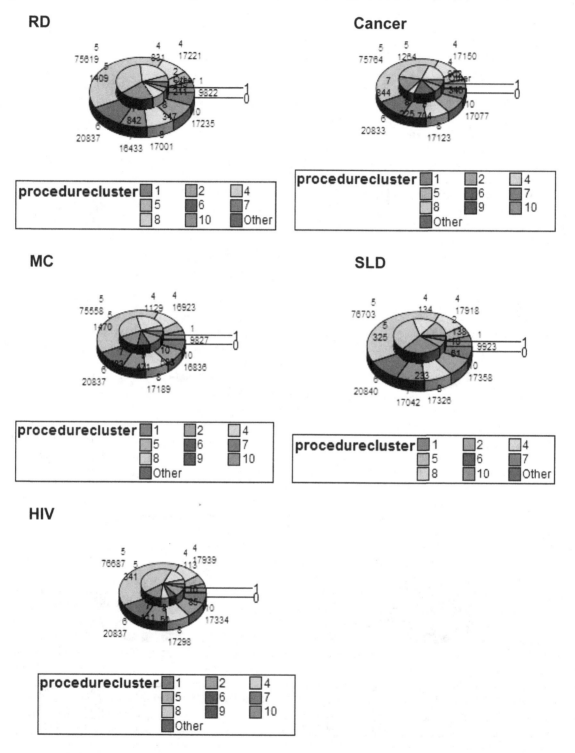

Table 9. APRDRG mortality index by diagnosis clusters

Table of diagnosescluster by APRDRG_Risk_Mortality						
diagnosescluster	APRDRG_Risk_Mortality(All Patient Refined DRG: Risk of Mortality Subclass)					Total
Frequency Row Pct Col Pct	0	1	2	3	4	
1	0 0.00 0.00	16780 99.55 12.86	68 0.40 0.15	6 0.04 0.03	2 0.01 0.03	16856
2	5 0.09 5.21	5359 94.98 4.11	249 4.41 0.55	27 0.48 0.15	2 0.04 0.03	5642
3	30 0.14 31.25	20486 98.38 15.71	186 0.89 0.41	59 0.28 0.33	62 0.30 1.03	20823
4	2 0.01 2.08	12109 82.63 9.28	1747 11.92 3.82	647 4.42 3.67	149 1.02 2.48	14654
5	31 0.43 32.29	5501 76.60 4.22	1027 14.30 2.25	487 6.78 2.76	135 1.88 2.24	7181
6	7 0.02 7.29	22833 71.35 17.51	7542 23.57 16.51	1357 4.24 7.69	263 0.82 4.37	32002
7	13 0.03 13.54	19414 50.00 14.88	12444 32.05 27.24	5099 13.13 28.89	1860 4.79 30.91	38830
8	4 0.07 4.17	5311 87.61 4.07	640 10.56 1.40	91 1.50 0.52	16 0.26 0.27	6062
9	2 0.00 2.08	13343 28.32 10.23	20609 43.74 45.12	9677 20.54 54.84	3491 7.41 58.02	47122
10	2 0.02 2.08	9299 86.87 7.13	1169 10.92 2.56	197 1.84 1.12	37 0.35 0.61	10704
Total	96	130435	45681	17647	6017	199876

USING TEXT MINER TO COMPARE PROVIDER QUALITY RANKINGS

Again, we want to use the definition of a patient severity index to examine the quality of care. We look to our examples of patients diagnosed with COPD, and also of patients undergoing cardiovascular bypass surgery. If we use text analysis with just the COPD patients and the selected hospitals, we get the results shown in Table 12. For this analysis, we restrict the number of our text clusters to just 5.

It is clear from table 12 that many of the patients suffer from heart conditions as well as COPD, and are placed in cluster 5. Patients in cluster 4 also have problems with chemical dependency, while patients in clusters 1 and 3 have pneumonia as well as COPD. In order to examine the data by hospital, we first have to determine which cluster is the least severe, and which is the most severe. Table 13 has

Figure 19. Graphical representation of APRDRG mortality index by diagnosis cluster

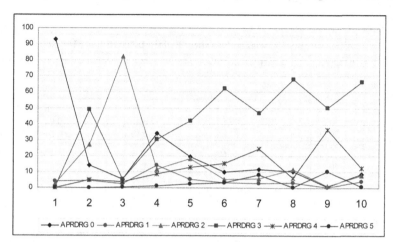

Figure 20. Decision tree to predict mortality index

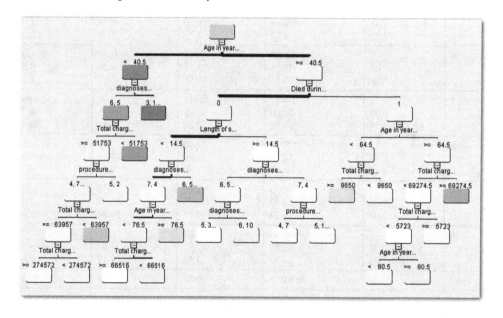

the relationship of cluster to mortality. Table 13 shows that cluster 3 has the least mortality while cluster 2 has the most. In order of mortality, 3<4<5<1<2.

We examine the relationship of cluster to length of stay and total charges using kernel density estimation (Figures 21 and 22). With the exception of cluster 4 dealing with drug dependency, there is a natural hierarchy in the length of stay with 3<1<5<2. It is somewhat understandable that cluster 4 might be a little different. However, with total charges, the ordering is 3<2<4<1<5.

The natural ordering in Figure 21 is 3<1<5<2. Again, cluster 4 is a little bit different, with the highest probability of a stay of between 4 and 8 days, again dealing with the dependency nature of the cluster. For Figure 22, the ordering is 3<2<4<1<5, which is slightly different compared to that for Figure 21. Cluster 2 has a high probability of a long length of stay but also a high probability of lower cost. Such

Table 10. Comparison of text clusters by mortality level

Table of diagnosescluster by DS_Mrt_Level							
diagnosescluster	DS_Mrt_Level(Disease Staging: Mortality Level)						Total
Frequency Row Pct Col Pct	0	1	2	3	4	5	
1	15662 92.93 46.65	695 4.12 9.96	454 2.69 1.61	42 0.25 0.05	1 0.01 0.00	0 0.00 0.00	16854
2	791 14.02 2.36	260 4.61 3.73	1530 27.12 5.42	2773 49.15 3.28	278 4.93 0.76	10 0.18 0.10	5642
3	1158 5.57 3.45	485 2.33 6.95	17132 82.35 60.67	1139 5.47 1.35	782 3.76 2.13	108 0.52 1.09	20804
4	4994 34.08 14.87	2076 14.17 29.75	1698 11.59 6.01	4422 30.18 5.24	1256 8.57 3.42	207 1.41 2.10	14653
5	1402 19.59 4.18	371 5.19 5.32	1294 18.09 4.58	2996 41.87 3.55	907 12.68 2.47	185 2.59 1.87	7155
6	3180 9.94 9.47	1068 3.34 15.30	1766 5.52 6.25	19931 62.29 23.60	4945 15.46 13.48	1105 3.45 11.19	31995
7	4443 11.45 13.23	1172 3.02 16.79	2207 5.69 7.82	18238 46.99 21.60	9564 24.64 26.07	3188 8.21 32.27	38812
8	635 10.48 1.89	192 3.17 2.75	710 11.72 2.51	4124 68.06 4.88	374 6.17 1.02	24 0.40 0.24	6059
9	392 0.83 1.17	225 0.48 3.22	619 1.31 2.19	23670 50.24 28.03	17267 36.65 47.07	4943 10.49 50.04	47116
10	920 8.59 2.74	435 4.06 6.23	826 7.72 2.93	7101 66.34 8.41	1313 12.27 3.58	109 1.02 1.10	10704
Total	33577	6979	28236	84436	36687	9879	199794

infections are ordinarily treated with antibiotics, but not by using surgery, which can be used to decrease the costs. Table 14 gives the relationship of cluster to hospital.

We now use a predictive model to examine the relationship of predicted to actual mortality. Table 15 compares the results to that of the previous indices.

Note that the rankings are different still compared to the APRDRG and the Demand Staging levels. It suggests that providers can move up or down in the ranking by changing the severity index used. For this analysis, the difference in the misclassification rate between the decision tree and regression is considerable (Figure 23).

Figure 24 gives the results of the memory based reasoning model, which was chosen as the best model. It shows a small false negative compared to the false positive rate for the training set and also for the validation set.

Table 11. Disease staging: mortality level by procedure clusters

Table of procedurecluster by DS_Mrt_Level							
procedurecluster	**DS_Mrt_Level(Disease Staging: Mortality Level)**						**Total**
Frequency Row Pct Col Pct	**0**	**1**	**2**	**3**	**4**	**5**	
1	205 8.30 2.41	194 7.85 10.84	147 5.95 2.10	1602 64.86 7.63	283 11.46 3.11	39 1.58 1.56	2470
2	186 7.33 2.19	67 2.64 3.75	98 3.86 1.40	1398 55.06 6.66	638 25.13 7.00	152 5.99 6.07	2539
3	877 63.92 10.31	14 1.02 0.78	102 7.43 1.46	368 26.82 1.75	10 0.73 0.11	1 0.07 0.04	1372
4	921 20.36 10.83	199 4.40 11.12	288 6.37 4.11	1944 42.97 9.26	937 20.71 10.29	235 5.19 9.38	4524
5	871 4.56 10.24	749 3.92 41.87	3477 18.21 49.64	9197 48.17 43.83	3958 20.73 43.46	839 4.39 33.51	19091
6	4628 88.20 54.43	250 4.76 13.97	341 6.50 4.87	23 0.44 0.11	5 0.10 0.05	0 0.00 0.00	5247
7	145 3.43 1.71	63 1.49 3.52	119 2.81 1.70	1749 41.36 8.34	1489 35.21 16.35	664 15.70 26.52	4229
8	105 2.39 1.23	59 1.34 3.30	155 3.52 2.21	3059 69.49 14.58	837 19.01 9.19	187 4.25 7.47	4402
9	360 21.47 4.23	121 7.22 6.76	85 5.07 1.21	845 50.39 4.03	224 13.36 2.46	42 2.50 1.68	1677
10	205 4.72 2.41	73 1.68 4.08	2192 50.51 31.30	798 18.39 3.80	727 16.75 7.98	345 7.95 13.78	4340
Total	8503	1789	7004	20983	9108	2504	49891

Table 12. Text clusters for patients with COPD

Cluster	Codes	Translation	Frequency
1	4661, 787, 466, 799, 2768, 486	Acute bronchiolitis, Symptoms involving the digestive system, Acute bronchitis, Senility without psychosis, Hypokalemia, Pneumonia	239
2	599, 5990, 518, 276, 2765, 5188	Other disorders of urethra and urinary tract, Urinary tract infection, Other diseases of lung, Disorders of fluic, electrolyte, and acid-base balance, Dehydration, Other diseases of the lung	299
3	4930, 493, 4939, 3829, 382, 486	Asthma, Otitis media, Pneumonia	59
4	3051, 305, 3050, 4912, 491, 2768	Nondependent tobacco use disorder, Nondependent abuse of drugs, Nondependent alcohol abuse, Obstructive chronic bronchitis, Chronic bronchitis, Hypokalemia	56
5	4140, 4019, 4273, 401, 427, 4912	Coronary atherosclerosis, Unspecified hypertension, Cardiac dysrhythmias, Essential hypertension, Atrial fibrillation, Obstructive chronic bronchitis	507

Table 13. COPD text cluster to mortality

Table of _CLUSTER_ by DIED				
CLUSTER		**DIED**		**Total**
Frequency Row Pct Col Pct	**0**	**1**		
1	231 96.65 20.70	8 3.35 18.18		239
2	280 93.65 25.09	19 6.35 43.18		299
3	59 100.00 5.29	0 0.00 0.00		59
4	55 98.21 4.93	1 1.79 2.27		56
5	491 96.84 44.00	16 3.16 36.36		507
Total	1116	44		1160

Figure 21. Kernel density of length of stay by cluster

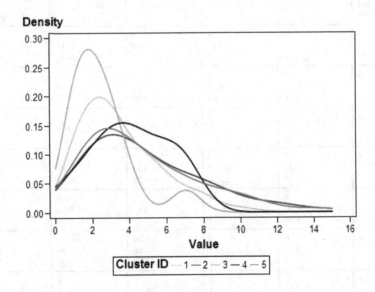

However, this model still misclassified almost 30% of the time, suggesting that there is still considerable random chance in the mortality of patients unaccounted for by the model.

We next use the example of cardiovascular surgery using procedure 36.1 to compare the results using Text Miner to those results from other measures. We use the diagnosis codes to define a severity index, again using just 5 classes. Once we define the classes, we need to determine how to rank the classes.

Figure 22. Kernel density of total charges by cluster

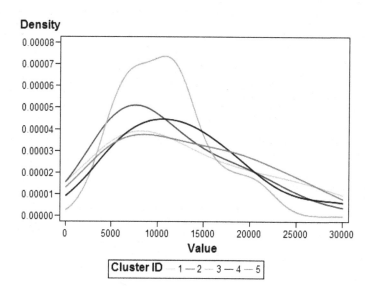

Table 14. Text cluster by hospital

Table of Hospital by Cluster						
Hospital	Cluster					Total
Frequency Row Pct Col Pct	1	2	3	4	5	
1	1 3.57 1.64	9 32.14 12.68	0 0.00 0.00	5 17.86 29.41	13 46.43 10.40	28
2	5 33.33 8.20	2 13.33 2.82	0 0.00 0.00	0 0.00 0.00	8 53.33 6.40	15
3	2 25.00 3.28	4 50.00 5.63	0 0.00 0.00	0 0.00 0.00	2 25.00 1.60	8
4	15 23.44 24.59	16 25.00 22.54	2 3.13 15.38	5 7.81 29.41	26 40.63 20.80	64
5	6 25.00 9.84	14 58.33 19.72	1 4.17 7.69	0 0.00 0.00	3 12.50 2.40	24
6	6 11.32 9.84	13 24.53 18.31	0 0.00 0.00	0 0.00 0.00	34 64.15 27.20	53
7	0 0.00 0.00	4 33.33 5.63	0 0.00 0.00	1 8.33 5.88	7 58.33 5.60	12
9	14 25.45 22.95	4 7.27 5.63	1 1.82 7.69	6 10.91 35.29	30 54.55 24.00	55
10	12 42.86 19.67	5 17.86 7.04	9 32.14 69.23	0 0.00 0.00	2 7.14 1.60	28
Total	61	71	13	17	125	287

Table 15. Rank comparisons between resource demand levels and APRDRG indices

Hospital	APRDRG Ranking	Demand Staging Ranking	Text Clusters
1	4	1	5
2	3	7	6
3	2	7	1
4	7	4	7
5	5	2	8
6	1	3	4
7	8	9	2
9	6	1	3
10	9	7	9

Figure 23. Results of predictive model

```
Fit Statistics
Model selection based on _TMISC_

                                Test:
Selected                  Misclassification
Model       Model Node          Rate

            AutoNeural3       0.46429
            DmineReg7         0.57143
Y           MBR8              0.28571
            Neural7           0.53571
            Reg7              0.39286
            Rule5             0.39286
            Tree7             0.42857
```

Then, we will compare the results to the hospitals. Table 16 gives the results of the text analysis.

We examine outcomes to define an order relationship to these clusters. Table 17 gives the comparison of mortality to cluster.

It is clear that 5>3>4>1>2 in terms of severity by actual mortality. We examine length of stay and total charges to see if that ordering holds. Note that none of the clusters has a high proportion of mortality, except possibly for cluster 5. Table 18 gives the summary statistics.

For length of stay, 5>4>1>2>3, and for total charges, 5>4>2>1>3. There is little difference between clusters 5 and 4, and between clusters 2 and 1. Therefore, the boundaries will be a little fuzzy and do switch the ordering. However, these changes are well within the margin of error as defined by the standard deviation. Table 19 gives the relationship of cluster to hospital.

Hospital 2, which has always ranked the lowest because of a zero mortality rate has most of its patients in clusters 2 and 5, which are on the extremes in terms of actual mortality. Hospital #7, which ranks high, has approximately 65% of its patients in the same two clusters. Therefore, the fact that Hospital #2 has

Figure 24. Predictive model using memory based reasoning

```
Classification Table

Data Role=TRAIN Target Variable=DIED

                        Target      Outcome               Total
Target    Outcome     Percentage   Percentage   Count   Percentage

   0         0         84.6154      64.7059       11      32.3529
   1         0         15.3846      11.7647        2       5.8824
   0         1         28.5714      35.2941        6      17.6471
   1         1         71.4286      88.2353       15      44.1176


Data Role=VALIDATE Target Variable=DIED

                        Target      Outcome               Total
Target    Outcome     Percentage   Percentage   Count   Percentage

   0         0         83.3333      38.4615        5      19.2308
   1         0         16.6667       7.6923        1       3.8462
   0         1         40.0000      61.5385        8      30.7692
   1         1         60.0000      92.3077       12      46.1538
```

a lower mortality rate should rank it higher compared to #7, if we can demonstrate that the patients in these two hospitals have approximately the same levels of severity.

USING PATIENT SEVERITY TO PREDICT OUTCOMES FOR INTERVENTION

Unlike the patient severity indices defined in Chapters 5-7, we can use Text Miner to predict more specific patient outcomes. We do not need to restrict attention to patient mortality. We demonstrate how such a prediction can work by examining the occurrence of resistant infection.

Table 16. Text analysis for cardiovascular surgery to compare ten hospitals

Cluster	Codes	Translation	Frequency
1	2766, 276, 2851, 285, 410, 4273	Fluid overload, Disorders of fluid, electrolyte, and acid-base balance, Acute posthemorrhagic anemia, Other and unspecified anemias, Acute myocardial infarction, Atrial fibrillation and flutter	323
2	272, v158, 4111, 401, 411, 2720	Disorders of lipoid metabolism, Other specified personal history presenting hazards to health, Intermediate coronary syndrome, Essential hypertension, Other acute and subacute forms of ischemic heart disease, Pure hypercholesterolemia	477
3	412, 413, 4130, v458, 401, 2724	Old myocardial infarction, Angina pectoris, Angina decubitus, Other postprocedural status, Essential hypertension, Other and unspecified hyperlipidemia	112
4	997, 9971, 4273, 3051, 496, 5119	Complications affecting specified body systems, not elsewhere classified, Cardiac complications, Atrial fibrillation and flutter, Tobacco use disorder, Chronic airway obstruction, not elsewhere classified, Unspecified pleural effusion	320
5	410, 318, 428, 4280, 4107, 2851	Acute myocardial infarction, Other specified mental retardation, Heart failure, Congestive heart failure, unspecified, Subendocardial infarction, Acute posthemorrhagic anemia	234

Table 17. Text cluster by mortality

Table of _CLUSTER_ by DIED			
Cluster Number	**DIED**		**Total**
	0	**1**	
1	320 99.07 22.25	3 0.93 10.71	323
2	476 99.79 33.10	1 0.21 3.57	477
3	110 98.21 7.65	2 1.79 7.14	112
4	315 98.44 21.91	5 1.56 17.86	320
5	217 92.74 15.09	17 7.26 60.71	234
Total	1438	28	1466

Table 18. Mean length of stay and total charges by cluster

Cluster ID	N Obs	Variable	Mean	Std Dev
1	323	LOS TOTCHG	10.1362229 121863.26	5.8192245 74192.26
2	477	LOS TOTCHG	7.6477987 129111.25	4.2998999 86952.70
3	112	LOS TOTCHG	7.0446429 90460.39	3.1519718 44919.65
4	320	LOS TOTCHG	10.9437500 134384.52	6.7515208 79940.11
5	234	LOS TOTCHG	13.0427350 172775.22	11.3907523 138952.94

Resistant infection is a serious nosocomial problem. There are few antibiotics that are effective in treating these infections, and the patient consequences can be significant, including amputation and death. Moreover, these infections add significantly to the cost of patient care and add to the patient length of stay. Medicare has just recently announced that they will no longer reimburse healthcare providers for the added cost of nosocomial infection, meaning that the provider will have to shoulder the complete cost of treating the infection.(Pear, 2007) One of the most difficult of the resistant infections is MRSA (Methicillin Resistant Staph), and we will use the term, MRSA, to represent the general category of resistant infections.

In the past, focus has been on general infection control procedures (Coia et al., 2006; Henderson, 2006), assuming a uniform patient risk, or on targeting patients using specific demographic and health parameters.(Roghmann, 2000; Lodise, McKinnon, & Rybak, 2003) In these studies, one patient location (for example, ICU)(Gerber et al., 2006; McBryde, Pettit, & McElwain, 2007) or one patient treatment

Table 19. Text cluster by hospital

Table of DSHOSPID by _CLUSTER_						
Hospital	_CLUSTER_(Cluster ID)					Total
	1	2	3	4	5	
1	70 21.54 21.67	109 33.54 22.85	45 13.85 40.18	66 20.31 20.63	35 10.77 14.96	325
2	1 9.09 0.31	6 54.55 1.26	0 0.00 0.00	3 27.27 0.94	1 9.09 0.43	11
3	22 19.64 6.81	42 37.50 8.81	6 5.36 5.36	23 20.54 7.19	19 16.96 8.12	112
4	43 17.00 13.31	86 33.99 18.03	16 6.32 14.29	90 35.57 28.13	18 7.11 7.69	253
5	11 12.50 3.41	44 50.00 9.22	1 1.14 0.89	20 22.73 6.25	12 13.64 5.13	88
6	44 25.14 13.62	41 23.43 8.60	9 5.14 8.04	37 21.14 11.56	44 25.14 18.80	175
7	105 37.10 32.51	38 13.43 7.97	21 7.42 18.75	45 15.90 14.06	74 26.15 31.62	283
8	4 8.89 1.24	14 31.11 2.94	5 11.11 4.46	14 31.11 4.38	8 17.78 3.42	45
9	10 12.82 3.10	41 52.56 8.60	4 5.13 3.57	7 8.97 2.19	16 20.51 6.84	78
10	13 13.54 4.02	56 58.33 11.74	5 5.21 4.46	15 15.63 4.69	7 7.29 2.99	96
Total	323	477	112	320	234	1466

was investigated.(Masaki et al., 2006) To date, the infections have not been controlled or prevented very successfully.(Bootsma, Diekmann, & Bonten, 2006; Loveday, Pellowe, Jones, & Pratt, 2006) Attempts to predict the infection have not been terribly successful, and without accurate prediction, preventive treatment cannot be targeted to those patients at highest risk.(Malde, Hardern, & Welch, 2006) If predictive modeling on a more general basis can be used to identify those patients most at risk for acquiring resistant infection, preventive measures can be targeted to reduce the likelihood of infection, reducing treatment costs while simultaneously improving patient care.(Thomas, Cantrill, Waghorn, & McIntyre, 2007)

In addition to predicting the occurrence of MRSA, we looked at treatment of the infection. While there is some suggestion that cutaneous infection can be treated with debridement and drainage for patients who are otherwise healthy, all other occurrences of resistant infection require some type of antibiotic treatment.(Gorwitz, Jernigan, Powers, & Jernigan, 2006) Unfortunately, we found that the use of antibiotics with MRSA occurred in only a small proportion of patients. This was an important,

Table 20. Twenty most frequent diagnoses and procedures for patients with MRSA

Diagnosis	Translation	Frequency	Procedure	Translation	Frequency
041.11	Staphylococcus aureus	3970	38.93	Venous catheterization, not elsewhere classified	1685
401.9	Unspecified hypertension	1637	86.04	Other incision with drainage of skin and subcutaneous tissue	764
599.0	Urinary tract infection, site not specified	1036	86.22	Excisional debridement of wound, infection, or burn	653
428.0	Congestive heart failure, unspecified	950			650
250.00	250.0 Diabetes mellitus without mention of complication, type unspecified	866	39.95	Hemodialysis	387
682.6	Other cellulitis and abscess, let except foot	699	96.04	Insertion of endotracheal tube	297
482.41	Pneumonia due to Staphylococcus aureus	695	96.72	Continuous mechanical ventilation for 96 consecutive hours or more	250
285.9	Anemia, unspecified	651	88.72	Diagnostic ultrasound of heart	216
427.31	Atrial fibrillation	626	99.21	Injection of antibiotic	204
496	Chronic airway obstruction, not elsewhere classified	604	38.95	Venous catheterization for renal dialysis	186
038.11	Staphylococcus aureus septicemia	585	86.28	Nonexcisional debridement of wound, infection or burn	167
276.5	Volume depletion	584	96.71	Continuous mechanical ventilation for less than 96 consecutive hours	143
305.1	Tobacco use disorder	552	33.24	Closed [endoscopic] biopsy of bronchus	
414.01	Coronary atherosclerosis of native coronary artery	472	96.6	Enteral infusion of concentrated nutritional substances	110
998.59	Other postoperative infection	464	43.11	Percutaneous [endoscopic] gastrostomy	98
538.01	Esophageal reflux	434	45.16	Esophagogastroduodenoscopy [EGD] with closed biopsy	95
403.91	Hypertensive kidney disease, unspecified	411	99.15	Parenteral infusion of concentrated nutritional substances	93
707.0	Decubitus ulcer	368	93.90	Continuous positive airway pressure	89
244.9	Unspecified hypothyroidism	363	34.91	Thoracentesis	86
311	Depressive disorder, not elsewhere classified	358	99.07	Transfusion of other serum	81

but completely unexpected find in the data.

Assuming that the Clusters are Interval Data

We use data from the National Inpatient Sample. We want to see if we can use treatment choices to find those with higher risk of infection compared to other treatments. Table 20 gives the 20 most frequent diagnoses and procedures associated with MRSA. There were a total of 5974 patients with a diagnosis of v09.0, or resistant infection, in the dataset. Code translations are also given.(Anonymous-ICD9)

Approximately 2/3 of the patients diagnosed with resistant infection are also diagnosed with Staphylococcus aureus, indicating MRSA; the remaining have other diagnoses, or none at all. Hypertension is identified in 27% of the patients followed by 17% with a urinary tract infection. Therefore, all but one of the 20 top diagnoses only occur in just a small proportion of patients; they can all be considered rare occurences. The procedures occur in an even smaller proportion of the patients, with 28% receiving venous catheterization followed by other incision with drainage of skin and subcutaneous tissue in 13%.

Since each individual diagnosis or procedure occurs in just a small proportion of patients, it is important to consider all possible combinations of diagnoses and procedures in order to identify all patients. Without some type of data compression to reduce these codes to a reasonable number of categories, they cannot be used in any predictive model. We use text mining to perform this task. Text mining can use the linkage between diagnoses and procedures to define categories of patients.(P. Cerrito, 2007; P. B. Cerrito, 2007) Again, in order to use text mining, we concatenate the fifteen columns of diagnosis codes into one text string, and then also concatenate the fifteen columns of procedure codes into a second text string. Then, we use the linkage in the text string between the concatenated codes to define a set of clusters of patient conditions, and a second set of clusters of procedures.

Another problem is that without some type of stratified sampling in the data, predictive models such as logistic regression cannot be used to predict the rare occurrence of infection. The constructed model will simply predict all patients, or nearly all patients in the non-occurrence group so that the model is accurate, but lacking in value. We use a stratified sample of 100% of the occurrence group and randomly select an equal number of non-occurrence patients for a 50/50 split in the resulting dataset. Then we use several predictive models, including logistic regression, neural networks, and decision trees to optimize results. While the overall model may lack in accuracy, we can use the defined lift to determine which patients should be treated prophylactically to reduce the occurrence of resistant infection. Lift allows us to find the patients at highest risk for occurrence, and with the greatest probability of accurate prediction. This is especially important since these are the patients we would want to take the greatest care for.

Given a lift function, we can decide on a decile cutpoint so that we can predict the high risk patients above the cutpoint, and predict the low risk patients below a second cutpoint, while failing to make a definite prediction for those in the center. In that way, we can dismiss those who have no risk, and aggressively treat those at highest risk. We can then decide somewhere in the center when to stop prophylactic treatment. That cutpoint will depend largely upon the differential in cost of treatment after infection versus cost of treatment to prevent infection. Lift allows us to distinguish between patients without assuming a uniformity of risk.

Table 21 gives a total of 32 clusters of patient diagnoses associated with MRSA; Table 22 gives a corresponding total of 31 clusters of patient procedures. Unlike the previous severity indices where we restricted the number of clusters, we can expand the number to investigate infection. We use a stratified sample of all patients with MRSA and a random sample of patients without MRSA to define the text clusters. Both clusters were identified using text mining.

Not every patient in a cluster will have all of the diagnoses listed in the cluster. These diagnoses are those that characterize the cluster. That means that the linkage between the diagnoses has a fairly high probably of occurring.

We will not label all of the clusters here. However, we consider some of the code combinations. For

Table 21. Clusters of diagnoses

Cluster #	Code Combinations	Translations	Frequency
1	303.91, 304.21, 291.81, 305.60, 305.20, 681.00	Other and unspecified alcohol dependence (continuous), Cocaine dependence (continuous), Alcohol withdrawal, Cocaine abuse (continuous), Cannabis abuse (continuous), Cellulitis and abscess, unspecified	335
2	272.0, 272.4, 401.9, 786.59, 600.00, 250.00	Pure hypercholesterolemia, Other and unspecified hyperlipidemia, Essential hypertension, Chest pain, Hypertrophy (benign) of prostate without urinary obstruction, Diabetes mellitus without mention of complication of unspecified type	370
3	648.21, 278.01, 285.9, 654.21, 663.31, 648.41	Anemia, Morbid obesity, Anemia, unspecified, Previous cesarean delivery, Other and unspecified cord entanglement, without mention of compression, Mental disorders (pregnancy delivered)	307
4	276.8, 275.2, 787.91, 276.5, 305.1, 285.9	Hypopotassemia, Disorders of magnesium metabolism, Diarrhea, Volume depletion, Tobacco use disorder, Anemia, unspecified	310
5	493.90, 301.83, 540.9, 530.81, 278.01, 682.0	Asthma, unspecified, Borderline personality disorder, Without mention of peritonitis, Esophageal reflux, Morbid obesity, Other cellulitis and abscess (face)	293
6	440.23, 707.15, 250.70, 250.82, 250.80, 731.8	Atherosclerosis of the extremities with ulceration, Ulcer of other part of foot (toes), Diabetes with peripheral circulatory disorders (unspecified type), Diabetes with other specified manifestations (Type II or unspecified uncontrolled), Diabetes with other specified manifestations (of unspecified type), Other bone involvement in diseases classified elsewhere	214
7	041.11, 683, 682.5, 616.4, 682.2, 608.4	Staphylococcus aureus, Acute lymphadenitis, Other cellulitis and abscess (buttock), Other abscess of vulva, Other cellulitis and abscess (hand except fingers and thumb), Other inflammatory disorders of male genital organs	416
8	V45.1, 294.10, 427.31, 996.62, 682.6, 403.91	Renal dialysis status, Dementia in conditions classified elsewhere without behavioral disturbance, Atrial fibrillation, Infection and inflammatory reaction due to internal prosthetic device, implant, and graft Due to vascular device, implant and graft, Other cellulitis and abscess (leg except foot), Hypertensive kidney disease (chronic)	965
9	041.11, 567.2, 998.59, 998.32, 682.2, 998.1	Staphylococcus aureus, Other suppurative peritonitis, Other postoperative infection, Disruption of external operation wound, Other cellulitis and abscess (trunk), Hemorrhage or hematoma or seroma complicating a procedure	270
10	278.00, 401.9, 780.57, 272.4, 250.00, 682.2	Obesity, unspecified, Essential hypertension, Unspecified sleep apnea, Other and unspecified hyperlipidemia, Diabetes mellitus without mention of complication (unspecified type), Other cellulitis and abscess (trunk)	260
11	596.54, 707.0, 907.2, 599.0, 344.1, 041.7	Neurogenic bladder NOS, Decubitus ulcer, Late effect of spinal cord injury, Urinary tract infection, site not specified, Paraplegia, Pseudomonas	338
12	319, 343.9, 780.3, v44.0, v44.1, 599.0	Unspecified mental retardation, Infantile cerebral palsy, unspecified, Convulsions, Tracheostomy, Gastrostomy, Urinary tract infection, site not specified	315
13	272.4, v45.01, 414.00, v45.81, 412, 428.0	Other and unspecified hyperlipidemia, Cardiac pacemaker, Of unspecified type of vessel, native or graft, Aortocoronary bypass status, Old myocardial infarction, Congestive heart failure, unspecified	439
14	V30.01, 770.89, 770.6, 770.81, 765.18, 779.3	Single liveborn, Other respiratory problems after birth, Transitory tachypnea of newborn, Primary apnea of newborn, Disorders relating to short gestation and low birthweight, Feeding problems in newborn	323
15	041.04, 644.03, 599.0, 646.63, 041.4, 041.3	Streptococcus (Group D [Enterococcus]), Threatened premature labor, Urinary tract infection, site not specified, Infections of genitourinary tract in pregnancy, Escherichia coli [E.coli], Friedländer's bacillus	274
16	263.9, 715.90, 294.8, 787.2, 599.0, 507.0	Unspecified protein-calorie malnutrition, Osteoarthrosis, unspecified whether generalized or localized, Other persistent mental disorders due to conditions classified elsewhere, Dysphagia, Urinary tract infection, site not specified, Pneumonitis due to solids and liquids due to inhalation of food or vomitus	505
17	276.1, 276.8, 276.7, 599.0, 491.21, 244.9	Hyposmolality and/or hyponatremia, Hypopotassemia, Hyperpotassemia, Urinary tract infection, site not specified, Obstructive chronic bronchitis with (acute) exacerbation, Unspecified hypothyroidism	358

Table 21. continued

Cluster #	Code Combinations	Translations	Frequency
18	382.9, 466.11, 558.9, 276.5, 458.9, 790.6	Unspecified otitis media, Acute bronchiolitis due to respiratory syncytial virus, Other and unspecified noninfectious gastroenteritis and colitis, Volume depletion, Hypotension, unspecified, Nonspecific findings on examination of blood (Other abnormal blood chemistry)	218
19	682.6, 916.5, 891.1, 916.1, 680.6, 041.11	Other cellulitis and abscess, leg other than foot, Insect bite, nonvenomous, infected, Open wound of knee, leg [except thigh], and ankle (complicated), Abrasion or friction burn, infected, Carbuncle and furuncle (leg except for foot), Staphylococcus aureus	191
20	785.52, 916.5, 891.1, 916.1, 680.6, 041.11	Septic shock, Insect bite, nonvenomous, infected, Open wound of knee, leg [except thigh], and ankle (complicated), Carbuncle and furuncle (leg except for foot)	399
21	530.81, 311, 553.3, 493.92, 786.50, 305.1	Esophageal reflux, Depressive disorder, not elsewhere classified, Diaphragmatic hernia, Asthma, unspecified, Chest pain, unspecified, Tobacco use disorder	284
22	244.9, 401.9, 733.00, v10.3, 272.4, v15.82	Unspecified hypothyroidism, Essential hypertension, Osteoporosis, unspecified, Personal history of malignant neoplasm (breast), Other and unspecified hyperlipidemia, History of tobacco use	326
23	913.5, 726.33, 682.4, 041.11, 682.3, 305.1	Insect bite, nonvenomous, infected, Olecranon bursitis, Other cellulitis and abscess (hand except fingers and thumb), Carbuncle and furuncle (leg except for foot), cellulitis and abscess (upper arm and forearm)	180
24	V05.3, 766.1, 767.8, 762.6, 774.6, v29.0	Viral hepatitis, Disorders relating to long gestation and high birthweight (Other "heavy-for-dates" infants), Other specified birth trauma, Other and unspecified conditions of umbilical cord, Unspecified fetal and neonatal jaundice, Observation for suspected infectious condition	398
25	583.81, 337.1, 250.40, 362.01, 357.2, 250.60	Nephritis and nephropathy, not specified as acute or chronic, in diseases classified elsewhere, Peripheral autonomic neuropathy in disorders classified elsewhere, Diabetes with renal manifestations of unspecified type, Background diabetic retinopathy, Polyneuropathy in diabetes, Diabetes with neurological manifestations of unspecified type	218
26	664.01, 659.61, 648.81, 658.11, 652.21, 642.31	First-degree perineal laceration, Elderly multigravida, Abnormal glucose tolerance, Premature rupture of membranes, Breech presentation without mention of version, Transient hypertension of pregnancy	508
27	427.31, 428.0, 507.0, 518.81, 496, 995.92	Atrial fibrillation, Congestive heart failure, unspecified, Pneumonitis due to solids and liquids (Due to inhalation of food or vomitus), Acute respiratory failure, Chronic airway obstruction, not elsewhere classified, Systemic inflammatory response syndrome due to infectious process with organ dysfunction	593
28	466.0, 491.21, 300.00, v15.82, 427.89, 428.0	Acute bronchitis and bronchiolitis, Obstructive chronic bronchitis (With (acute) exacerbation), Anxiety states, unspecified, History of tobacco use, Other specified cardiac dysrhythmias, Congestive heart failure, unspecified	399
29	626.2, v57.89, 285.1, v43.65, 280.0, 562.10	Excessive or frequent menstruation, Other specified rehabilitation procedure, Acute posthemorrhagic anemia, Organ or tissue replaced by other means, knee joint, Iron deficiency anemias, secondary to blood loss, Diverticulosis of colon (without mention of hemorrhage)	952
30	443.9, 401.9, 250.00, 997.62, 682.6, 682.7	Peripheral vascular disease, unspecified, Essential hypertension, Diabetes mellitus without mention of complication of unspecified type, Infection (chronic), Other cellulitis and abscess, leg except foot, Other cellulitis and abscess, foot except toes	181
31	V02.59, 311, 715.90, 300.00, 733.00, 682.2	Other specified bacterial diseases, Depressive disorder, not elsewhere classified, Osteoarthrosis, unspecified whether generalized or localized, Anxiety states, unspecified, Osteoporosis, unspecified, Other cellulitis and abscess, trunk	292
32	412, 428.0, 411.1, v45.82, 272.4, v45.01	Old myocardial infarction, Congestive heart failure, unspecified, Intermediate coronary syndrome, Percutaneous transluminal coronary angioplasty status, Other and unspecified hyperlipidemia, Cardiac pacemaker	515

Table 22. Clusters of procedures

Cluster #	Code Combinations	Translations	Frequency
1	39.95, 40.0, 39.43, 38.95, 39.42, 97.49	Hemodialysis, Incision of lymphatic structures, Removal of arteriovenous shunt for renal dialysis, Venous catheterization for renal dialysis, Revision of arteriovenous shunt for renal dialysis, Removal of other device from thorax	203
2	81.02, 84.51, 81.62, 81.08, 80.51, 77.79	Other cervical fusion, anterior technique, Insertion of interbody spinal fusion device, Fusion or refusion of 2-3 vertebrae, Lumbar and lumbosacral fusion, posterior technique, Excision of intervertebral disc, Excision of bone for graft (other)	45
3	93.89, 99.59, 93.24, 87.21, 86.03, 85.91	Rehabilitation, not elsewhere classified, Other vaccination and inoculation, Training in use of prosthetic or orthotic device, Contrast myelogram, Incision of pilonidal sinus or cyst, Aspiration of breast	4290
4	81.91, 80.26, 80.6, 81.83, 77.81, 80.16	Arthrocentesis, Arthroscopy of knee, Excision of semilunar cartilage of knee, Other repair of shoulder, Other partial ostectomy of ribs and sternum, Other arthrotomy of knee	144
5	88.72, 42.23, 89.44, 37.99, 81.11, 39.95	Diagnostic ultrasound of heart, Other esophagoscopy, Other cardiovascular stress test, Other operations on heart and pericardium, Ankle fusion, Hemodialysis	135
6	74.1, 75.34, 03.95, 99.48, 66.32, 66.39	Low cervical cesarean section, Other fetal monitoring, Spinal blood patch, Administration of measles-mumps-rubella vaccine, Other bilateral ligation and division of fallopian tubes, Other bilateral destruction or occlusion of fallopian tubes	171
7	79.36, 33.27, 22.19, 33.24, 86.11, 96.04	Open reduction of fracture with internal fixation of knee, Closed endoscopic biopsy of lung, Other diagnostic procedures on nasal sinuses, Closed [endoscopic] biopsy of bronchus, Biopsy of skin and subcutaneous tissue, Insertion of endotracheal tube	150
8	65.61, 54.59, 68.59, 68.29, 68.39, 70.92	Other removal of both ovaries and tubes at same operative episode, Laparoscopic lysis of peritoneal adhesions, Other vaginal hysterectomy, Other excision or destruction of lesion of uterus, Other subtotal abdominal hysterectomy, NOS, Other operations on cul-de-sac	170
9	87.74, 68.51, 59.8, 60.29, 56.0, 56.31	Retrograde pyelogram, Laparoscopically assisted vaginal hysterectomy, Ureteral catheterization, Other transurethral prostatectomy, Transurethral removal of obstruction from ureter and renal pelvis, Ureteroscopy	144
10	37.22, 88.56, 88.53, 37.94, 88.72, 36.12	Left heart cardiac catheterization, Coronary arteriography using two catheters, Angiocardiography of left heart structures, Implantation or replacement of automatic cardioverter/defibrillator, total system, Diagnostic ultrasound of heart, (Aorto)coronary bypass of two coronary arteries	192
11	88.76, 51.22, 54.91, 88.38, 51.23, 51.85	Diagnostic ultrasound of abdomen and retroperitoneum, Cholecystectomy, Percutaneous abdominal drainage, Other computerized axial tomography, Laparoscopic cholecystectomy, Endoscopic sphincterotomy and papillotomy	261
12	94.68, 86.3, 86.74, 86.28, 86.59, 86.22	Combined alcohol and drug detoxification, Other local excision or destruction of lesion or tissue of skin and subcutaneous tissue, Attachment of pedicle or flap graft to other sites, Nonexcisional debridement of wound, infection or burn, Closure of skin and subcutaneous tissue of other sites, Excisional debridement of wound, infection, or burn	715
13	03.09, 81.61, 93.54, 77.79, 99.02, 81.63	Other exploration and decompression of spinal canal, Other procedures on spine, Application of splint, Excision of bone for graft (other), Transfusion of previously collected autologous blood, Fusion or refusion of 4- 8 vertebrae	101
14	99.20, 88.53, 37.22, 88.57, 36.07, 36.01	Injection or infusion of platelet inhibitor, Angiocardiography of left heart structures, Left heart cardiac catheterization, Other and unspecified coronary arteriography, Insertion of drug-eluting coronary artery stent(s), Removal of coronary artery obstruction and insertion of stent(s)	192
15	96.6, 97.02, 99.99, 97.03, 43.11, 96.72	Enteral infusion of concentrated nutritional substances, Replacement of gastrostomy tube, Leech therapy, Replacement of tube or enterostomy device of small intestine, Percutaneous [endoscopic] gastrostomy, Continuous mechanical ventilation for 96 consecutive hours or more	157

Table 22. continued

Cluster #	Code Combinations	Translations	Frequency
16	45.23, 45.13, 42.92, 45.42, 45.25, 43.41	Colonoscopy, Other endoscopy of small intestine, Dilation of esophagus, Endoscopic polypectomy of large intestine, Closed [endoscopic] biopsy of large intestine, Biopsy, closed, of unspecified intestinal site, Other local excision of lesion of duodenum	117
17	99.19, 99.18, 99.17, 99.29, 99.23, 89.52	Injection of anticoagulant, Injection or infusion of electrolytes, Injection of insulin, Injection or infusion of other therapeutic or prophylactic substance, Injection of steroid, Electrocardiogram	163
18	75.62, 73.01, 72.71, 73.4, 73.59, 73.09	Repair of current obstetric laceration of rectum and sphincter ani, Induction of labor by artificial rupture of membranes, Vacuum extraction with episiotomy, Medical induction of labor, Other manually assisted delivery, Other artificial rupture of membranes	437
19	99.07, 86.05, 93.90, 94.65, 84.17, 86.0	Transfusion of other serum, Incision with removal of foreign body or device from skin and subcutaneous tissue, Continuous positive airway pressure, Drug detoxification, Amputation above knee, Incision of skin and subcutaneous tissue	437
20	73.4, 74.1, 03.91, 73.09, 96.49, 75.34	Medical induction of labor, Low cervical cesarean section, Injection of anesthetic into spinal canal for analgesia, Other artificial rupture of membranes, Other genitourinary instillation, Other fetal monitoring	600
21	95.47, 54.21, 99.83, 38.92, 45.76, 47.09	Hearing examination, not otherwise specified, Laparoscopy, Other phototherapy, Umbilical vein catheterization, Sigmoidectomy, Other appendectomy	91
22	38.93, 80.82, 54.3, 85.0, 82.01	Venous catheterization, not elsewhere classified, Other local excision or destruction of lesion of joint (elbow), Excision or destruction of lesion or tissue of abdominal wall or umbilicus, Mastotomy, Exploration of tendon sheath of hand	475
23	96.71, 96.72, 96.04, 38.91, 31.1, 38.93	Continuous mechanical ventilation for less than 96 consecutive hours, Continuous mechanical ventilation for 96 consecutive hours or more, Insertion of endotracheal tube, Arterial catheterization, Temporary tracheostomy, Venous catheterization, not elsewhere classified	602
24	86.27, 94.27, 34.04, 79.35, 94.62, 37.83	Debridement of nail, nail bed, or nail fold, Other electroshock therapy, Insertion of intercostal catheter for drainage, Open reduction of fracture with internal fixation (femur), Alcohol detoxification, Initial insertion of dual-chamber device	323
25	86.04, 83.19, 86.22, 38.93, 78.63, 86.66	Other incision with drainage of skin and subcutaneous tissue, Other division of soft tissue, Excisional debridement of wound, infection, or burn, Venous catheterization, not elsewhere classified, Removal of implanted devices from bone (radius and ulna), Homograft to skin	352
26	45.42, 44.22, 45.23, 45.16, 45.25, 44.43	Endoscopic polypectomy of large intestine, Endoscopic dilation of pylorus, Colonoscopy, Esophagogastroduodenoscopy [EGD] with closed biopsy, Closed [endoscopic] biopsy of large intestine, Endoscopic control of gastric or duodenal bleeding	251
27	39.50, 39.29, 39.90, 88.49, 88.48, 38.12	Angioplasty or atherectomy of other non-coronary vessel(s), Other (peripheral) vascular shunt or bypass, Insertion of non-drug-eluting peripheral vessel stent(s), Arteriography of other specified sites, Arteriography of femoral and other lower extremity arteries, Endarterectomy (other vessels of head and neck)	325
28	95.46, 25.91, 99.55, 64.0, 95.47, 95.41	Other auditory and vestibular function tests, Lingual frenotomy, Prophylactic administration of vaccine against other diseases, Circumcision, Hearing examination, not otherwise specified, Audiometry	251
29	99.05, 99.25, 86.05, 88.91, 86.07, 03.31	Transfusion of platelets, Injection or infusion of cancer chemotherapeutic substance, Incision with removal of foreign body or device from skin and subcutaneous tissue, Magnetic resonance imaging of brain and brain stem, Insertion of totally implantable vascular access device, Spinal tap	325
30	93.75, 94.44, 93.81, 94.39, 94.25, 94.38	Other speech training and therapy, Other group therapy, Recreation therapy, Other individual psychotherapy, Other psychiatric drug therapy, Supportive verbal psychotherapy	102
31	86.04, 21.1, 71.09	Other incision with drainage of skin and subcutaneous tissue, Incision of nose, Other incision of vulva and perineum	387

example, cluster 20 contains insect bite in addition to conditions related to wounds. Often, a community-acquired infection is first diagnosed as an insect bite. Additional clusters are listed below.

Cluster 6 is related to patients with diabetes who have problems with diabetic foot ulcers:

440.23: atherosclerosis of the extremities with ulceration
707.15: ulcer of toes
250.70: diabetes with peripheral circulatory disorder
250.80: diabetes with other specified manifestations
682.7: cellulitis of foot
730.07: acute osteomyelitis of ankle and foot

Cluster 19 is related to bursitis and wounds:

916.5: insect bite, nonvenomous, infected
891.1: complicated open wounded of knee
916.1: abrasion or friction burn, infected
680.6: carbuncle and furuncle
726.65: prepatellar bursitis
989.5: venom

Cluster 22 is related to severe infection:

785.52: septic shock
996.62: complications of reattached hand
403.91: hypertensive kidney disease
996.73: complications of renal dialysis device
584.9: acute renal failure
036.9: meningococcal infection

Cluster 23 is related to abuse as well as to infection:

913.5: insect bite, infected
726.33: olecranon bursitis
682.4: cellulitis of hand
682.3: cellulitis, upper arm
305.1: tobacco use disorder
305.60: cocaine abuse
305.70: amphetamine abuse
305.90: unspecified drug abuse

We list some of the procedure clusters below.
Cluster 1:

39.95: Hemodialysis

40.0: Incision of lymphatic structures

39.43: Removal of arteriovenous shunt for renal dialysis

38.95: Venous catheterization for renal dialysis

39.42: Revision of arteriovenous shunt for renal dialysis

Cluster 22:

39.93: Insertion of vessel-to-vessel cannula

80.82: Other local excision or destruction of lesion of joint (elbow)

54.3: Excision or destruction of lesion or tissue of abdominal wall or umbilicus

85.0: Mastotomy

82.01: Exploration of tendon sheath of hand

Both of these clusters (as shown in Table 1) have a high incidence rate of MRSA. Contrast these with cluster 2 with a low incidence rate of MRSA:

81.02 Other cervical fusion, anterior technique

84.51 Insertion of interbody spinal fusion device

81.62 Fusion or refusion of 2-3 vertebrae

81.08 Lumbar and lumbosacral fusion, posterior technique

81.51 Total hip replacement

Another cluster with a high proportion of MRSA is 31:

86.04: Other incision with drainage of skin and subcutaneous tissue

21.1: Incision of nose

71.09: Other incision of vulva and perineum

Similarly, cluster 25 starts in the same way, with procedures related to wounds:

86.04: Other incision with drainage of skin and subcutaneous tissue

83.19: Other division of soft tissue

86.22: Excisional debridement of wound, infection, or burn

38.93: Venous catheterization, not elsewhere classified

78.6: Removal of implanted devices from bone

86.66: Homograft to skin

Figure 25 shows a representation of the patients classified into Cluster 6. The multiple diagnosis codes for diabetes are very prominent, as are the diagnosis codes for osteomyelitis (730). However, there are also a number of patients with diagnoses 681 and 682 (Cellulitis and abscess of finger and toe, Other cellulitis and abscess). These two diagnoses commonly accompany a diagnosis of osteomyelitis. For this reason, they are given a lower weight when there is also a diagnosis of osteomyelitis and are not used to characterize the cluster when using text analysis.

Similarly, Figure 26 shows some of the patients classified into cluster 7. In this cluster, diagnosis 681 is again quite prominent. However, in contrast to cluster 6, there is no accompanying diagnosis of 730 for osteomyelitis. Therefore, 681 has higher weight when determining the characteristics of the cluster.

In addition, the specific codes that appear are 682.2 (cellulitis in the trunk) and 682.5 (cellulitis in the buttock), indicating that these patients are also characterized by the specific location of the condition. These conditions are more likely to occur from sexual practices rather than from diabetes. This is in contrast to Figure 25, which is more likely to have 682.7, or cellulitis in the foot.

Figure 27 shows the proportion of MRSA cases per diagnosis cluster; Figure 28 shows the proportion per procedure cluster. As Figure 27 shows, clusters 6,7,9,19,20, and 23 have the highest rates of resistant infection. Cluster 6 suggests foot ulcers and cellulitis that are commonly associated with diabetes; cluster 9 suggests nosocomial resistant infection from childbirth. Clusters 19, 20, and 23 suggest a community acquired infection that was initially diagnosed as an insect bite.(Gorwitz et al., 2006) Cluster 7 appears to be the result of male-on-male sexual practices.(Beck, 2008; Erskine, 2008) Because diagnoses cannot distinguish between nosocomial and community acquired MRSA, diagnoses will not be sufficient to predict the occurrence of nosocomial infection. Cluster 14, focused primarily on childbirth, has a very low occurrence of MRSA, as do clusters 24 and 26. These two clusters are also focused on childbirth. The fact that the occurrence is low indicates that prophylactic treatment is probably not necessary for labor and delivery, nor is it necessary when treating the newborns.

Figure 28 indicates that there is a considerable difference in the rate of MRSA by procedure cluster.

Figure 25. Patients in cluster 6

DIAGNOSES
6827 25002 73017 68110 4019 5939 28529
25080 70715 40391 68110 04111 V090 2859 41401 4264
68110 04111 V090
73027 6827 70715 04111 25000 4019 44023 71590 V090
25080 70714 7318 7854 40391 73027 3569 04111 V090
70713 5990 04111 V090 44023 73027 2989 25080 7318
25080 6827 V090 V4972 3051 4019 V0259 4439 70715
6827 04111 V090 042
6827 04111 V090 042
25070 6827 V1259 78701 53081 2859 311 2761 4019 04111 V4973 V090 44023 2449 70715
6827 V090 04184 04111
V5849 V4972 2724 25050 4019 V090 25070 73007 2809 7318 04111 V4971
25081 6827 28529 0416 04104 4439 40391 2749 78820 2724 53081 60001 V090 70715
25071 25081 04104 58381 25041 4019 7318 V1259 04111 V1581 V090 73027 2859 44024
70715 6827 3441 V090 34461 04111 6826
73017 6827 71590 73390 4439 04111 V090 7242 71107
25071 7070 V090 25081 2948 4019 7318 6827 73027 70719 04111 7854 70714 V441 5990
25080 7318 04111 41401 V090 V1259 70715 3051 496 25070 6827 V4975 73027
486 4280 71906 73027 V090 04111 2859 70715 27800 25080 V5861 7318 4512 4019 51882
5990 6827 25080 V090 04111 70715
44024 6827 5533 V090 3051 70715 04111 78099 4019 73007
99762 68110 V5867 V090 25080 4019 2724 04111 70715
6827 04111 V090 9173
68110 V090 04111
7907 25082 V1582 51889 04102 7318 04111 V090 73027 70715
25082 7318 73027 04111 04102 68110 6827
70715 04111 3004 70705 25000 V090 40391 73300 7100 68110
70715 04111 V090 2859 49390 4019 6827
99762 7318 V090 73027 V4975 04111 311 25080
6827 V090 04111
6827 04111 3004 V155 V090 7295 2859 49320 4019 70715

Figure 26. Patients in cluster 7

DIAGNOSES
68100 6822 04111 V090 3051 V642
67434 6822 7907 64894 7098 65484 6248 04111 V090
68100 04111 V090
7821 4730 04111 V090 V4589
6820 6822 6800 6825 04111 V090 7840
6805 6825 04111 V090 6930
6825 04111 V090
6822 04111 V090
6822 7907 6802 04111 V090
566 04111 V090
9195 04111 V090
6822 25001 04111 V090 4019
6822 6850 70583 04111 V090 25000 4019 71690
68100 04111 V090
6825 04111 V090
6822 25081 04111 V090 4019
0542 3829 04111 V090 3480 7422
68100 73098 04111 V090 72789
475 04111 V090 V08
6826 6823 6822 6806 6803 25081 04111 V090 70583
6822 04111 V090
6822 6802 04111 V090 V453
6822 99811 04111 V090
6084 04111 V090
6822 25003 04111 V090
6829 04111 V090
6822 V090 3051
38001 38013 684
6822 V090 04111
6820 V090 04111
042 04111 69010 V090 78791 5368 29690 6822

Figure 27. Rate of MRSA by diagnosis cluster

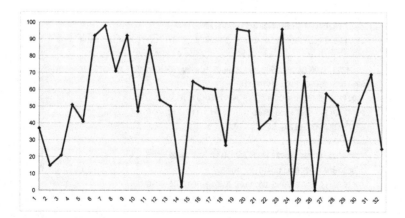

Figure 28. Rate of MRSA by procedure cluster

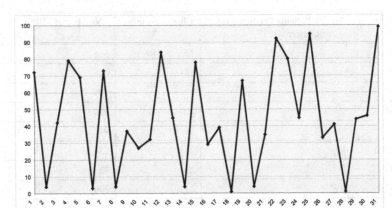

Figure 29. Scoring text clusters

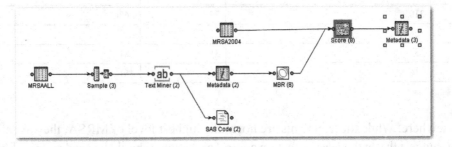

There are some clusters that have extremely high rates and these high rates suggest that patients in those clusters should be treated prophylactically to reduce the rate of resistant infection. Clusters 22, 25, and 31 have the highest rates of infection. These suggest that there is a relationship between infection and surgical wounds with debridement, joint destruction, and wound drainage.

In contrast, procedure clusters 6, 8, and 18 have low rates of resistant infection. Clusters 6 and 18 relate to childbirth, reinforcing the discovery from the diagnosis clusters that childbirth has a low occurrence of MRSA. Cluster 8 has to do with hysterectomies. Patients in these clusters do not seem to need prophylactic treatment.

We want to determine the robustness of the defined clusters of diagnoses. Figure 29 shows the model using new data from the National Inpatient Sample. We used 2005 data to define the text clusters; we use 2004 data to score them.

Table 23 gives the frequency count for both the 2004 and 2005 data by cluster to see if the distribution is relatively similar. In particular, we want to determine whether there are any patients in cluster 7 in the year 2004, dealing with MRSA infection from homosexual sexual practices. Approximately 447 patients are predicted into that cluster, indicating that the trend started as early as 2004.

The vast majority of patients were predicted into cluster #6, with diagnoses: Atherosclerosis of the extremities with ulceration, Ulcer of other part of foot (toes), Diabetes with peripheral circulatory disorders (unspecified type), Diabetes with other specified manifestations (Type II or unspecified uncontrolled), Diabetes with other specified manifestations (of unspecified type), Other bone involvement in diseases

Table 23. Scored diagnosis clusters for 2004 data

Cluster Number	Number of MRSA Patients Predicted into Cluster	Cluster Number	Number of MRSA Patients Predicted into Cluster
1	98	17	365
2	623	18	64
3	66	19	100
4	191	20	320
5	71	21	94
6	48496	22	134
7	447	23	72
8	1971	24	700
9	86	25	78
10	225	26	469
11	260	27	546
12	145	28	477
13	210	29	2680
14	105	30	27
15	55	31	181
16	316	32	451

classified elsewhere. While these patients are not at the highest level of MRSA, they are at a very high level. It does suggest that at the least, infection control procedures should be used on this class of patients to reduce the occurrence of MRSA. Another large number of infections are predicted into cluster 29, Excessive or frequent menstruation, Other specified rehabilitation procedure, Acute posthemorrhagic anemia, Organ or tissue replaced by other means, knee joint, Iron deficiency anemias, secondary to blood loss, Diverticulosis of colon (without mention of hemorrhage). These patients, however, have a much lower occurrence of MRSA and prophylactic treatment is probably unnecessary.

We next use predictive modeling. First, we need to define a profit/loss matrix to determine the difference between a positive prediction of MRSA, and a negative prediction. Then, we need to partition the sampled dataset into training, validation, and testing subsets. We also use several models to determine the model of best fit.(P. B. Cerrito, 2007) Since we have over-sampled the occurrence of MRSA, we also need to set the prior probabilities of occurrence and non-occurrence to those that exist in the population. In this first example, the procedure and diagnosis clusters are defined as interval variables.

The use of a profit/loss matrix will not change the model results; it will change the choice of which model is optimal. The default for "best" fit is the misclassification rate; this can be modified to finding the model with the highest profit (or minimal loss). Therefore, by changing the profit/loss matrix, we can perform a sensitivity analysis to determine when the optimal model choice will change. We use the available patient demographics as well as the categories of patient diagnoses and procedures. Using just the misclassification, the optimal model is a regression with a 50% misclassification rate. Since we used a 50/50 split in the data, 50% misclassification is a poor fit. If the cost of treatment is 10 times the cost for prophylactic treatment, the best model is a neural network with an overall average cost less than 1/10 of the cost of prophylactic treatment per patient. If the cost of treatment is 100 times the cost for prophylactic treatment, then the best model is a decision tree with an average cost that is ½ of the cost of prophylactic treatment per patient. In other words, as the cost of treatment of MRSA increases, more patients are targeted for prophylactic treatment. The decision tree is given in Figure 30. Note that because the procedure clusters and diagnosis clusters are defined as interval variables, the splits occur based upon a numbered level.

Note that the procedure clusters are more prominent compared to the diagnosis clusters when defining the decision tree. Note also that there is a combination of procedure cluster and diagnosis cluster used in determining risk for MRSA. Only one patient demographic, age, is used in the tree, and then, only on one branch. In other words, it is the diagnosis and procedure more than the demographics that are important in determining patient risk. The corresponding ROC curve is given in Figure 31. It appears to be a good fit in terms of both specificity and sensitivity.

This decision tree shows that it is possible to get a model even while mis-identifying variables. The

Figure 30. Decision tree with a cost of treatment that is 100 times the cost of prophylactic treatment

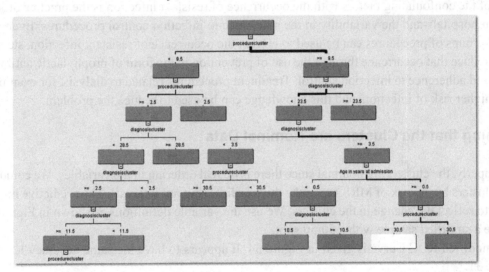

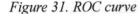

Figure 31. ROC curve

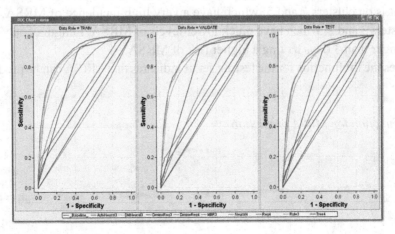

diagnosis and procedure clusters are nominal data, and should more properly be identified as nominal. Once the inequalities are noted in the decision tree, it should be corrected and redone.

However, if this model is used, almost 95% of the patients are treated prophylactically. That is not a reasonable result, so we look to find the patients at highest risk. For this, we use the lift function, shown in Figure 32.

Figure 32 indicates that the lift is two or higher for the first decile of patients. The highest lift in this decile comes from a regression model. It shows that approximately 10% of the patients should very definitely be treated prophylactically.

While the National Inpatient Sample does not include prescription information, there are two procedures related to antibiotics: 99.21 (infusion of antibiotic) and 00.14 (infusion of linezolid). Surprisingly, only 58 of the MRSA patients had either of these procedures listed in any of the 15 columns of procedure codes. This was an unexpected finding in the data. Either the patients are not treated with antibiotics, or the use of antibiotics is substantially under-reported in the hospital environment. Data mining can help you to investigate results that you do not anticipate. The use of antibiotics for resistant infection requires additional study.

One of the confounding factors with the occurrence of resistant infection is the practice of infection control in hospitals-and the variability in the adherence to infection control procedures. Even so, once different groups of procedures can be used to predict the occurrence of resistant infection, steps can be taken to reduce that occurrence through the use of prevention in the form of prophylactic antibiotics, or in increased adherence to infection control. Treatment procedures related to dialysis, for example, have a much higher risk of infection, and this knowledge can be used to reduce the problem.

Assuming that the Clusters are Nominal Data

More properly, the clusters are nominal since there is no real ordering in the variables. We could renumber the clusters by the risk of MRSA to make them ordinal (but not interval). The predictive model then changes to reflect the change in the clusters. We use the variable definitions as shown in Figure 33. We again use a stratified sample with a 50/50 split.

The modified ROC Curve is given in Figure 34. It appears to have the same accuracy level as that in Figure 31.

The corresponding decision tree is given in Figure 35. Note that the clusters are separated individually in the tree in contrast to the tree shown in Figure 30. It is also a simpler tree compared to that in Figure 30. The first split is on clusters 7 and 5, which have a very high incidence of MRSA. The next split is on diagnosis clusters 3 and 2, which have much lower levels of MRSA. Length of stay also contributes, with a stay of longer than 3 days having a higher risk of MRSA.

Figure 36 gives the lift function for the testing set. It indicates that MRSA can be predicted for the first

Figure 32. Lift Function for MRSA prediction

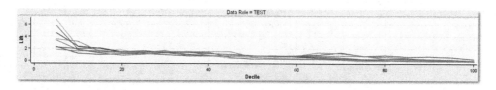

Figure 33. Variable definitions

Name	Role	Level
AGE	Input	Interval
ASOURCE	Input	Nominal
FEMALE	Input	Nominal
KEY	ID	Nominal
LOS	Input	Interval
RACE	Input	Nominal
TOTCHG	Input	Interval
ZIPInc_Qrtl	Input	Ordinal
diagnosescluster	Input	Nominal
mrsa	Target	Binary
procedurecluster	Input	Nominal

Figure 34. ROC for modified predictive model

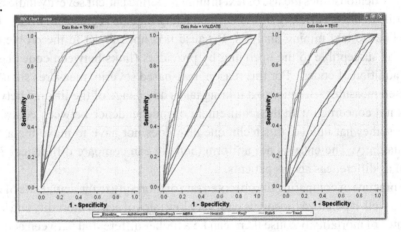

Figure 35. Decision tree results

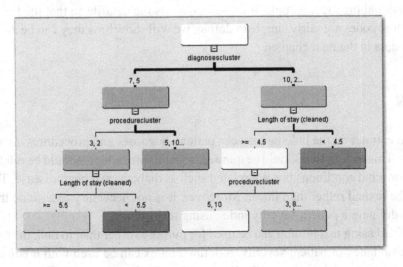

Figure 36. Lift function for revised prediction model

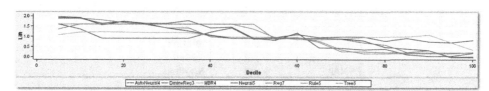

4 deciles. Therefore, we can now identify the high risk patients in the first four deciles. Moreover, the patients in the last 3 deciles have a low risk of MRSA and would not require any prophylactic treatment.

FUTURE TRENDS

This chapter clearly demonstrates the use of text mining to define patient severity indices. It gives results that are far superior to those currently in use defined using logistic regression. Future trends will be to convert more indices to text mining analysis. Because it is not subject to the problems of regression models, it is not as susceptible to the upcoding by providers (links between codes become more important than the addition of codes). For this reason, text-based severity measures should take the place of regression-based measures. Because text mining takes advantage of the linkage between conditions, this procedure is not concerned with the requirement of independence between codes. Because text is considered to be somewhat unique, this technique also does not have to make the assumption of the uniformity of data entry. The entry is not uniform, and we can compare differences in coding across providers as well as differences across patients.

However, the practice of comparing the observed rate of mortality to the actual rate of mortality should be reconsidered as well. It penalizes hospitals with very low rates of actual mortality and rewards hospitals with very high rates of mortality because there can be a higher differential between actual and predicted rates when the actual rate is high. While it can be very satisfactory to develop a "scorecard" to rank providers, quality of care is multi-dimensional, and it should be examined in multiple dimensions.

While the National Inpatient Sample, used here, defines the datafile so that the text strings of diagnosis and procedure codes are fairly simple to define, we will show how they can be defined using more complex claims data in the next chapter.

DISCUSSION

Text mining concentrates on the linkage between patient diagnoses and procedures, assuming that there are relationships. This assumption should be quite reasonable-procedures should be related to diagnoses, and there are co-morbid conditions that are related such as diabetes and heart disease. The relationships are assumed to be textual rather than linear. Moreover, it is not necessary to assume the uniformity of data entry when defining a patient severity index using text mining.

An index defined using text mining can be used for purposes other than to rank the quality of providers and to define an index of patient severity. A defined index can be used with predictive modeling to determine patients most at risk for a specific disease; in particular, we can predict for a specific nosocomial illness in order to prevent the outcome from occurring. We showed one example here; others can be considered as well. In particular, text mining can be used to predict the risk of patient falls, and of medication errors so that prevention can also be used to reduce such adverse events.

One of the biggest problems with defining such indices is that they do not give similar or consistent results. Therefore, the use of the technique of text mining to define patients at highest risk for nosocomial infection allows validation by comparing the index to outcomes. In addition, the relationship of a severity index to patient outcomes allows for validation when the outcomes are not used to define the index, as is the case with text mining techniques.

REFERENCES

Anonymous-ICD9. Version. icd9.chrisendres.com

Beck, A. (2008). Drug-resistant staph found to be passed in gay sex. *Thomson Reuters*.

Bootsma, M., Diekmann, O., & Bonten, M. (2006). Controlling methicillin-resistant Staphylococcus aureus: quantifying the effects of interventions and rapid diagnostic testing. *Proceedings of the National Academy of Sciences of the United States of America, 103*(14), 5620–5625.doi:10.1073/pnas.0510077103

Cerrito, P. (2007). Text Mining Coded Information. In H. A. D. Prado & E. Ferneda (Eds.), *Emerging Technologies of Text Mining: Techniques and Applications*. New York: IGI Global.

Cerrito, P. B. (2007). *Introduction to Data Mining with Enterprise Miner*. Cary, NC: SAS Press.

Coia, J., Duckworth, G., Edwards, D., Farrington, M., Fry, C., & Humphreys, H. (2006). Guidelines for the control and prevention of meticillin-resistant Staphylococcus aureus in healthcare facilities. *The Journal of Hospital Infection, 63*(Suppl 1), S1–S44.doi:10.1016/j.jhin.2006.01.001

Erskine, R. (2008). Study shows stronger MRSA strain spreading among homosexual men [Electronic Version]. *WCSH6, January 21, 2008* from http://www.wcsh6.com/news/article.aspx?storyid=78949.

Feldman, R., & Sanger, J. (2006). *The Text mining Handbook: Advanced Approaches in Analyzing Unstructured Data*. Cambridge, UK: Cambridge University Press.

Gerber, S. I., Jones, R. C., Scott, M. V., Price, J. S., Dworkin, M. S., & Filippell, M. B. (2006). Management of outbreaks of methicillin-resistant Staphylococcus aureus infection in the neonatal intensive care unit: a consensus statement. *Infection Control and Hospital Epidemiology, 27*(2), 139–145. doi:10.1086/501216

Gorwitz, R. J., Jernigan, D. B., Powers, J. H., & Jernigan, J. A. (2006). *Strategies for clinical management of MRSA in the community: summary of an experts' meeting convened by the Centers for Disease Control and Prevention*.

Henderson, D. K. (2006). Managing methicillin-resistant staphylococci: A paradigm for preventing nosocomial transmission of resistant organisms. *The American Journal of Medicine, 119*(6Suppl 1), S45–S52.doi:10.1016/j.amjmed.2006.04.002

Kao, A., & Poteet, S. R. (2006). *Natural Language Processing and Text Mining*. Berlin: Springer.

Lodise, T., McKinnon, P. S., & Rybak, M. (2003). Prediction model to identify patients with Staphylococcus aureus bacteremia at risk for methicillin resistance. *Infection Control & Epidemiology, 24*(9), 655–661. doi:10.1086/502269

Loveday, H., Pellowe, C., Jones, S., & Pratt, R. (2006). A systematic review of the evidence for interventions for the prevention and control of methicillin-resistant Staphylococcus aureus (1996-2004): report to the Joint MRSA Working Party. *The Journal of Hospital Infection, 63*(Suppl 1), S45–S70. doi:10.1016/j.jhin.2006.01.002

Malde, D., Hardern, L., & Welch, M. (2006). Is it possible to predict outcome in MRSA positive patients undergoing arterial reconstruction. *International Angiology, 25*(1), 78–83.

Masaki, H., Nagatake, T., Asoh, N., Yoshimine, H., Watanbe, K., & Watanabe, H. (2006). Significant reduction of nosocomial pneumonia after introduction of disinfection of upper airways using providone-iodone in geriatric wards. *Dermatology (Basel, Switzerland), 212*(Suppl 1), 98–102. doi:10.1159/000089206

McBryde, E., Pettit, A., & McElwain, D. (2007). A stochastic mathematical model of methicillin resistant Staphylococcus aureus transmission in an intensive care unit: predicting the impact of interventions. *Journal of Theoretical Biology, 245*(3), 470–481.doi:10.1016/j.jtbi.2006.11.008

Pear, R. (2007, August 19, 2007). Medicare Says It Won't Cover Hospital Errors. *New York Times*.

Roghmann, M. (2000). Predicting methicillin resistance and the effect of inadequate empiric therapy on survival in patients with Staphylococcus aureus bacteremia. *Archives of Internal Medicine, 160*(7), 1001–1004. doi:10.1001/archinte.160.7.1001

Thomas, S., Cantrill, S., Waghorn, D., & McIntyre, A. (2007). The role of screening and antibiotic prophylaxis in the prevention of percutaneous gastrostomy site infection caused by methicillin-resistant Staphylococcus aureus. *Alimentary Pharmacology & Therapeutics, 25*(5), 593–597.

Weiss, S., Indurkhya, N., Zhang, T., & Damerau, F. (2004). *Text Mining: Predictive Methods for Analyzing Unstructured Information*. Berlin: Springer.

Chapter 9
Working from Claims Data

INTRODUCTION

Claims data are more difficult to work with to extract the necessary information about patient conditions in relationship to costs. There can be multiple claims for the same patient episode from different sources. A physician visit after an inpatient claim can be followed up for the inpatient stay rather than to consider the inpatient stay as the start of a new patient episode or a new patient problem. Therefore, in addition to analyzing patient conditions as represented by ICD9 codes, we must also attempt to define an episode and to distinguish between new problems and follow up of old problems.

The second major difference in using claims data as opposed to the data we have been using up to this point is that there exists a one-to-many relationship in the data that must be taken care of. For example, one inpatient stay may have several follow up visits, and one or two of those visits may be classified as outpatient stays while others are classified as physician visits. We need to find a way to convert the one-to-many relationship to a one-to-one so that we can investigate outcomes. Another difference is that not all medical services are necessarily allowable, so that the medical record may be incomplete. For example, until recently, Medicare disallowed almost all medications. Therefore, such information

DOI: 10.4018/978-1-60566-752-2.ch009

would not be recoverable. However, inpatient medications are usually not identified separately in the billing record, so such information would still remain incomplete.

Moreover, although hospital providers tend to use ICD9 codes, physicians are more likely to use the CPT coding system. Therefore, in addition to defining episodes, it is necessary to be able to use multiple coding systems. In this chapter, we will discuss the means of working with such data to determine patient severity. Because of the nature of text mining, it is very well equipped to use multiple coding systems since it mostly relies upon the linkage between codes instead of relying on a specific list of codes. It is the linkage between codes that is used in text mining to define patient clusters.

BACKGROUND

Claims data are used to identify general trends concerning patient treatment. (Smith-Bindman, Quale, Chu, Rosenberg, & Kerlikowske, 2006; Wilkinson, Askew, & Dixon, 2006) Claims data are also used to make cross-references to different treatments. In Ceratti, Roger France, and Beguin, claims information was compared to the hospital clinical database to determine if treatment and diagnosis were related, or whether treatment was absent given a diagnosis. (Ceratti, France, & Beguin, 2008) Such observational studies relating billing data to clinical outcomes are fairly common.(Kaushal, Bates, Franz, Soukup, & Rothschild, 2007) Billing charges for prophylactic medication can also be compared to average costs of disease treatment.(Collinet-Adler et al., 2007)

Another study cross-referenced billing data from general practice to that of hospital emergency departments to see if patient visits for infection in the general practice could predict near term increases in emergency room utilization for similar infections.(Sloane et al., 2006) Another use of claims data has been to determine whether appropriate testing is conducted for patients with chronic illnesses. For example, claims are used to determine if patients with diabetes are administered regular A1C tests or to determine if patients with heart conditions are prescribed an ace inhibitor. (Philipneri et al., 2008)

Since multiple providers treat the same patients, the development of a patient severity index will not be as useful to rank the quality of providers since it will become difficult to separate the contribution of each provider. Instead, it can be used to find patterns of treatment and to find those treatment patterns that lead to the best patient outcomes. It can be used to find the relationship between different treatments and different outcomes for the same patient conditions.

First, the data have to be examined to define separate episodes, and to investigate episodes in relationship to patient outcomes. Solutions under the general category of episode grouper have been developed specifically to fuse claims data. The methodology is difficult to find since it is mostly proprietary, and little exists in the research literature.(P. Claus, P. Carpenter, C. Chute, D. Mohr, & P. Gibbons, 1997; Forthman, Dove, & Wooster, 2000; Rosen & Mayer-Oakes, 1999) A brief summary is given in Forthman, Dove and Wooster.(Forthman et al., 2000) The main purpose of these groupers is to identify homogeneous groups of patients so that cost comparisons and summaries can be made. These "episode groupers" are used in analysis with little understanding as to how episodes are defined or how patients are grouped.(Bassin, 1999; Currie et al., 2005; Kerr, McGlynn, Vorst, & Wickstrom, 2000; Thomas, 2005; Wan, Crown, Berndt, Finkelstein, & Ling, 2002) However, it is known that the groupers do not take into consideration the severity of an individual patient's condition.(Thomas, 2005)

One method of grouping is to examine medications of a similar nature, and to define the end of an episode if there is at least one day between prescriptions.(Bonetto, Nose, & Barbui, 2006) The Medicare

Claims Processing Manual defines an episode of care as having a maximum time period of 60 days or until discharge, although episodes of care can be overlapping.(Anonymous, 2006b) Another study defined episodes as 30-day periods while a third compared 4-month to 9-month absence of treatment as the end of an episode.(Ritzwoller, Crounse, Shetterly, & Rublee, 2006; Thomas, 2006) There are still other definitions of episodes, including one per year.(Hong et al., 1998) However, such fixed time intervals do not take into consideration the nature and requirement of follow up to major treatment events.

The main method used to define an episode of care is a variable timeframe, or "washout" period, defined as a continuous time period with an absence of treatment; that time period changes with the definition of the patient's condition.(Anonymous, 2006a; P. L. Claus, P. C. Carpenter, C. G. Chute, D. N. Mohr, & P. S. Gibbons, 1997; Hall & Llinas, 2001) Such a method assumes the existence of a washout period. This may not exist in the treatment of chronic diseases.

Unfortunately, it is not always clear just what that time period should be. For example, when a bone gets infected with the superbug known as MRSA, recurrence can occur up to a year after treatment is completed. Should this year be the definition of an episode, or should a period of say, six months be used to end the episode? One study that attempted to define an episode concluded that the duration was approximately 5 weeks for treatment of diabetic foot ulcers, excluding all patients who had a bone infection or amputation.(Mehta, Suzuki, Glick, & Schulman, 1999) Yet most clinical studies of the same problem consider 8-12 weeks as a minimum time period for healing of the wounds, almost twice the length of the defined episode.(Jude, Apelqvist, Spraul, & Martini, 2006; Xu et al., 2007; Sheehan, Jones, Giurini, Caselli, & Veves, 2006) As another example, chronic diseases that are physician managed will have ongoing treatment if periodic testing and monitoring occur. In that case, an episode has to be defined differently for different treatments for the same patient condition.

Once a patient episode is defined, it is usually examined independently of other episodes for the same patient.(Jonsson, Bolinder, & Lundkvist, 2006) The main measure of an episode is its total cost. (Peltokorpi & Kujala, 2006) However, that means that the likelihood that a treatment pathway in episode one can lead to episode two is not examined.(Horn, 2001) In particular, we want to determine whether treatment choices lead to additional episodes of care. For example, suppose a treatment standard decreases inpatient stays from 5 days to 4 days, but at the cost of doubling the readmission rate.(Koh & Leong, 2001) Without examining the sequence of admissions, the 1-day reduction would be considered a cost effective outcome, especially if an episode is defined as the time from admission to discharge.(Kujala, Lillrank, Kronstrom, & Peltokorpi, 2006) In addition to variability in patient response to treatments, there are competing risks that result in different choices of treatment made either by the physician or the patient.(Keen, Moore, & West, 2006) (Jonsson et al., 2006)Treatment variability is very characteristic of psychiatric treatment, even more so than for physical ailments.(Singh & Grange, 2005)

Another consideration is the pathway itself, defined by compliance with and the continuity of care, especially to determine the effectiveness of disease management.(Greenberg & rosenheck, 2005; Solz & Gilbert, 2001) We need to create a definition of compliance with care, and to rank compliance with treatment. We also need to ensure that all treatments (including prescribed medications) are included in the pathway, and are used to define episodes of care.

Relying on claims data, which is combined in one database from multiple sources, a date of care is included in each claim. However, if a patient is treated in the hospital, there can be several different physicians giving different types of care on the same day. It becomes a major challenge to relate these together into one episode. At a minimum, claims from the same episode should have the same diagnosis related group (DRG) code. However, this code may be entered inaccurately. Claims for medications may not contain this code at all. Each claim will have a service date. We start by creating a clustering for each patient based upon date and DRG codes. Not every patient claim will be clustered successfully. From there, predictive modeling will be used for the unclustered values to predict membership into each cluster.(Putten, Kok, & Gupta, 2002; Xue, 2006)

To examine the sequence of episodes, we can define a time series with multiple time endpoints. The initial time point will define the initial treatment and beginning of a chronic problem. The additional time points will be defined as either the end of the episode, or a change in condition, where the chronic illness gets better, or worse. We can use both fixed and dynamic regressors to investigate the patient outcomes. These regressors can represent a different medication, or a decision to perform surgery, or a change from outpatient to inpatient status. They can also represent a new, ongoing treatment. The fixed regressors will represent patient demographic information, and the initial severity of the patient's condition. The time series will be transactional in nature as the changes in treatment will not necessarily occur at fixed intervals. We can start by defining a time series for each patient, and then consolidating them into a series of forecasted outcomes. Once we have the likelihood of various outcomes defined by the time series, we can create a decision tree to look at the probability of each outcome given treatment choices.

In addition, it will be important to detect outliers either as they occur, or before they occur in terms of both cost and outcomes. Therefore, the claims data can be considered streaming data, with changes in treatments indicative of future outcomes that can be costly either to payer or patient. Once the model is developed, it can be scored and used in future data. In that way, we can continue to examine treatment pathways for optimal choices even as treatments and protocols change with the development of new drugs, devices, and procedures.

What we will focus on in the chapter is the necessary SAS preprocessing code that is needed to define episodes in the claims data so that the data can be investigated as discussed in chapters 2-8. In particular, we will discuss ways to convert the one-to-many to a one-to-one relationship for examination.

MEPS DATA

We will first examine the MEPS dataset. It has one major difference compared to more general claims data in that it has translated all patient encounters into ICD9 codes. Therefore, we do not have to worry about conversion of codes, nor do we need to consider multiple coding systems. However, we do have to consider the fact that different types of patient utilization of the healthcare system is contained within different datasets. It has an additional advantage in that there is extensive information on patients, including employment, income, and geographic region.

We will start with a problem first discussed in Chapter 2. We investigated patient compliance with medication prescriptions for osteoporosis. We did not examine which of the medications prescribed optimize outcomes because the medications file contains no outcome measures. However, we can consider the inpatient, outpatient, and physician visits files to determine which of the patients suffered from orthopedic-related injuries, specifically fractures. Then we can see if there is a relationship between compliance, patient severity, medications, and adverse events to see if one of the medications reduces the occurrence of these events. We use the measure defined in Chapter 2 relating patient compliance to the number of prescriptions. Since we discussed the inpatient and outpatient episodes, and showed that patients with higher levels of medication compliance in fact had more episodes of treatment, we examine the relationship of medications to physician visits here. In this example, we investigate the tests performed in physician offices by the medication choice to see if treatment decisions are related to medications. The following code merges the dataset containing the medications by patient and the physician visits, file H94G. The description of this physician visit dataset is located at http://www.meps. ahrq.gov/mepsweb/data_stats/download_data_files_codebook.jsp?PUFId=H94G. Then we can examine the physician orders in relationship to physician choice for medications.

```
PROC SQL;
CREATE TABLE SASUSER.medsandvisits AS SELECT      QUERY1_FOR_SUMMARY_STATISTI_00.Revise-
dRXName,
    QUERY1_FOR_SUMMARY_STATISTI_00.RXSTRENG,
    QUERY1_FOR_SUMMARY_STATISTI_00.DUPERSID,
    QUERY1_FOR_SUMMARY_STATISTI_00._WAY_,
    QUERY1_FOR_SUMMARY_STATISTI_00._TYPE_,
    QUERY1_FOR_SUMMARY_STATISTI_00._FREQ_,
    QUERY1_FOR_SUMMARY_STATISTI_00.RXQUANTY_Mean,
    QUERY1_FOR_SUMMARY_STATISTI_00.RXQUANTY_StdDev,
    QUERY1_FOR_SUMMARY_STATISTI_00.RXQUANTY_Min,
    QUERY1_FOR_SUMMARY_STATISTI_00.RXQUANTY_Max,
    QUERY1_FOR_SUMMARY_STATISTI_00.RXQUANTY_Sum,
    QUERY1_FOR_SUMMARY_STATISTI_00.RXQUANTY_N,
    QUERY1_FOR_SUMMARY_STATISTI_00.DUID,
    QUERY1_FOR_SUMMARY_STATISTI_00.PID,

        .
        .
        .

    QUERY1_FOR_SUMMARY_STATISTI_00.VARSTR,
    QUERY1_FOR_SUMMARY_STATISTI_00.VARPSU,
    H94G.DUID AS DUID1,
    H94G.PID AS PID1,
    H94G.DUPERSID AS DUPERSID2,
    H94G.EVNTIDX AS EVNTIDX1,
    H94G.EVENTRN AS EVENTRN1,
    H94G.FFEEIDX AS FFEEIDX1,
    H94G.PANEL AS PANEL1,
    H94G.MPCELIG,
    H94G.MPCDATA AS MPCDATA1,
    H94G.OBDATEYR,
    H94G.OBDATEMM,
    H94G.OBDATEDD,
    H94G.SEETLKPV AS SEETLKPV1,
    H94G.MVPLACE,
    H94G.SEEDOC AS SEEDOC1,
    H94G.DRSPLTY AS DRSPLTY1,
    H94G.MEDPTYPE AS MEDPTYPE1,
```

Table 1. Treatment performed in physician visit by medication (percent of patients)

Treatment Performed	IV Therapy	Lab Tests	X-Rays	MRI/CATSCAN	Medication Prescribed
Actonel®	1.20	13.08	10.94	15.97	3.38
Boniva®	0	13.54	3.09	3.09	4.64
Evista®	0	22,49	4.54	13.84	6.51
Fosamax®	0.22	18.88	6.72	11.58	4.22
	EKG	**EEG**	**Other Test**	**Surgical Procedure**	
Actonel®	3.45	0.26	16.34	7.45	
Boniva®	2.04	0	4.51	6.80	
Evista®	3.30	0	24.21	21.51	
Fosamax®	2.24	0.50	20.72	11.84	

```
H94G.DOCATLOC,
    H94G.VSTCTGRY AS VSTCTGRY1,
    H94G.VSTRELCN AS VSTRELCN1,
    H94G.PHYSTH AS PHYSTH1,
    H94G.OCCUPTH AS OCCUPTH1,
    H94G.SPEECHTH AS SPEECHTH1,
    H94G.CHEMOTH AS CHEMOTH1,
    H94G.RADIATTH AS RADIATTH1,
    H94G.KIDNEYD AS KIDNEYD1,
    H94G.IVTHER AS IVTHER1,
    H94G.DRUGTRT AS DRUGTRT1,
    H94G.RCVSHOT AS RCVSHOT1,
    H94G.PSYCHOTH AS PSYCHOTH1,
    H94G.LABTEST AS LABTEST1,
    H94G.SONOGRAM AS SONOGRAM1,
    H94G.XRAYS AS XRAYS1,
    H94G.MAMMOG AS MAMMOG1,
    H94G.MRI AS MRI1,
    H94G.EKG AS EKG1,
    H94G.EEG AS EEG1,
    H94G.RCVVAC AS RCVVAC1,
    H94G.ANESTH AS ANESTH1,
    H94G.OTHSVCE AS OTHSVCE1,
    H94G.SURGPROC AS SURGPROC1,
    H94G.MEDPRESC AS MEDPRESC1,
    H94G.VAPLACE AS VAPLACE1,
        .
        .
        .
```

```
   H94G.VARPSU AS VARPSU1
FROM SASUSER.medications AS sasuser.medsandvisits
   LEFT JOIN sasuser.H94G AS H94G ON sasuser.medications.DUPERSID = H94G.DUPERSID);
QUIT;
```

Once we merge the files, we can examine the relationship of physician orders to medications (Table 1).

There are considerable differences in the type of treatment given the differerent medications. Patients taking Actonel® are much more likely to have an X-Ray or an MRI; those taking Boniva® are much less likely. It could be that patients with more serious conditions are given Actonel® while Boniva® is used more for prevention-or it could be that physicians prescribing Actonel® are more knowledgeable about needed follow up to guard against side effects. Data mining can identify the issue that will require drill down to investigate the reasons for the outcomes. However, without data mining, the differential between medications and additional tests would not be identified, and you would have no way of understanding that drill down is required. In other words, data examinations such as these allow us to formulate questions to investigate.

MEDPAR DATA

We next examine some claims data that are relatively public. Medpar gives the billing information for Medicare. It is publicly available, although there can be a small cost affiliated with data acquisition. In fact, many of the public companies that define patient severity indices rely upon Medpar because it is so readily available. In addition, The Centers for Medicare and Medicaid maintain a data warehouse consisting of patients with a defined chronic disease, and this information, too, is available for a fee. There are multiple forms in Medicare data and we provide the SAS code on how to "unpack" the different forms for use in analysis. We are using the 2005 version of the data.

```
Libname Medpar "F:\Medpar Data\";
Data Medpar.customer Medpar.accommodations Medpar.ancillary_services
Medpar.diagnosis Medpar.outpatient;
Infile 'F:\Medpar Data\Suburban-DFU-V6-Q4-2006.txt' TRUNCOVER;
Input @1 type $2. @;
Select;
When (type='20') do;
Input @5 patient_control_no $20.
   @55 sex $1.
   @56 birthdate $8.
   @64 marital_status $1.
   @65 admission_source $2.
   @123 start_date $8.
   @131 admission_hour $2.
   @133 START_DATE $8.
   @141 END_DATE $8.
```

```
    @149 patient_status $2.
    @151 discharge_hour $2.
    @153 payment_received $10.
    @163 estimated_due $10.
    @173 med_record_no $17.
;
format birthdate start_date START_DATE END_DATE yymmdd8.;
output Medpar.customer;
```

The form identified as '20' contains demographic and general admission information about the patient.

```
end;
when (type='50') do;
input @2 sequence_number $3.
    @6 Patient_control_no $20.
    @29 accom_revenue_code $4.
    @33 accom_rate $9.
    @42 accom_days $4.
    @46 accom_total_charges $10.
    @56 accom_non_covered_charges $10.
    @66 form_locater $4.
    @70 accom_revenue_code_2 $4.
    @74 accom_rate_2 $9.
    @83 accom_days_2 $4.
    @87 accom_total_charges_2 $10.
    @97 accom_non_covered_2 $10.
    @111 accom_revenue_code_2 $4.
    @115 accom_rate_3 $9.
    @124 accom_days_3 $4.
    @128 accom_total_charges_3 $10.
    @138 accom_non_covered_3 $10.
    @152 accom_revenue_code_4 $4.
    @156 accom_rate_4 $9.
    @164 accom_days_4 $4.
    @168 accom_total_charges_4 $10.
    @178 accom_non_covered_4 $10.
;
output Medpar.accommodations;
end;
```

Type '50' gives the overall information about the patient's admission and the rate per day.

```
when (type='60') do;
input @3 Patient_control_no $20.
   @28 ancillary_revenue_code $4.
   @32 HCPCS_Procedure_code $5.
   @37 Modifier_1_HCPCS_CPT $2.
   @39 Modifier_2_HCPCS_CPT $2.
   @41 ancillary_Units_of_service $7.
   @48 ancillary_total_charges $10.
   @55 ancillary_non_covered_charges $10.
   @68 form_locater $4.
   @72 assessment_date $8.
   @83 ancillary_revenue_code_2 $4.
   @87 HCPCS_Procedure_code_2 $5.
   @92 Modifier_1_HCPCS_CPT_2 $2.
   @94 Modifier_2_HCPCS_CPT_2 $2.
   @96 ancillary_Units_of_service_2 $7.
   @103 ancillary_total_charges_2 $10.
   @111 ancillary_non_covered_charges_2 $10.
   @127 assessment_date_2 $8.
   @138 ancillary_revenue_code_3 $4.
   @142 HCPCS_Procedure_code_3 $5.
   @147 Modifier_1_HCPCS_CPT_3 $2.
   @149 Modifier_2_HCPCS_CPT_3 $2.
   @151 ancillary_Units_of_service_3 $7.
   @158 ancillary_total_charges_3 $10.
   @168 ancillary_non_covered_charges_3 $10.
   @182 assessment_date_3 $8.
;
output Medpar.ancillary_services;
end;
```

Type '60 gives information using HCPCS codes instead of ICD9 codes and gives ancillary services.

```
when (type='70') do;
input @3 sequence $2.
   @5 patient_control_no $20.
   @25 principal_diagnosis $6.
   @31 code2 $6.
   @37 code3 $6.
   @43 code4 $6.
   @49 code5 $6.
   @55 code6 $6.
   @61 code7 $6.
```

```
@67 code8 $6.
@73 code9 $6.
@79 principal_procedure $7.
@86 principal_procedure_date $8.
@94 other_procedure_1 $7.
@101 other_procedure_1date $8.
@109 other_procedure_2 $7.
@116 other_procedure_2date $8.
@124 other_procedure_3 $7.
@131 other_procedure_3date $8.
@139 other_procedure_4 $7.
@146 other_procedure_4date $8.
@154 other_procedure_5 $7.
@161 other_procedure_5date $8.
@169 admitting_diagnosis $6.
@175 external_E_code $6.
@181 procedure_coding_method $1.
;
output Medpar.diagnosis;
end;
```

This datasheet gives the ICD9 procedure and diagnosis codes for the patient. Up to 6 of each are allowed.

```
when (type='61') do;
input @3 sequence $2.
   @5 Patient_control_no $20.
   @28 revenue_center $4.
   @32 HCPCS_procedure_code $5.
   @37 modifier_1 $2.
   @39 modifier_2 $2.
   @41 units_of_service $7.
   @48 form_locater $6.
   @54 outpatient_total_charges $6.
   @64 outpatient_non_covered $10.
   @83 revenue_center_2 $4.
   @87 HCPCS_procedure_code_2 $5.
   @92 modifier_1_2 $2.
   @94 modifier_2_2 $2.
   @96 units_of_service_2 $7.
   @109 outpatient_total_charges_2 $6.
   @119 outpatient_non_covered_2 $10.
   @138 revenue_center_3 $4.
   @142 HCPCS_procedure_code_3 $5.
```

```
    @147 modifier_1_3 $2.
    @149 modifier_2_3 $2.
    @151 units_of_service_3 $7.
    @164 outpatient_total_charges_3 $6.
    @174 outpatient_non_covered_3 $10.
    @184 date_of_service $8.
;
output Medpar.outpatient;
end;
end;
run;
```

Dataset '61' gives outpatient information, and again, shifts to HCPCS codes. There can be multiple '61' sheets for each inpatient encounter. Therefore, as in more standard claims data, we have to concern ourselves with two or more different coding schemes. This provides little problem if the severity index relies only upon a small subset of patient conditions while ignoring the rest.

Once the data have been separated, they need to be re-merged depending upon the data examination. Dataset '70' contains information related to diagnosis and procedure codes. We can use the CATX statement defined previously to combine them into text strings for analysis purposes. We will want to merge the dataset information containing the episode date, the diagnosis and procedure codes from '70' and then we want to collect summary statistics concerning costs, and merge the two pieces of information together on a one-on-one basis. We use the following code to combine the data:

```
Data medpar.newdata;
Set medpar.diagnosis;
Procedures=catx(' ',principal.procedure, other.procedure_1, …,other_procedure_5);
Diagnoses=catx (' ', principal_diagnosis, code2 code3,…,code9);
```

This code is followed by

```
Proc sort data=medpar.newdata ;
by patient_control_no;
proc sort data=medpar.outpatient;
by patient_control_no;
proc merge;
set medpar.newdata medpar.outpatient;
by patient_control_no;
```

Once we have these datasets merged, we investigate them in the same way as we have in previous chapters.

CLAIMS DATA

We also have data from a claims dataset to examine repeat procedures for cardiovascular surgery. In this example, we want to work with dates, costs, and codes to define an episode. We first look at the number of claims for each patient, and examine the number of days between claims. Clearly, claims that have the same ICD9 codes and occur within a certain amount of time after an inpatient visit will define follow up visits for that inpatient episode. We use the following code:

```
Proc sort data=sasuser.claims;
By identifier date;
Run;
Data sasuser.countbyday;
Set sasuser.claims;
By identifier;
If first.identifier then numdays=1;
Else numdays+1;
Run;
```

Then we define a variable as the difference in time between claims by using the following code:

```
Data sasuser.differencebyclaims;
Set sasuser.countbyday;
By identifier date;
Differenceindays=dif(date);
If first.identifier then differenceindays=0;
Run;
```

If the difference in days is zero, then the claim is related to the first day of treatment for the patient; otherwise, it is the difference in days from the time of the specific treatment claim to the time of the first day of treatment. We next filter the patients who have just one date of treatment, and the patients who have multiple dates of treatment.

```
Data sasuser.onetreatment;
Set sasuser.differencebyclaims;
By identifier date;
If (last.identifier and numdays=1);
Run;
```

For multiple treatments:

```
Data sasuser.multipletreatments;
Set sasuser.differencebyclaims;
By identifier date;
```

```
If (last.identifier and numdays=1) then delete;
Run;
```

We also want to eliminate repeat observations:

```
Data sasuser.norepeats;
Set multipletreatments;
By identifier;
   If (not first.identifier and differenceindays=0) then delete;
Run;
```

Then we filter out the first observation so that we can use it to determine the number of episodes per patient, and look at the recurrence in episodes.

```
Data sasuser.episodes;
Set sasuser.norepeats;
By identifier data;
If first.identifier;
Run;
```

We can then append the dataset created above (called sasuser.episodes) to the dataset with only one entry (sasuser.onetreatment). In this way, we can compare patients with and without repeat episodes in relationship to the ICD9 (or CPT) codes identifying treatment to see if some decisions are more likely to be related to particular outcomes. In this respect, we are going beyond looking at actual versus predicted mortality to examining real outcomes. For example, we can look at bypass surgery versus angioplasty with a stent, and looking at the values of a drug-eluting stent. We can also examine the relationship between medications prescribed for diabetes and time to disease progression to see if some medications prolong the time to disease progress over others. We can also take into consideration patient compliance with medications by using pharmacy claims data.

FUTURE TRENDS

Insurers will hold providers more and more accountable with how healthcare dollars are spent. Moreover, insurers will be less willing to pay for errors and for poor treatment. They will be relying on their own claims databases to investigate the quality of care, and will start disallowing claims from providers residing at the bottom of the quality list. For this reason alone, providers need to understand how such claims information is used to define the quality of care.

DISCUSSION

While more difficult to work with, claims data are routinely available. Because such data are proprietary, most health insurers are reluctant to make such information available. The Medpar claims are available through the Centers for Medicare and Medicaid. Moreover, there are private companies that combine information from multiple insurers and make the data available, although the cost can be quite high. One such is the Thomson Medstat Marketscan data. It is extremely useful, but highly expensive. However, Thomson Medstat does have a dissertation program available for PhD students who want to use the data to examine health outcomes. Students individually have to request access to the data.

REFERENCES

Anonymous. (2006a). *episode treatment groups* [Electronic Version], 1-8. Retrieved 2007 from www.ingenix.com.

Anonymous. (2006b). *Medicare Claims Processing Manual.* Retrieved 2007, from http://www.cms.hhs.gov/manuals/downloads/clm104c10.pdf

Bassin, E. (1999). Episodes of care: a tool for measuring the impact of healthcare services on cost and quality. *Disease Management & Health Outcomes, 6,* 319–325. doi:10.2165/00115677-199906060-00002

Bonetto, C., Nose, M., & Barbui, C. (2006). Generating psychotropic drug exposure data from computer-based medical records. *Computer Methods and Programs in Biomedicine, 83,* 120–124.doi:10.1016/j.cmpb.2006.06.004

Ceratti, A., France, F. R., & Beguin, C. (2008). Health data quality improvement by comparing administrative medical data and billing data. *International Journal of Medical Informatics, 77*(8), 527–533. doi:10.1016/j.ijmedinf.2007.10.003

Claus, P., Carpenter, P., Chute, C., Mohr, D., & Gibbons, P. (1997). Clinical care management and workflow by episodes. *Proceedings of the AMIA Annual Fall Symposium, 1997,* 91–95.

Claus, P. L., Carpenter, P. C., Chute, C. G., Mohr, D. N., & Gibbons, P. S. (1997). *Clinical care management and workflow by episodes.* Retrieved 2007, from http://www.amia.org/pubs/symposia/D004137.PDF

Collinet-Adler, S., Stauffer, W. M., Boulware, D. R., Rogers, K. L., Rogers, T. B., & Williams, D. N. (2007). Financial implications of refugee malaria: the impact of pre-departure presumptive treatment with anti-malarial drugs. *The American Journal of Tropical Medicine and Hygiene, 77*(3), 458–463.

Currie, C. J., Morgan, C. L., Dixon, S., McEwan, P., Marchant, N., Bearne, A., et al. (2005). The financial costs of hospital care for people with diabetes who have single and multiple macrovascular complications. *diabetes Research and Clinical Practices, 67,* 144-151.

Forthman, M. T., Dove, H. G., & Wooster, L. D. (2000). Episode treatment groups (ETGs): a patient classification system for measuring outcomes performance by episode of illness. *Topics in Health Information Management, 21*(2), 51–61.

Greenberg, G. A., & Rosenheck, R. A. (2005). Continuity of care and clinical outcomes in a national health system. *Psychiatric Services (Washington, D.C.), 56*(4), 427–433. doi:10.1176/appi.ps.56.4.427

Hall, D. L., & Llinas, J. (2001). *Handbook of Multisensor Data Fusion*. Cleveland, OH: CRC.

Hong, W., Rak, I., Ciuryia, V., Wilson, A., Kylstra, J., & Meltzer, H. (1998). Medical-claims databases in the design of a health-outcomes comparison of quetiapine. *Schizophrenia Research, 32*(1), 51–58. doi:10.1016/S0920-9964(98)00040-1

Horn, S. D. (2001). Quality, clinical practice improvement, and the episode of care. *Managed Care Quarterly, 9*(3), 10–24.

Jonsson, L., Bolinder, B., & Lundkvist, J. (2006). Cost of hypoglycemia in patients with Type 2 diabetes in Sweden. *Value in Health, 9*(3), 193–198.doi:10.1111/j.1524-4733.2006.00100.x

Jude, E., Apelqvist, J., Spraul, M., & Martini, J. (2006). Prospective randomized controlled study of Hydrofiber dressing containing ionic silver or calcium alginate dressings in non-ischaemic diabetic foot ulcers. *Diabetic Medicine, 24*, 280–288. doi:10.1111/j.1464-5491.2007.02079.x

Kaushal, R., Bates, D. W., Franz, C., Soukup, J. R., & Rothschild, J. M. (2007). Costs of adverse events in intensive care units. *Critical Care Medicine, 35*(11), 2479–2483.doi:10.1097/01. CCM.0000284510.04248.66

Keen, J., Moore, J., & West, R. (2006). Pathways, networks and choice in health care. *International Journal of Health Care Quality Assurance, 19*(4), 316–327. doi:10.1108/09526860610671373

Kerr, E., McGlynn, E., Vorst, K. V., & Wickstrom, S. (2000). Measuring antidepressant prescribing practice in a healthcare system using administrative data: implications for quality measurement and improvement. *The Joint Commission Journal on Quality Improvement, 265*(4), 203–216.

Koh, H., & Leong, S. (2001). Data mining applications in the context of casemix. *Annals of the Academy of Medicine, Singapore, 30*(4Suppl), 41–49.

Kujala, J., Lillrank, P., Kronstrom, V., & Peltokorpi, A. (2006). Time-based management of patient processes. *Journal of Health Organization and Management, 20*(6), 512–524.doi:10.1108/14777260610702262

Mehta, S., Suzuki, S., Glick, H., & Schulman, K. (1999). Determining an episode of care using claims data: diabetic foot ulcer. *Diabetes Care, 22*(7), 1110–1115.doi:10.2337/diacare.22.7.1110

Peltokorpi, A., & Kujala, J. (2006). Time-based analysis of total cost of patient episodes. *International Journal of Health Care Quality Assurance, 19*(2), 136–143. doi:10.1108/09526860610651672

Philipneri, M. D., Rey, L. A. R., Schnitzler, M. A., Abbott, K. C., Brennan, D. C., & Takemoto, S. K. (2008). Delivery patterns of recommended chronic kidney disease care in clinical practice: administrative claims-based analysis and systematic literature review. *Clinical and Experimental Nephrology, 12*(1), 41–52.doi:10.1007/s10157-007-0016-3

Putten, P. d., Kok, J. N., & Gupta, A. (2002). Data fusion through statistical matching. 2007, from http://papers.ssrn.com/sol3/papers.cfm?abstract_id=297501#

Ritzwoller, D. P., Crounse, L., Shetterly, S., & Rublee, D. (2006). The association of comorbidities, utilization and costs for patients identified with low back pain. *BMC Musculoskeletal Disorders, 7*, 72. doi:10.1186/1471-2474-7-72

Rosen, A., & Mayer-Oakes, A. (1999). Episodes of care: theoretical frameworks versus current operational realities. *Joint Commission on Quality Improvement, 25*(3), 111–138.

Sheehan, P., Jones, P., Giurini, J. M., Caselli, A., & Veves, A. (2006). Percent change in wound area of diabetic foot ulcers over a 4-week period is a robust predictor of complete healing in a 12-week prospective trial. *Plastic and Reconstructive Surgery, 117*(Suppl), 239S–244S.doi:10.1097/01.prs.0000222891.74489.33

Singh, S. P., & Grange, T. (2005). Measuring pathways to care in first-episode psychosis: a systematic review. *Schizophrenia Research, 81*, 75–82.doi:10.1016/j.schres.2005.09.018

Sloane, P. D., MacFarquhar, J. K., Sickbert-Bennett, E., Mitchell, C. M., Akers, R., & Weber, D. J. (2006). Syndromic surveillance for emergency infections in office practice using billing data. *Annals of Family Medicine, 4*(4), 351–358.doi:10.1370/afm.547

Smith-Bindman, R., Quale, C., Chu, P. W., Rosenberg, R., & Kerlikowske, K. (2006). Can Medicare billing claims data be used to assess mammography utilization among women ages 65 and older? *Medical Care, 44*(5), 463–470.doi:10.1097/01.mlr.0000207436.07513.79

Solz, H., & Gilbert, K. (2001). Health claims data as a strategy and tool in disease management. *The Journal of Ambulatory Care Management, 24*(2), 69–85.

Thomas, J. W. (2005). Should episode-based economic profiles be risk adjusted to account for differences in patients' health risks? *Health Research and Educational Trust, April, 2006*, 581-590.

Thomas, J. W. (2006). Economic profiling of physicians: does omission of pharmacy claims bias performance measurement? *The American Journal of Managed Care, 12*, 341–351.

Wan, G., Crown, W., Berndt, E., Finkelstein, S., & Ling, D. (2002). Healthcare expenditure in patients treated with vaniafaxine or selective serotonin reuptake inhibitors for depression and anxiety. *International Journal of Clinical Practice, 56*(6), 434–439.

Wilkinson, D., Askew, D. A., & Dixon, A. (2006). Skin cancer clinics in Australia: workload profile and performance indicators from an analysis of billing data. *MJA, 184*(4), 162–164.

Xu, L., McLennan, S. V., Lo, L., & Natfajl, A. (2007). Bacterial load predicts healing rate in neuropathic diabetic foot ulcers. *Diabetes Care, 30*(2), 378–380.doi:10.2337/dc06-1383

Xue, S. (2006). *A fault diagnosis system based on data fusion algorithm.* Paper presented at the First international conference on innovative computing information and control, Beijing, China.

Chapter 10
Use of Risk Adjustment Models for Provider Reimbursements

INTRODUCTION

In this chapter, we will focus on the use of patient severity indices to determine the reimbursement to healthcare providers. In order to do this, we must first examine the standard practice of reimbursing hospitals for specific DRG codes, and for reimbursing other providers based upon a point system that designates the level of service. We especially want to investigate the problem of upcoding, or "gaming" in more detail to determine if it can be detected and corrected, so that providers are reimbursed based upon the actual level of care, and not upon better coding practices.

Each hospital has a contract with a healthcare provider that designates the level of reimbursement. The reimbursement is based upon a general formula, with consideration of locat costs. However, these formulas are linear, suggesting that the standard assumption is made that the patient costs are normally distributed. As discussed in Chapter 3, this assumption is not valid. Therefore, we will also examine the issue of reimbursement based upon the normal distribution to determine whether such reimbursements are reasonable, or whether providers are losing money because of the need to treat patients who need extraordinary care. Unfortunately, regression assumes that the relationship of cost to need is linear; if the distribution is gamma or exponential, the relationship will not be linear and the cost will be skewed.

DOI: 10.4018/978-1-60566-752-2.ch010

Therefore, fewer patients are identified as extraordinary if the assumption of normality is made, and there will be a group of patients who require costly treatment, but for whom providers will only receive standard reimbursement. Approximately 5% are identified as outliers when the proportion of outliers is more in the neighborhood of 10-15%.

BACKGROUND

Report Cards to Influence Providers

Insurers have considerable leverage to influence providers to change policies and to comply with guidelines and benchmarks.(Hollingsworth, Krein, Miller, DeMonner, & Hollenbeck, 2007) Reimbursements are now often linked to the quality of care. This is known as value-based purchasing, or pay for performance, often abbreviated as P4P. Such models assume, for example, that better care will reduce surgical complications, length of stay, and readmission rates.(Lewis & Friesen, 2006) Currently, the Centers for Medicare and Medicaid have established a voluntary system for physicians to report 16 measures of quality outcomes. Hospitals report on 10 measures. Although voluntary, hospitals not reporting can suffer a financial penalty, which tends to make it mandatory. In other words, reporting is "voluntary" in the same way that federal income tax is defined as "voluntary".

In the Medicare Prescription Drug, Improvement, and Modernization Act of 2003, Congress directed the Institute of Medicine to identify options for pay-for-performance to be implemented through Medicare reimbursement.(Anonymous-Medicare, 2003) Other insurers are expected to follow. However, instead of penalizing providers for poor performance, the approach has been to reward high performance with bonuses. (Bhattacharyya, Priyesh, & Freiberg, 2008; Hazelwood & Cook, 2008) The impact is the same. Higher ranked providers get more money.

Unfortunately, physicians are now being taught how to "game" the system to optimize their ranking while not actually improving patient care. In this respect, scarce resources are devoted to documentation to maximize reimbursement rather than to provide actual improvements in healthcare.(Bodrock & Mion, 2008) In addition, it is possible that resources will be focused on the patient conditions that are included in the reporting, neglecting other patient conditions that are not.

Consider, for example, some advice provided to physicians (Hayward & Kent, 2008) specifically on how to "game" the system, including providing incorrect blood pressure readings for hard to treat patients. It also suggests that adults can always be diagnosed with something, and these diagnoses can be used to increase reimbursements.

All too often clinicians are stingy in diagnosing patients with disease. These physicians carelessly mislabel many patients as "healthy," overlooking more subtle signs of disease, giving patients a false and dangerous sense of security. In the era of P4P, this is virtually malpractice. Fortunately, experts are beginning to recognize what simple common sense tells us: people are either diseased or prediseased, since good health is always temporary. Thankfully, it's now quite difficult for an adult patient to avoid having at least one of the following diseases: diabetes/prediabetes, hypertension/prehypertension, obesity/ overweight/flabby thighs, or a detectable LDL level.... This one little activity can (1) lower costs per diseased patient (since your "diagnosed" cases are now less sick on average), (2) make your patients appear more ill (since they will now have more comorbid conditions), while (3) improving your quality measures (since it's much easier to control hypertension if the patient rarely had BPs above 130/80 to begin with). Your average control of these diseases and costs per patient will soon run circles around those of physicians who allow themselves to be hamstrung by more old-fashioned diagnostic criteria. So, screen aggressively and diagnose generously!... Wouldn't it be better for all involved to just keep taking her blood pressure until the blood pressure goal is met? If 2 or 3 checks don't do the trick, a conscientious physician should be willing to sacrifice a Korotkoff sound or two for the sake of quality. We have found that ultrarapid cuff deflation can be an equally effective nonpharmacologic remedy for these resistant cases, and improve patient comfort at the same time. Be creative—you will find a way to reach the recommended goal!

For example, patients were diagnosed with diabetes if fasting glucose values were above 140 mg/dl. Then it was redefined at 126 mg/dl. Now 100 mg/dl is defined as pre-diabetes. Similarly, patients were treated for high cholesterol at 220 mg/dl. Then it became 200 mg/dl and now it is moving to 170 mg/dl. Each time the standard is lowered, more patients are diagnosed and treated. The number of diagnoses for each patient increases.

Another concern with pay-for-performance is "adverse selection", or restricting access to the most severely ill, the uninsured, or the elderly with complex medical problems. (Bodrock & Mion, 2008) Indeed, the above quote in Hayward & Kent goes on to suggest that a physician should refuse to treat such patients, recommending another provider to the patient, who would be willing to treat the patient. One study examining the unintended consequences of pay for performance indicated that providers with a large minority patient population are penalized under the system either because minority patients are harder to treat, or because they are more likely to be uninsured or to wait until their condition worsened. (Karve, Ou, Lytle, & Peterson, 2008) This study also showed that hospitals with large minority populations were less likely to deliver evidence-based care, reducing their performance on input measures as well as outcome measures. The question is, then, whether payers will take the patient's socioeconomic status into consideration when defining reimbursements. There is no question that patient compliance is an important issue, and more affluent patients are far more likely to comply with treatment requirements compared to those who are less affluent.

Currently, reimbursement measures have focused on inputs into the system. For example, performance measures proposed for surgeons include:(Lewis & Friesen, 2006)

- Prophylactic antibiotics delivered within one hour before surgery
- The prophylactic antibiotic as an appropriate cephalosporin
- Prophylactic antibiotics are discontinued within 24 hours of surgery ending
- Appropriate venous thromboembolism prophylaxis was ordered

While these are reasonable goals, there is no measure as to whether the surgeon is better at surgery compared to other surgeons. Since the first three measures listed above involve antibiotic delivery, it would be worthwhile to measure the infection rates of surgical patients to determine if there is a difference across surgeons, and whether there is a small misclassification rate in predicting infection just using the input measures listed above.

Another contract for performance measures utilized by a private insurer included the following measures, again focusing on inputs rather than outcomes: (Collier, 2007)

Figure 1. Comparison of infection rates across hospitals

Facility / City	Rate
STATEWIDE	0.28%
Brandon Regional Hospital 100243 Brandon	Higher than Expected 0.37%
H Lee Moffitt Cancer Center & Research Institute 110009 Tampa	As Expected 0.4%
Memorial Hospital of Tampa 100206 Tampa	As Expected 0.38%
Saint Joseph's Hospital 100075 Tampa	As Expected 0.26%
South Bay Hospital 100259 Sun City Center	As Expected 0.22%
South Florida Baptist Hospital 100132 Plant City	As Expected 0.26%
Tampa General Hospital 100128 Tampa	Higher than Expected 0.33%
Town & Country Hospital 100255 Tampa	As Expected 0.15%
University Community Hospital 100173 Tampa	Lower than Expected 0.19%
University Community Hospital at Carroll 100069 Tampa	As Expected 0.29%

- Access to care (24/7 in house care)
- Less than 18:1 physician to patient ratio
- Medical records available within 12 hours
- Discharge summary within 24 hours
- Attendance at monthly hospitalist meetings
- JCAHO and National Patient Safety Goals met
- Self Directed Learning through the Society of Hospitalist Medicine membership

Suppose all of the above goals are met. Are there still differences in treatment outcomes? How does monthly attendance at meetings improve the quality of care? For example, many hospitalists work in hospital emergency departments. Do the hospitalists have different admission rates? Do they have different treatment costs for similar patients? None of these outcomes would be reflected in the above inputs.

Because of the problem in assessing the quality of care based upon patient diagnoses, some payers are considering using clinical lab values such as hematocrit levels to rank the quality of providers.(Thornton & Hakim, 1997) However, as the above quote in Hayward & Kent suggests, even clinical values can be "gamed". In fact, reporting of clinical values gives physicians reasons to exclude patients from reporting if these patients do not meet clinical targets.(Doran, Fullwood, Reeves, Gravelle, & Roland, 2008) Without some measure or definition of patient compliance with treatment, such measures will not truly reflect the quality of care.

Public Reporting of Outcomes

Another outcome of interest is the degree and proportion of patients with nosocomial infections and adverse events that should be preventable. While there are 21 states that require some reporting of nosocomial infections, only four make the information available to the public: Florida, Pennsylvania, Missouri, and Vermont. More states, however, are expected to follow. Medicare will no longer pay for the costs of patient care related to such infections or to medical errors. Therefore, hospitals with high rates of one or both will have their costs increase significantly since they will not be able to pass them

Figure 2. Vermont report card

Data Report Period: Discharges October 1, 2005 through September 30, 2006				
	Prophylactic Antibiotic Received within 1 Hour Prior to Surgery	Prophylactic Antibiotic Selection for Surgical Patients* (*Data for this measure was collected 7/1/06 - 9/30/06)	Prophylactic Antibiotic Discontinued within 24 hours after Surgery	Composite Score
Click "Define" for expanded explanation of the category above it	Define	Define	Define	Define
National Average	84.8% 221,496/261,151	91.6% 238,739/260,545	75.1% 188,490/250,937	n/a
State Average	87.86% 2,019/2.298	92.6% 413/446	85.01% 1,894/2,228	75.53% 1747/2313
Achievable Benchmark(Represents the average performance achieved by the top hospitals in the U.S.)	97.7% 25,540/26,138	99.2% 26,060/26,275	95.6% 24,171/25,293	n/a
Brattleboro Memorial Hospital	94.16% 129/137	93.94% 31/33	91.6% 120/131	86.86% 119/137
Central Vermont Medical Ctr.	89.14% 197/221	97.37% 37/38	90.05% 190/211	80.44% 181/225
Copley Hospital	67.31% 70/104	100% 14/14	76.47% 78/102	55.66% 59/106

along to payers.(Arias, 2008) Preventive measures will also add to costs, but not to reimbursements without some negotiations between providers and payers. Figure 1 shows one such comparison provided by Florida.(Anonymous-Floridareporting, 2008)

Note that Brandon Regional Hospital is identified as higher than expected at 0.37% whereas the H Lee Moffitt Cancer Center has a higher rate of 0.40%, but is identified as expected. Does the H Lee Moffitt Cancer Center have sicker patients, or is it just better at "gaming" the reporting? Given that it is exclusively a cancer center that treats many with terminal conditions, the H Lee Moffitt Center undoubtedly has sicker patients, many of them terminal, and it can have a higher expected mortality rate.

Florida is the only state to offer such comprehensive information. Pennsylvania limits reporting to infections that are device-related and publicizes reports based upon peer groups rather than individual providers (Anonymous-Penn, 2008); Missouri limits reporting to central line-associated bloodstream infections using a three-point scale of higher than expected, as expected, and lower than expected. The rates are adjusted by patient severity, but the severity measure is not identified. (Anonymous-Missouri, 2008) Vermont reports central-line infections, and also surgical infection prevention measures. Vermont, too, focuses upon inputs rather than infection rates (Figure 2). (Anonymous-Vermont, 2008)

However, mandatory reporting will only increase. As of 2007, the Centers for Medicare and Medicaid required the submission of specific data in order for the hospital provider to receive full Medicare payments. Thus, it is no longer "voluntary".

Healthgrades.com uses the Medpar data (publicly available for a fee) to provide information to the public on quality ranking of providers. It will provide more details about the public information, but at a small cost. Such public reporting will continue to increase as well. Therefore, providers must learn to deal with this type of reporting.

Table 1. Physician reimbursement by medication for treatment of osteoporosis

RevisedRXName	N Obs	Variable	Mean	Std Dev
Actonel®	6214	SUM OF REIMBURSEMENT TOTAL CHARGE	139.4900000 261.0492787	634.5592923 892.4160990
Boniva®	1702	SUM OF REIMBURSEMENT TOTAL CHARGE	98.6538977 211.6433980	182.7933705 1215.17
Evista®	2915	SUM OF REIMBURSEMENT TOTAL CHARGE	138.7793274 346.3469526	414.3256163 1678.43
Fosamax®	11555	SUM OF REIMBURSEMENT TOTAL CHARGE	154.8413638 286.5861503	307.8532491 729.2619202

Reimbursement Formulas

It is very difficult to find information concerning reimbursement formulas. However, information on Medicare reimbursements is readily available, and we will discuss it in detail. In addition, the MEPS data provides actual reimbursement information as well as actual payments from different providers. For this reason, it is extremely valuable information. We can use this information to see if we can estimate the relationship of payment to charges. We can also look at the cost-to-charge ratio to see which hospitals greatly inflate their charges, and see if these are the same hospitals that shift patients into higher categories of severity.

Another aspect of reimbursement is that approximately 5-6% of the patient population is designated as outlier and the provider is eligible for an additional payment; the formulas for payment only allow for 5-6% of the population to be so designated. As we noted in chapter 3, this percentage assumes that the population is normally distributed. However, if the true distribution is more likely to be gamma, a considerably higher proportion of the population should have this designation. (Anonymous-CMS, 2006) Since it is fairly reasonable to assume a gamma distribution instead of a normal distribution, providers

Figure 3. Kernel density of reimbursements by medication

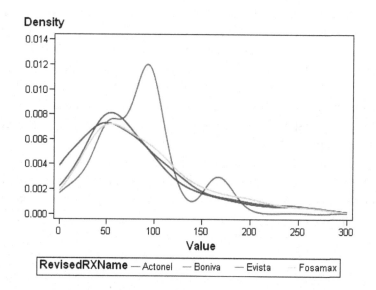

Figure 4. Kernel density of physician charges by medication

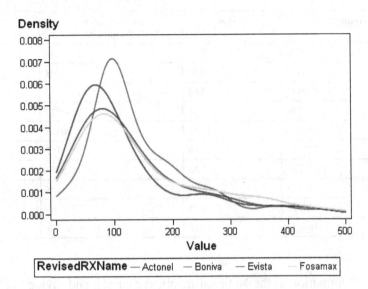

are substantially under-paid for the proportion of outlier patients encountered. In addition, the outlier cost can be exponentially higher compared to the more typical patient, but the outlier reimbursement is just a linear increase over standard payments.

We consider again our example with osteoporosis and medications. As we saw in Chapter 9, there is a considerable difference in the use of diagnostic tests given the different medications. We again examine the difference by medication to examine the physician reimbursements. Table 1 gives the average reimbursement by medication as well as the total charges; Figures 3 and 4 give the kernel density distributions.

It appears that patients prescribed Boniva® yield lower average reimbursements compared to the other three drugs, with Fosamax® having the highest reimbursement. Actonel® has the highest level of variabililty. However, the kernel density estimations show something slightly different.

In both cases, patients prescribed Boniva® have higher charges and higher reimbursements compared to the other three medications, even though patients prescribed Actonel® have more diagnostic tests. Because the users of Boniva® have a lower probability of extreme outliers, the average cost is actually less compared to the other three medications.

EXAMINATION OF THE NUMBER AND IMPORTANCE OF DIAGNOSIS CODES

One of the things that is important to payers and to patients is to be able to determine which providers are gaming the system. In order to do so, we need to examine the severity index of a provider in relationship to the codes used to define the patient's condition. In particular, we start with examining which providers use the maximum number of codes to identify patient co-morbidities. Certainly, a provider who identifies 9 or 10 conditions will tend to have a sicker patient compared to a provider who identifies 4 or 5 conditions, and it is to the provider's advantage to increase the number of diagnoses. More diagnoses will have a higher probability of including those that are used to define the severity index.

Table 2. Frequency for class variable

class	Frequency	Percent	Cumulative Frequency	Cumulative Percent
1	930	0.01	930	0.01
2	649478	9.32	650408	9.33
3	950622	13.64	1601030	22.97
4	867899	12.45	2468929	35.43
5	801427	11.50	3270356	46.92
6	744191	10.68	4014547	57.60
7	651332	9.35	4665879	66.95
8	578229	8.30	5244108	75.25
9	539992	7.75	5784100	82.99
10	1185273	17.01	6969373	100.00

We start with the information in the National Inpatient Sample, and divide the patient population by the number of ICD9 diagnosis codes for each patient. Then we compare the patient severity indices that are included with the data to see if there is a difference based just upon the number of codes. We will then examine the least significant codes and compare their severity to the most significant codes (recall that the codes are to be listed in their order of importance). We will truncate the number of codes to compare the severity of the other Indices based upon the number of codes used.

First, we define a class based just upon the number of codes listed in the National Inpatient Sample. We use the following code:

```
data nis.numberofcodes;
set nis.addseverity;
if (dx10 eq ' ') then class=10;
if (dx9 eq ' ') then class=9;
if (dx8 eq ' ') then class=8;
if (dx7 eq ' ') then class=7;
if (dx6 eq ' ') then class=6;
if (dx5 eq ' ') then class=5;
if (dx4 eq ' ') then class=4;
if (dx3 eq ' ') then class=3;
if (dx2 eq ' ') then class=2;
if (dx1 eq ' ') then class=1;
run;
```

The results are given in Table 2. Next, we perform a table analysis of the number of codes without any reference to the severity and compare it to the severity indices as discussed in Chapters 5-7.

The distribution of these class values is relatively uniform. Note, however, that the largest class contains ten diagnosis codes. We restricted our attention to just the first ten codes. Tables 3 and 4 compare the classes defined above in Table 2 with the APRDRG mortality and severity indices. We want to see

Table 3. APRDRG mortality index by class variable

Table of class by APRDRG_Risk_Mortality						
class	APRDRG_Risk_Mortality(All Patient Refined DRG: Risk of Mortality Subclass)					Total
Frequency Row Pct Col Pct	0	1	2	3	4	
1	930 100.00 24.41	0 0.00 0.00	0 0.00 0.00	0 0.00 0.00	0 0.00 0.00	930
2	654 0.10 17.17	645843 99.44 12.84	2159 0.33 0.15	525 0.08 0.12	297 0.05 0.25	649478
3	343 0.04 9.00	929442 97.77 18.48	18951 1.99 1.36	1247 0.13 0.30	639 0.07 0.55	950622
4	353 0.04 9.27	812750 93.65 16.16	49930 5.75 3.57	3006 0.35 0.71	1860 0.21 1.59	867899
5	295 0.04 7.74	699659 87.30 13.91	91469 11.41 6.55	8014 1.00 1.90	1990 0.25 1.70	801427
6	279 0.04 7.32	580017 77.94 11.53	140953 18.94 10.09	19269 2.59 4.56	3673 0.49 3.13	744191
7	212 0.03 5.56	448453 68.85 8.92	170053 26.11 12.17	28312 4.35 6.70	4302 0.66 3.67	651332
8	190 0.03 4.99	337481 58.36 6.71	192737 33.33 13.80	41684 7.21 9.87	6137 1.06 5.23	578229
9	198 0.04 5.20	253043 46.86 5.03	215182 39.85 15.40	60843 11.27 14.41	10726 1.99 9.15	539992
10	356 0.03 9.34	322144 27.18 6.41	515706 43.51 36.91	259449 21.89 61.43	87618 7.39 74.73	1185273
Total	3810	5028832	1397140	422349	117242	6969373

if there is a shift to a more severe category as the number of diagnosis codes increases, independent of the actual severity of the patient's condition.

An APRDRG code of 0 indicates that the patient cannot be classified. Note that 99% of all patients with just one diagnosis code are in APRDRG code 1, regardless of the actual severity of that code. The probability of APRDRG class 4 increases to a high of 7+% if the patient has all ten diagnosis codes, regardless of what those codes represent. Similarly, the probability of codes 2,3, and 4 increase as the number of diagnosis codes increases. In fact, 75% of all patients in APRDRG class 4 have ten codes identified. While it might be assumed that patients with more codes are more severe, we will examine this level in detail.

For the severity index, the trend is even more pronounced with the severity class 1 ranging from a high of 94% for two diagnosis codes to a low of 9% for all ten diagnosis codes with 76% of all patients

Table 4. APRDRG severity index by class variable

Table of class by APRDRG_Severity						
class	APRDRG_Severity(All Patient Refined DRG: Severity of Illness Subclass)					Total
Frequency Row Pct Col Pct	0	1	2	3	4	
1	930 100.00 24.41	0 0.00 0.00	0 0.00 0.00	0 0.00 0.00	0 0.00 0.00	930
2	654 0.10 17.17	614605 94.63 18.99	32569 5.01 1.24	1648 0.25 0.18	2 0.00 0.00	649478
3	343 0.04 9.00	776844 81.72 24.01	163713 17.22 6.22	9491 1.00 1.02	231 0.02 0.14	950622
4	353 0.04 9.27	563970 64.98 17.43	278324 32.07 10.57	24449 2.82 2.63	803 0.09 0.48	867899
5	295 0.04 7.74	420551 52.48 13.00	335343 41.84 12.74	43313 5.40 4.66	1925 0.24 1.14	801427
6	279 0.04 7.32	306483 41.18 9.47	364172 48.94 13.84	68382 9.19 7.36	4875 0.66 2.89	744191
7	212 0.03 5.56	210954 32.39 6.52	349317 53.63 13.27	84826 13.02 9.13	6023 0.92 3.58	651332
8	190 0.03 4.99	143002 24.73 4.42	320313 55.40 12.17	105725 18.28 11.38	8999 1.56 5.34	578229
9	198 0.04 5.20	95844 17.75 2.96	291390 53.96 11.07	136117 25.21 14.65	16443 3.05 9.76	539992
10	356 0.03 9.34	103579 8.74 3.20	496976 41.93 18.88	455191 38.40 48.99	129171 10.90 76.67	1185273
Total	3810	3235832	2632117	929142	168472	6969373

in severity class 4 having all ten codes. To examine the three disease staging levels, we use Tables 5-7.

Here, too, patients have a higher probability of a higher category in length of stay as the number of diagnosis codes changes from 1 to 10; 62% of the patients in level 5 have 10 codes.

While sicker patients will have more diagnosis codes, it is also true that those who are "gamed" will have a higher number of codes. Moreover, if there is a strong relationship between the number of codes and the level of severity, any hospital can start increasing the amount of coding in order to shift patients into a higher category.

Table 8 gives the relationship between the Charlson Index and the number of diagnosis codes. The triangular nature of the matrix in Table 8 shows that the Charlson Index increases as the number of diagnosis codes increases.

Table 5. Disease staging: length of stay

Table of class by DS_LOS_Level						
class	DS_LOS_Level(Disease Staging: Length of Stay Level)					Total
Frequency Row Pct Col Pct	1	2	3	4	5	
1	0 0.00 0.00	1 1.79 0.00	25 44.64 0.00	19 33.93 0.00	11 19.64 0.00	56
2	64270 9.91 21.31	428448 66.04 30.54	137036 21.12 3.56	15887 2.45 1.36	3147 0.49 1.29	648788
3	62363 6.56 20.68	344927 36.30 24.59	505198 53.16 13.13	32262 3.39 2.76	5531 0.58 2.26	950281
4	54398 6.27 18.04	230048 26.51 16.40	523408 60.33 13.61	51847 5.98 4.43	7921 0.91 3.24	867622
5	44449 5.55 14.74	143974 17.97 10.26	526888 65.76 13.70	76220 9.51 6.51	9696 1.21 3.96	801227
6	33418 4.49 11.08	94964 12.76 6.77	508666 68.37 13.22	95605 12.85 8.16	11341 1.52 4.64	743994
7	21663 3.33 7.18	62883 9.66 4.48	448357 68.85 11.66	105128 16.14 8.98	13178 2.02 5.39	651209
8	12694 2.20 4.21	42605 7.37 3.04	386724 66.90 10.05	119191 20.62 10.18	16879 2.92 6.90	578093
9	6732 1.25 2.23	28916 5.36 2.06	334139 61.89 8.69	145169 26.89 12.40	24915 4.61 10.19	539871
10	1592 0.13 0.53	25952 2.19 1.85	475913 40.16 12.37	529637 44.69 45.23	151930 12.82 62.13	1185024
Total	301579	1402718	3846354	1170965	244549	6966165

For a Charlson Index of 12, 62% of the patients have ten diagnosis codes. The largest percentage of patients with ten codes is 70% for a Charlson Index of 11. Recall that as the Charlson Index increases to 12 and 13, the overall severity as identified by patient outcomes actually decreases because the weights for HIV are too great.

While we know the relationship of the number of codes to the severity indices, we also need to examine the relationship to the patient outcomes. In particular, we want to determine the relationship between the number of codes and mortality, length of stay, and total charges. Table 9 examines the number of codes to mortality. Figures 5 and 6 examine the kernel density estimates of charges and stay by the number of diagnosis codes.

The highest proportion of patients who died had no diagnosis codes. Beyond that, the mortality rate increases with the number of diagnosis codes, suggesting that the number of codes is representative of the patient's severity.

Table 6. Disease staging: mortality level

Table of class by DS_Mrt_Level							
class	DS_Mrt_Level(Disease Staging: Mortality Level)						Total
Frequency Row Pct Col Pct	0	1	2	3	4	5	
1	0 0.00 0.00	2 3.57 0.00	3 5.36 0.00	32 57.14 0.00	18 32.14 0.00	1 1.79 0.00	56
2	119109 18.35 8.99	49427 7.62 17.68	355267 54.75 31.98	119793 18.46 3.99	5186 0.80 0.50	153 0.02 0.07	648935
3	339135 35.68 25.61	55948 5.89 20.02	295841 31.13 26.63	243454 25.62 8.10	14941 1.57 1.45	1092 0.11 0.51	950411
4	282584 32.57 21.34	56781 6.54 20.31	161778 18.64 14.56	322487 37.17 10.73	40383 4.65 3.91	3687 0.42 1.72	867700
5	218607 27.28 16.51	43056 5.37 15.40	95251 11.89 8.57	375107 46.81 12.48	63349 7.91 6.14	5896 0.74 2.76	801266
6	151577 20.37 11.45	29371 3.95 10.51	65653 8.82 5.91	400156 53.78 13.31	86952 11.69 8.42	10318 1.39 4.82	744027
7	95487 14.66 7.21	18977 2.91 6.79	47682 7.32 4.29	374958 57.58 12.48	100387 15.42 9.72	13735 2.11 6.42	651226
8	57081 9.87 4.31	11889 2.06 4.25	34762 6.01 3.13	337417 58.37 11.23	118475 20.49 11.47	18485 3.20 8.64	578109
9	33223 6.15 2.51	7299 1.35 2.61	25435 4.71 2.29	303104 56.14 10.09	144562 26.78 14.00	26255 4.86 12.27	539878
10	27533 2.32 2.08	6766 0.57 2.42	29332 2.48 2.64	528838 44.63 17.60	458214 38.67 44.38	134348 11.34 62.79	1185031
Total	1324336	279516	1111004	3005346	1032467	213970	6966639

Note that both figures show that missing values and class 1 with no diagnosis codes have the greatest variance with respect to patient outcome. For length of stay, class 4 (with 4 diagnosis codes) has the highest probability of a short length of stay with classes 2 and 3 having the next highest probability. For total charges (which are entirely controlled by the provider), the probability is ranked in the exact order as the number of diagnosis codes. It is reasonable that the charges relate to the number of patient conditions; however, reimbursements and charges are not necessarily the same thing. Length of stay, however, is usually determined by the physician rather than the hospital, so the hospital has limited control over costs while being held accountable for them. What is not known is whether patients with a higher number of diagnoses also have more critical diseases, and are, in fact, sicker. Therefore, we also consider the classification codes once we restrict all patients to the same number of codes. In this example, we will remove all patients with fewer than five codes, and we will truncate all codes beyond

Table 7. Disease staging: resource demand level

Table of class by DS_RD_Level						
class	DS_RD_Level(Disease Staging: Resource Demand Level)					Total
Frequency Row Pct Col Pct	1	2	3	4	5	
1	0 0.00 0.00	4 7.14 0.00	31 55.36 0.00	21 37.50 0.00	0 0.00 0.00	56
2	318258 49.05 79.50	143313 22.09 9.54	157849 24.33 4.55	28625 4.41 2.14	744 0.11 0.29	648789
3	75289 7.92 18.81	520571 54.78 34.66	291351 30.66 8.40	60766 6.39 4.54	2308 0.24 0.90	950285
4	5925 0.68 1.48	366778 42.27 24.42	399557 46.05 11.52	90580 10.44 6.77	4791 0.55 1.86	867631
5	678 0.08 0.17	218745 27.30 14.56	458848 57.27 13.22	114716 14.32 8.58	8245 1.03 3.20	801232
6	117 0.02 0.03	123952 16.66 8.25	475322 63.89 13.70	132058 17.75 9.88	12550 1.69 4.88	743999
7	18 0.00 0.00	67788 10.41 4.51	435412 66.86 12.55	132405 20.33 9.90	15589 2.39 6.06	651212
8	8 0.00 0.00	36216 6.26 2.41	387727 67.07 11.18	133492 23.09 9.98	20651 3.57 8.03	578094
9	5 0.00 0.00	18810 3.48 1.25	345482 63.99 9.96	145324 26.92 10.87	30251 5.60 11.76	539872
10	9 0.00 0.00	5785 0.49 0.39	517993 43.71 14.93	499057 42.11 37.33	162182 13.69 63.03	1185026
Total	400307	1501962	3469572	1337044	257311	6966196

the first five. The most critical codes should be listed first, so this truncation is reasonable.

But then, how do we determine whether patients with truncated codes are more severe compared to patients who only have 5 codes to begin with? First, we look at the difference in primary diagnosis between the two groups: less than 4 codes and 5 codes or more. Next, we use text mining to examine the subgroup of patients with 5 or more codes, and compare the text clusters to patients who have 4 or fewer codes. First, we look at the most frequent codes for both groups to determine if patients with 5 or more codes have more severe problems. To simplify the analyses, we use a random sample of both groups. Table 10 gives the frequency list for the two groups.

At first glance, the two sets of codes look quite different. Yet, once the codes related to childbirth are eliminated, 401.9 is first in both groups followed by 428.0. In other words, it appears that if we treat childbirth, labor, and delivery as very different from the remaining reasons to be hospitalized, the codes

Table 8. Charlson index and number of diagnosis codes

Table of charlson by class

charlson Frequency Row Pct Col Pct	1	2	3	4	5	6	7	8	9	10	Total
0	892 0.02 95.91	622839 14.39 95.90	868837 20.08 91.40	723479 16.72 83.36	585252 13.53 73.03	459120 10.61 61.69	339642 7.85 52.15	251426 5.81 43.48	193041 4.46 35.75	282315 6.52 23.82	4326843
1	20 0.00 2.15	21596 1.51 3.33	62054 4.35 6.53	108325 7.59 12.48	155232 10.88 19.37	188672 13.23 25.35	189985 13.32 29.17	181077 12.69 31.32	171238 12.00 31.71	348263 24.41 29.38	1426462
2	10 0.00 1.08	4959 0.73 0.76	14779 2.17 1.55	23022 3.38 2.65	38150 5.61 4.76	59907 8.81 8.05	74735 10.99 11.47	87015 12.79 15.05	99704 14.66 18.46	277931 40.86 23.45	680212
3	6 0.00 0.65	75 0.02 0.01	2799 0.88 0.29	8368 2.62 0.96	14620 4.58 1.82	23383 7.33 3.14	29626 9.28 4.55	36563 11.46 6.32	46243 14.49 8.56	157456 49.34 13.28	319139
4	1 0.00 0.11	0 0.00 0.00	78 0.06 0.01	737 0.61 0.08	2591 2.14 0.32	6092 5.04 0.82	9062 7.49 1.39	12434 10.28 2.15	17661 14.61 3.27	72256 59.76 6.10	120912
5	1 0.00 0.11	0 0.00 0.00	1474 2.78 0.16	2334 4.40 0.27	2781 5.24 0.35	3189 6.01 0.43	3871 7.30 0.59	4808 9.06 0.83	6470 12.20 1.20	28115 53.00 2.37	53043
6	0 0.00 0.00	9 0.03 0.00	547 1.88 0.06	1367 4.70 0.16	2181 7.50 0.27	2782 9.57 0.37	3014 10.37 0.46	3204 11.02 0.55	3562 12.25 0.66	12402 42.67 1.05	29068
7	0 0.00 0.00	0 0.00 0.00	31 0.37 0.00	167 1.98 0.02	377 4.47 0.05	651 7.72 0.09	851 10.10 0.13	1053 12.49 0.18	1280 15.19 0.24	4018 47.67 0.34	8428
8	0 0.00 0.00	0 0.00 0.00	23 0.62 0.00	94 2.52 0.01	206 5.52 0.03	314 8.42 0.04	403 10.81 0.06	475 12.74 0.08	557 14.94 0.10	1657 44.44 0.14	3729
9	0 0.00 0.00	0 0.00 0.00	0 0.00 0.00	6 0.56 0.00	32 3.01 0.00	67 6.31 0.01	111 10.45 0.02	116 10.92 0.02	165 15.54 0.03	565 53.20 0.05	1062
10	0 0.00 0.00	0 0.00 0.00	0 0.00 0.00	0 0.00 0.00	2 0.61 0.00	12 3.65 0.00	24 7.29 0.00	45 13.68 0.01	49 14.89 0.01	197 59.88 0.02	329
11	0 0.00 0.00	0 0.00 0.00	0 0.00 0.00	0 0.00 0.00	3 2.65 0.00	2 1.77 0.00	6 5.31 0.00	10 8.85 0.00	14 12.39 0.00	78 69.03 0.01	113
12	0 0.00 0.00	0 0.00 0.00	0 0.00 0.00	0 0.00 0.00	0 0.00 0.00	0 0.00 0.00	2 6.90 0.00	2 6.90 0.00	7 24.14 0.00	18 62.07 0.00	29
13	0 0.00 0.00	0 0.00 0.00	0 0.00 0.00	0 0.00 0.00	0 0.00 0.00	0 0.00 0.00	0 0.00 0.00	1 25.00 0.00	1 25.00 0.00	2 50.00 0.00	4
Total	930	649478	950622	867899	801427	744191	651332	578229	539992	1185273	6969373

Table 9. Mortality by number of diagnosis codes

Table of class by DIED			
class	DIED(Died during hospitalization)		Total
Frequency Row Pct Col Pct	0	1	
1	826 94.62 0.01	47 5.38 0.05	873
2	648327 99.83 9.44	1105 0.17 1.07	649432
3	948760 99.82 13.82	1723 0.18 1.67	950483
4	863970 99.56 12.59	3777 0.44 3.67	867747
5	796429 99.40 11.60	4806 0.60 4.67	801235
6	736908 99.05 10.74	7054 0.95 6.86	743962
7	643236 98.79 9.37	7846 1.21 7.62	651082
8	568825 98.42 8.29	9136 1.58 8.88	577961
9	528067 97.84 7.69	11660 2.16 11.33	539727
10	1128970 95.29 16.45	55748 4.71 54.18	1184718
Total	6864318	102902	6967220

are quite similar. This is not unreasonable, since most women who are hospitalized for childbirth are, in fact, quite healthy and do not have many co-morbidities. Healthier women are more likely to become pregnant and to give birth, especially since women with severe diseases such as cancer are often advised to terminate the pregnancy in order to treat their own diseases.

Therefore, we will remove all patients related to childbirth and re-evaluate the remaining patients. In order to do this, we first look to the procedure codes. Codes from 72 through 75 represent obstetric procedures; we filter out all patients with these procedures. Then we again examine the most frequent codes in the two groups of patients, those with four or fewer listed, and those with five or more. Table 11 shows the revised list of diagnosis codes. For patients with five or more codes, the list in Table 11 changes only slightly; for 4 or fewer codes, it changes considerably.

Figure 5. Length of stay by number of clusters

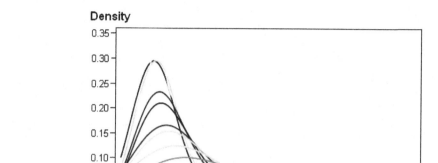

Figure 6. Total charges by number of clusters

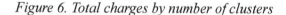

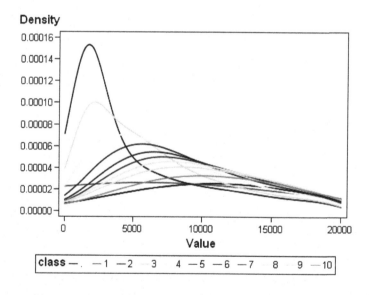

Most of the codes are relatively similar in the two groups, indicating that the patients may not be that far apart in terms of severity. After examining the most common codes, we use text mining to cluster the codes separately for each group to see if they generate similar clusters. Diabetes is higher on the frequency list for patients with 5 or more diagnosis codes compared to patients with 4 or fewer as is the condition of COPD. These suggest partially that patients with 5 or more codes are sicker compared to those with fewer than 5 codes. However, as many appear to have similar conditions, it seems that quite a few patients were shifted into higher categories by adding codes.

Table 10. Most frequent codes for patients with 5 or more clusters compared to patients with fewer than 5 clusters

Fewer Than 5 Codes	Translation of Codes	Frequency	5 Or More Codes	Translation of Codes	Frequency
V3000	Single liveborn without C-section	5388	4019	Unspecified hypertension	10153
V270	Singe liveborn	5360	4280	Congestive Heart Failure	4721
4019	Unspecified hypertension	4478	25000	Diabetes Mellitus	3846
4280	Congestive Heart Failure	2719	41401	Coronary atherosclerosis	3652
V3001	Single liveborn With C-section	2211	42731	Atrial fibrillation	3599
42731	Atrial fibrillation	2011	496	Chronic airway obstruction, not elsewhere classified	2828
V053	Viral hepatitis	1960	5990	Urinary tract infection, site not specified	2633
486	Pneumonia, organism unspecified	1637	2724	Other and unspecified hyperlipidemia	2573
2765	Disorders of fluid, electrolyte, and acid-base balance, Volume depletion	1627	486	Pneumonia, organism unspecified	2278
3051	Tobacco use disorder	1562	2765	Disorders of fluid, electrolyte, and acid-base balance, Volume depletion	2245
5990	Urinary tract infection, site not specified	1548	53081	Esophageal reflux	2171
25000	Diabetes mellitus	1510	3051	Tobacco use disorder	2129
41401	Coronary atherosclerosis	1504	2449	Unspecified hypothyroidism	1720
496	Chronic airway obstruction, not elsewhere classified	1492	V270	Singe liveborn	1671
7746	Unspecified fetal and neonatal jaundice	1259	2859	Anemia, unspecified	1499
53081	Esophageal reflux	1044	2720	Pure hypercholesterolemia	1395
2724	Other and unspecified hyperlipidemia	974	40391	Hypertensive chronic kidney disease	1373
40391	Hypertensive chronic kidney disease	910	78039	Convulsions	1343
5849	Acute renal failure, unspecified	855	2761	Hyposmolality and/or hyponatremia	1263

Table 12 has the clusters from 4 or fewer codes; and also the clusters for 5 or more codes. These clusters were defined using text analysis.

We need to consider how the clusters differ, compared by the number of classes. Consider cluster 11 in both groups. For fewer than five codes:

- Other cellulitis and abscess (Upper arm and forearm)
- Other cellulitis and abscess (Trunk)
- Staphylococcus aureus
- Other cellulitis and abscess (Foot, except toes)

Table 11. Most frequent codes for patients with 5 or more clusters compared to patients with fewer than 5 clusters excluding labor, deliver, and newborn conditions

Fewer Than 5 Codes	Translation of Codes	Frequency	5 Or More Codes	Translation of Codes	Frequency
4019	Unspecified hypertension	3567	4019	Unspecified hypertension	7545
4280	Congestive Heart Failure	2198	4280	Congestive Heart Failure	3249
42731	Atrial fibrillation	1830	25000	Diabetes Mellitus	2875
V053	Viral hepatitis	1337	41401	Coronary atherosclerosis	2639
41401	Coronary atherosclerosis	1275	42731	Atrial fibrillation	2514
2765	Disorders of fluid, electrolyte, and acid-base balance, Volume depletion	1250	496	Chronic airway obstruction, not elsewhere classified	1986
5990	Urinary tract infection, site not specified	1246	2724	Other and unspecified hyperlipidemia	1944
25000	Diabetes mellitus	1231	5990	Urinary tract infection, site not specified	1777
486	Pneumonia, organism unspecified	1637	486	Pneumonia, organism unspecified	1571
496	Chronic airway obstruction, not elsewhere classified	1136	53081	Esophageal reflux	1549
3051	Tobacco use disorder	1116	2765	Disorders of fluid, electrolyte, and acid-base balance, Volume depletion	1509
2724	Other and unspecified hyperlipidemia	756	3051	Tobacco use disorder	1505
53081	Esophageal reflux	730	2449	Unspecified hypothyroidism	1246
40391	Hypertensive chronic kidney disease	637	2859	Anemia, unspecified	1111
5849	Acute renal failure, unspecified	631	2720	Pure hypercholesterolemia	1088
78039	Convulsions	627	40391	Hypertensive chronic kidney disease	975
49390	Asthma, unspecified	573	78039	Convulsions	948
2449	Unspecified hypothyroidism	560	2761	Hyposmolality and/or hyponatremia	923
2859	Anemia, unspecified	551	41400	Coronary atherosclerosis	897

- Other postoperative infection
- Other cellulitis and abscess (Buttock)

and for five or more codes:

- Infection with microorganisms resistant to penicillins
- Other cellulitis and abscess (leg, except foot and ankle)
- Intramural leiomyoma of uterus
- Other cellulitis and abscess (foot,except toes)
- Staphylococcus aureus
- Mitral valve disorders

Table 12. Clusters of diagnoses

Cluster Codes for 4 or Fewer Codes	Translation of Codes	Cluster Codes for 5 or More Codes	Translation of Codes
V1582, 7802, 27800, 2768, 27651, 5180	History of tobacco use, Syncope and collapse, Obesity, unspecified, Hypopotassemia, Dehydration, Pulmonary collapse	2761, 486, 51881, 0389, 4280, 78659	Hyposmolality and/or hyponatremia, Pneumonia, organism unspecified, Unspecified septicemia, Congestive heart failure, unspecified, Chest pain
2720, 4019, 2724, v4581, 41401, 25000	Pure hypercholesterolemia, Essential hypertension, Other and unspecified hyperlipidemia, Aortocoronary bypass status, Coronary atherosclerosis, Diabetes mellitus	41400, 42731, 4111, 4280, v4582	Coronary atherosclerosis, Atrial fibrillation, Intermediate coronary syndrome, Congestive heart failure, Percutaneous transluminal coronary angioplasty status
496, 2765, 0389, 486, 42731, 49121	Chronic airway obstruction, not elsewhere classified, Volume depletion, Unspecified septicemia, Pneumonia, organism unspecified, Atrial fibrillation, Obstructive chronic bronchitis with (acute) exacerbation	73300, 71590, 2720, 49390, 53081, 4019	Osteoporosis, unspecified, Osteoarthrosis, unspecified whether generalized or localized, Pure hypercholesterolemia, Asthma, unspecified, Esophageal reflux, Essential hypertension
41401, 42731, v5789, 40391, 5849, 4254	Coronary atherosclerosis, Atrial fibrillation, Other specified rehabilitation procedure, Hypertensive chronic kidney disease, Acute renal failure, unspecified, Other primary cardiomyopathies	42789, 27800, 7802, 496, 2449, 3051	Other specified cardiac dysrhythmias, Obesity, unspecified, Syncope and collapse, Chronic airway obstruction, not elsewhere classified, Unspecified hypothyroidism, Tobacco use disorder
30500, 29620, 30560, 49390, 2989, 30391	Alcohol abuse, Major depressive disorder, single episode, Cocaine abuse, Asthma, unspecified, Unspecified psychosis, Other and unspecified alcohol dependence	2449, 2720, 25000, 53081, 2724, 3051	Unspecified hypothyroidism, Pure hypercholesterolemia, Diabetes mellitus, Esophageal reflux, Other and unspecified hyperlipidemia, Tobacco use disorder
2189, 5770, 27800, 6262, 5601, 2181	Leiomyoma of uterus, unspecified, Acute pancreatitis, Obesity, unspecified, Excessive or frequent menstruation, Paralytic ileus, Intramural leiomyoma of uterus	30560, 30391, 30500, 78039, 29181, 29680	Cocaine abuse, Other and unspecified alcohol dependence, Alcohol abuse, Other convulsions, Alcohol withdrawal, Bipolar disorder, unspecified
30520, 72210, 3051, 49390, 30401, 5409	Cannabis abuse, Lumbar intervertebral disc without myelopathy, Tobacco use disorder, Asthma, unspecified, Opioid type dependence, Appendicitis without mention of perforation, peritonitis, or rupture	2800, 1977, 1985, 9974, 1970, 27651	Iron deficiency anemias (secondary to blood loss), Secondary malignant neoplasm of respiratory and digestive systems (secondary to liver), Secondary malignant neoplasm of other specified sites (bone and bone marrow), Digestive system complications, Secondary malignant neoplasm of respiratory and digestive systems (secondary to lung), Dehydration
2449, 2859, 2720, 4019, 25000, 5990	Unspecified hypothyroidism, Anemia, unspecified, Pure hypercholesterolemia, Unspecified hypertension, Diabetes Mellitus, Urinary tract infection, site not specified	4241, 4240, 4271, 42732, 41071, 4280	Aortic valve disorders, Mitral valve disorders, Paroxysmal ventricular tachycardia, Atrial flutter, Subendocardial infarction, Congestive heart failure, unspecified
7470, v053, 6851, 79099, 7852	Patent ductus arteriosus, Viral hepatitis, Pilonidal cyst, Other nonspecific findings on examination of blood, Undiagnosed cardiac murmurs	29410, 3310, 0414, 2765, 5990, 5589	
46610, 008, 2765, 00861, 07999	Acute bronchiolitis, Intestinal infections due to other organisms, Volume depletion, Rotavirus, Unspecified viral infection	29410, 3310, 0414, 2765, 5990, 5589	Dementia in conditions classified elsewhere without behavioral disturbance, Alzheimer's disease, Escherichia coli [E.coli], Volume depletion, Urinary tract infection, site not specified, Other and unspecified noninfectious gastroenteritis and colitis

Table 12. continued

Cluster Codes for 4 or Fewer Codes	Translation of Codes	Cluster Codes for 5 or More Codes	Translation of Codes
6823, 6822, 04111, 6827, 99859, 6825	Other cellulitis and abscess (Upper arm and forearm), Other cellulitis and abscess (Trunk), Staphylococcus aureus, Other cellulitis and abscess (Foot, except toes), Other postoperative infection, Other cellulitis and abscess (Buttock)	V090, 6826, 2181, 6827, 04111, 4240	Infection with microorganisms resistant to penicillins, Other cellulitis and abscess (leg, except foot and ankle), Intramural leiomyoma of uterus, Other cellulitis and abscess (foot,except toes), Staphylococcus aureus, Mitral valve disorders
2761, 2768, 5990, 5849, 42731, 49121	Hyposmolality and/or hyponatremia, Hypopotassemia, Urinary tract infection, site not specified, Acute renal failure, unspecified, Atrial fibrillation, Obstructive chronic bronchitis	V4385, v5481, 43820, v5789, 7812, v4364	Organ or tissue replaced by other means, Aftercare following joint replacement, Hemiplegia affecting unspecified side, Other specified rehabilitation procedure, Abnormality of gait, Organ or tissue replaced by other means (hip)

For the first group, the cellulitis is likely to be from staph, but not resistant staff; in the second group, the infection is from resistant staph. In addition, the first group is more likely to have the infection in the arm, trunk, or buttocks whereas the second group has the infection in the foot and leg. The locations indicate that the first group has more community-acquired infection in addition to hospital acquired postoperative infection while the second group is more likely to have hospital-acquired infection. Moreover, the second group has related heart problems.

Table 12 shows that patients with 5 or more codes are quite simllar to patients with 4 or fewer codes, with just slight differences in the actual codes themselves. More drill down to examine the nature of these codes in more detail will find the nature of the gaming.

EXAMPLE OF CARDIOVASCULAR SURGERY

To further examine the aspect of "gaming", we look at the number of diagnoses by hospital when restricted to the cardiovascular procedures in 36.1. Table 13 shows the proportion of patients with the number of diagnosis codes for each procedure. Note that the proportion skews towards a higher number of codes. Procedure 3615 has the highest proportion of patients with 15 diagnosis codes.

Table 14 gives the relationship of number of codes to hospital. Hospital #1 has almost 60% of the patients with all 15 diagnosis codes while hospital #7 has none; the most these patients have is 14 at 65%. As we have already shown, hospitals that "game" the system tend to identify more codes per patient.

We use a predictive model to see if the number of codes increases the proportion of predicted mortality. Table 15 gives the proportion of patients who died by the number of diagnoses. Note that all of these patients have at least 12 different diagnoses. Since the diagnosis codes are assigned at discharge, it is possible that the number of diagnoses was increased after death.

Figure 7 gives the results of the predictive model, which includes hospital, procedure, and number of diagnoses without any patient demographics; the memory based reasoning node is the best model.

Table 16 gives the quality ranking based upon the number of diagnosis codes. Table 17 compares the

Table 13. Number of diagnosis codes by procedure

Table of Number of Diagnoses by Procedures								
Number of Diagnoses	**Principal Procedure**							**Total**
Frequency Row Pct Col Pct	3611	3612	3613	3614	3615	3616	3619	
2	0 0.00 0.00	0 0.00 0.00	0 0.00 0.00	0 0.00 0.00	3 100.00 0.80	0 0.00 0.00	0 0.00 0.00	3
4	0 0.00 0.00	0 0.00 0.00	1 33.33 0.25	0 0.00 0.00	2 66.67 0.53	0 0.00 0.00	0 0.00 0.00	3
6	1 7.14 0.93	2 14.29 0.69	3 21.43 0.75	4 28.57 1.52	4 28.57 1.07	0 0.00 0.00	0 0.00 0.00	14
8	3 8.33 2.78	7 19.44 2.43	9 25.00 2.24	7 19.44 2.65	6 16.67 1.60	4 11.11 14.29	0 0.00 0.00	36
10	7 10.29 6.48	18 26.47 6.25	20 29.41 4.98	8 11.76 3.03	13 19.12 3.47	2 2.94 7.14	0 0.00 0.00	68
11	8 7.27 7.41	18 16.36 6.25	38 34.55 9.45	14 12.73 5.30	31 28.18 8.27	1 0.91 3.57	0 0.00 0.00	110
12	10 8.47 9.26	17 14.41 5.90	30 25.42 7.46	20 16.95 7.58	39 33.05 10.40	2 1.69 7.14	0 0.00 0.00	118
13	10 5.59 9.26	34 18.99 11.81	42 23.46 10.45	38 21.23 14.39	51 28.49 13.60	4 2.23 14.29	0 0.00 0.00	179
14	33 7.89 30.56	94 22.49 32.64	121 28.95 30.10	91 21.77 34.47	68 16.27 18.13	10 2.39 35.71	1 0.24 100.00	418
15	36 6.96 33.33	98 18.96 34.03	138 26.69 34.33	82 15.86 31.06	158 30.56 42.13	5 0.97 17.86	0 0.00 0.00	517
Total	108	288	402	264	375	28	1	1466

ranking using the number of codes to the rankings from the predictive models in the previous models.

For the first time, the hospital with zero mortality (hospital #2) does not have the lowest rank. There are three hospitals with zero difference between the actual and predicted values. Overall, this model more accurately predicts the mortality by hospital than do any of the previous models.

NOSOCOMIAL INFECTION

Because nosocomial infection is such a problem, and because providers are reducing or eliminating payments to treat such infection, we want to look at specific reporting issues related to it. In particular, we want to see if hospitals are under-reporting a nosocomial rate by looking to the proportion of procedures

Table 14. Number of diagnosis codes by hospital

Number of diagnosis codes	Hospital										Total
Frequency Row Pct Col Pct	1	2	3	4	5	6	7	8	9	10	
2	2 66.67 0.62	0 0.00 0.00	0 0.00 0.00	0 0.00 0.00	0 0.00 0.00	0 0.00 0.00	0 0.00 0.00	0 0.00 0.00	1 33.33 1.28	0 0.00 0.00	3
4	0 0.00 0.00	0 0.00 0.00	2 66.67 1.79	0 0.00 0.00	0 0.00 0.00	0 0.00 0.00	0 0.00 0.00	0 0.00 0.00	0 0.00 0.00	1 33.33 1.04	3
6	1 7.14 0.31	0 0.00 0.00	1 7.14 0.89	3 21.43 1.19	2 14.29 2.27	0 0.00 0.00	4 28.57 1.41	1 7.14 2.22	2 14.29 2.56	0 0.00 0.00	14
8	6 16.67 1.85	1 2.78 9.09	2 5.56 1.79	1 2.78 0.40	2 5.56 2.27	2 5.56 1.14	5 13.89 1.77	4 11.11 8.89	5 13.89 6.41	8 22.22 8.33	36
10	15 22.06 4.62	1 1.47 9.09	3 4.41 2.68	17 25.00 6.72	4 5.88 4.55	6 8.82 3.43	9 13.24 3.18	2 2.94 4.44	9 13.24 11.54	2 2.94 2.08	68
11	26 23.64 8.00	1 0.91 9.09	7 6.36 6.25	19 17.27 7.51	8 7.27 9.09	16 14.55 9.14	16 14.55 5.65	5 4.55 11.11	6 5.45 7.69	6 5.45 6.25	110
12	26 22.03 8.00	0 0.00 0.00	13 11.02 11.61	16 13.56 6.32	9 7.63 10.23	13 11.02 7.43	19 16.10 6.71	6 5.08 13.33	7 5.93 8.97	9 7.63 9.38	118
13	33 18.44 10.15	1 0.56 9.09	22 12.29 19.64	27 15.08 10.67	11 6.15 12.50	25 13.97 14.29	46 25.70 16.25	2 1.12 4.44	8 4.47 10.26	4 2.23 4.17	179
14	30 7.18 9.23	4 0.96 36.36	7 1.67 6.25	34 8.13 13.44	7 1.67 7.95	113 27.03 64.57	184 44.02 65.02	25 5.98 55.56	5 1.20 6.41	9 2.15 9.38	418
15	186 35.98 57.23	3 0.58 27.27	55 10.64 49.11	136 26.31 53.75	45 8.70 51.14	0 0.00 0.00	0 0.00 0.00	0 0.00 0.00	35 6.77 44.87	57 11.03 59.38	517
Total	325	11	112	253	88	175	283	45	78	96	1466

that have higher rates of nosocomial, or more specifically, of resistant infection. In this case, we also need to identify which patients are entering the hospital with the infection, and which patients acquired it while there. We extend the work given in Chapter 8 that discussed the relationship between MRSA, patient diagnoses, and patient procedures. This, too, will allow us to investigate the possible occurrence of gaming in the reported data. Patients, for example, with an initial diagnosis of "insect bite" are more likely to have acquired the infection in the community rather than in the hospital, as are patients with osteomyelitis and diabetic foot ulcers. However, patients undergoing orthopedic procedures who also have resistant infection undoubtedly received it while in the hospital. While it would be helpful to know how well the hospital follows infection control protocols, such information will not always be available. However, high infection rates for resistant infection might warrant an examination of infection control procedures.

Unfortunately, studies that have considered the reliability of reporting nosocomial infection indicate

Table 15. Mortality by number of diagnosis codes for cardiovascular patients

Table of Number of Codes by DIED

Number of Codes	DIED(Died during hospitalization)		Total
Frequency Row Pct Col Pct	0	1	
2	3 100.00 0.21	0 0.00 0.00	3
4	3 100.00 0.21	0 0.00 0.00	3
6	14 100.00 0.97	0 0.00 0.00	14
8	36 100.00 2.50	0 0.00 0.00	36
10	68 100.00 4.73	0 0.00 0.00	68
11	110 100.00 7.65	0 0.00 0.00	110
12	117 99.15 8.14	1 0.85 3.57	118
13	178 99.44 12.38	1 0.56 3.57	179
14	408 97.61 28.37	10 2.39 35.71	418
15	501 96.91 34.84	16 3.09 57.14	517
Total	1438	28	1466

that the error rate is extremely high. An early study examined the lack of accuracy in relationship to lost revenue to treat the infection. Now that providers are reducing or eliminating reimbursements for such treatment, the reliability must be questioned even more. (Massanari, Wilkerson, Streed, & Walter J Hierholzer, 1987) There will be every incentive to under-report such infections.

A study performed almost fifteen years after that of Massanari, et. al. indicates that accuracy is still an issue in the reporting of nosocomial infection. (Vegni et al., 2004) Both studies found that just slightly more than 50% of nosocomial infections were accurately reported. A specific ICD9 code does not exist for a diagnosis of nosocomial infection. The question, then, is how can a nosocomial infection be identified through billing data? Table 18 reproduces the diagnosis clusters from Chapter 8, modifying the last column to identify the potential for a nosocomial infection. If it is not nosocomial, it is community acquired. However, this information is provided by a domain expert as a nosocomial infection

Figure 7. Results of predictive model

```
Fit Statistics
Model selection based on _TMISC_


                                 Test:
          Selected           Misclassification
          Model    Model Node       Rate

                   AutoNeural11     0.50000
                   DMNeural10       0.50000
                   DmineReg11       0.50000
             Y     MBR11            0.44444
                   Neural11         0.50000
                   Reg10            0.50000
                   Rule6            0.50000
                   Tree11           0.55556
```

Table 16. Predictive mortality versus actual mortality based upon number of codes

Hospital	Actual Mortality	Predictive Mortality	Difference	Rank
1	1.23	2.46	1.23	3
2	0	0	0	6
3	4.46	3.57	-0.89	9
4	0.79	6.32	5.53	1
5	1.14	3.41	2.27	2
6	0.57	1.14	0.57	4
7	3.53	3.89	0.36	5
8	2.22	2.22	0	6
9	1.28	1.28	0	6
10	3.13	1.04	-2.09	10

Table 17. Comparison of ranks using other models

Hospital	APRDRG Rank	Resource Demand Rank	Number of Codes
1	6	8	3
2	10	10	6
3	1	9	9
4	7	6	1
5	2	3	2
6	3	5	4
7	4	1	5
8	9	4	6
9	5	2	6
10	8	7	10

Table 18. Diagnosis codes related to MRSA

Cluster #	Code Combinations	Translations	Nosocomial?
1	303.91, 304.21, 291.81, 305.60, 305.20, 681.00	Other and unspecified alcohol dependence (continuous), Cocaine dependence (continuous), Alcohol withdrawal, Cocaine abuse (continuous), Cannabis abuse (continuous), Cellulitis and abscess, unspecified	No
2	272.0, 272.4, 401.9, 786.59, 600.00, 250.00	Pure hypercholesterolemia, Other and unspecified hyperlipidemia, Essential hypertension, Chest pain, Hypertrophy (benign) of prostate without urinary obstruction, Diabetes mellitus without mention of complication of unspecified type	No
3	648.21, 278.01, 285.9, 654.21, 663.31, 648.41	Anemia, Morbid obesity, Anemia, unspecified, Previous cesarean delivery, Other and unspecified cord entanglement, without mention of compression, Mental disorders (pregnancy delivered)	Yes
4	276.8, 275.2, 787.91, 276.5, 305.1, 285.9	Hypopotassemia, Disorders of magnesium metabolism, Diarrhea, Volume depletion, Tobacco use disorder, Anemia, unspecified	Yes
5	493.90, 301.83, 540.9, 530.81, 278.01, 682.0	Asthma, unspecified, Borderline personality disorder, Without mention of peritonitis, Esophageal reflux, Morbid obesity, Other cellulitis and abscess (face)	No
6	440.23, 707.15, 250.70, 250.82, 250.80, 731.8	Atherosclerosis of the extremities with ulceration, Ulcer of other part of foot (toes), Diabetes with peripheral circulatory disorders (unspecified type), Diabetes with other specified manifestations (Type II or unspecified uncontrolled), Diabetes with other specified manifestations (of unspecified type), Other bone involvement in diseases classified elsewhere	No
7	041.11, 683, 682.5, 616.4, 682.2, 608.4	Staphylococcus aureus, Acute lymphadenitis, Other cellulitis and abscess (buttock), Other abscess of vulva, Other cellulitis and abscess (hand except fingers and thumb), Other inflammatory disorders of male genital organs	Yes
8	V45.1, 294.10, 427.31, 996.62, 682.6, 403.91	Renal dialysis status, Dementia in conditions classified elsewhere without behavioral disturbance, Atrial fibrillation, Infection and inflammatory reaction due to internal prosthetic device, implant, and graft Due to vascular device, implant and graft, Other cellulitis and abscess (leg except foot), Hypertensive kidney disease (chronic)	Yes
9	041.11, 567.2, 998.59, 998.32, 682.2, 998.1	Staphylococcus aureus, Other suppurative peritonitis, Other postoperative infection, Disruption of external operation wound, Other cellulitis and abscess (trunk), Hemorrhage or hematoma or seroma complicating a procedure	Yes
10	278.00, 401.9, 780.57, 272.4, 250.00, 682.2	Obesity, unspecified, Essential hypertension, Unspecified sleep apnea, Other and unspecified hyperlipidemia, Diabetes mellitus without mention of complication (unspecified type), Other cellulitis and abscess (trunk)	No
11	596.54, 707.0, 907.2, 599.0, 344.1, 041.7	Neurogenic bladder NOS, Decubitus ulcer, Late effect of spinal cord injury, Urinary tract infection, site not specified, Paraplegia, Pseudomonas	Yes
12	319, 343.9, 780.3, v44.0, v44.1, 599.0	Unspecified mental retardation, Infantile cerebral palsy, unspecified, Convulsions, Tracheostomy, Gastrostomy, Urinary tract infection, site not specified	Yes
13	272.4, v45.01, 414.00, v45.81, 412, 428.0	Other and unspecified hyperlipidemia, Cardiac pacemaker, Of unspecified type of vessel, native or graft, Aortocoronary bypass status, Old myocardial infarction, Congestive heart failure, unspecified	Yes
14	V30.01, 770.89, 770.6, 770.81, 765.18, 779.3	Single liveborn, Other respiratory problems after birth, Transitory tachypnea of newborn, Primary apnea of newborn, Disorders relating to short gestation and low birthweight, Feeding problems in newborn	Yes
15	041.04, 644.03, 599.0, 646.63, 041.4, 041.3	Streptococcus (Group D [Enterococcus]), Threatened premature labor, Urinary tract infection, site not specified, Infections of genitourinary tract in pregnancy, Escherichia coli [E.coli], Friedländer's bacillus	Yes
16	263.9, 715.90, 294.8, 787.2, 599.0, 507.0	Unspecified protein-calorie malnutrition, Osteoarthrosis, unspecified whether generalized or localized, Other persistent mental disorders due to conditions classified elsewhere, Dysphagia, Urinary tract infection, site not specified, Pneumonitis due to solids and liquids due to inhalation of food or vomitus	Yes

Table 18. continued

Cluster #	Code Combinations	Translations	Nosocomial?
17	276.1, 276.8, 276.7, 599.0, 491.21, 244.9	Hyposmolality and/or hyponatremia, Hypopotassemia, Hyperpotassemia, Urinary tract infection, site not specified, Obstructive chronic bronchitis with (acute) exacerbation, Unspecified hypothyroidism	Yes
18	382.9, 466.11, 558.9, 276.5, 458.9, 790.6	Unspecified otitis media, Acute bronchiolitis due to respiratory syncytial virus, Other and unspecified noninfectious gastroenteritis and colitis, Volume depletion, Hypotension, unspecified, Nonspecific findings on examination of blood (Other abnormal blood chemistry)	Yes
19	682.6, 916.5, 891.1, 916.1, 680.6, 041.11	Other cellulitis and abscess, leg other than foot, Insect bite, nonvenomous, infected, Open wound of knee, leg [except thigh], and ankle (complicated), Abrasion or friction burn, infected, Carbuncle and furuncle (leg except for foot), Staphylococcus aureus	No
20	785.52, 916.5, 891.1, 916.1, 680.6, 041.11	Septic shock, Insect bite, nonvenomous, infected, Open wound of knee, leg [except thigh], and ankle (complicated), Carbuncle and furuncle (leg except for foot)	No
21	530.81, 311, 553.3, 493.92, 786.50, 305.1	Esophageal reflux, Depressive disorder, not elsewhere classified, Diaphragmatic hernia, Asthma, unspecified, Chest pain, unspecified, Tobacco use disorder	No
22	244.9, 401.9, 733.00, v10.3, 272.4, v15.82	Unspecified hypothyroidism, Essential hypertension, Osteoporosis, unspecified, Personal history of malignant neoplasm (breast), Other and unspecified hyperlipidemia, History of tobacco use	No
23	913.5, 726.33, 682.4, 041.11, 682.3, 305.1	Insect bite, nonvenomous, infected, Olecranon bursitis, Other cellulitis and abscess (hand except fingers and thumb), Carbuncle and furuncle (leg except for foot), cellulitis and abscess (upper arm and forearm)	No
24	V05.3, 766.1, 767.8, 762.6, 774.6, v29.0	Viral hepatitis, Disorders relating to long gestation and high birthweight (Other "heavy-for-dates" infants), Other specified birth trauma, Other and unspecified conditions of umbilical cord, Unspecified fetal and neonatal jaundice, Observation for suspected infectious condition	Yes
25	583.81, 337.1, 250.40, 362.01, 357.2, 250.60	Nephritis and nephropathy, not specified as acute or chronic, in diseases classified elsewhere, Peripheral autonomic neuropathy in disorders classified elsewhere, Diabetes with renal manifestations of unspecified type, Background diabetic retinopathy, Polyneuropathy in diabetes, Diabetes with neurological manifestations of unspecified type	No
26	664.01, 659.61, 648.81, 658.11, 652.21, 642.31	First-degree perineal laceration, Elderly multigravida, Abnormal glucose tolerance, Premature rupture of membranes, Breech presentation without mention of version, Transient hypertension of pregnancy	Yes
27	427.31, 428.0, 507.0, 518.81, 496, 995.92	Atrial fibrillation, Congestive heart failure, unspecified, Pneumonitis due to solids and liquids (Due to inhalation of food or vomitus), Acute respiratory failure, Chronic airway obstruction, not elsewhere classified, Systemic inflammatory response syndrome due to infectious process with organ dysfunction	Yes
28	466.0, 491.21, 300.00, v15.82, 427.89, 428.0	Acute bronchitis and bronchiolitis, Obstructive chronic bronchitis (With (acute) exacerbation), Anxiety states, unspecified, History of tobacco use, Other specified cardiac dysrhythmias, Congestive heart failure, unspecified	Yes
29	626.2, v57.89, 285.1, v43.65, 280.0, 562.10	Excessive or frequent menstruation, Other specified rehabilitation procedure, Acute posthemorrhagic anemia, Organ or tissue replaced by other means, knee joint, Iron deficiency anemias, secondary to blood loss, Diverticulosis of colon (without mention of hemorrhage)	Yes
30	443.9, 401.9, 250.00, 997.62, 682.6, 682.7	Peripheral vascular disease, unspecified, Essential hypertension, Diabetes mellitus without mention of complication of unspecified type, Infection (chronic), Other cellulitis and abscess, leg except foot, Other cellulitis and abscess, foot except toes	No

Table 18. continued

Cluster #	Code Combinations	Translations	Nosocomial?
31	V02.59, 311, 715.90, 300.00, 733.00, 682.2	Other specified bacterial diseases, Depressive disorder, not elsewhere classified, Osteoarthrosis, unspecified whether generalized or localized, Anxiety states, unspecified, Osteoporosis, unspecified, Other cellulitis and abscess, trunk	No
32	412, 428.0, 411.1, v45.82, 272.4, v45.01	Old myocardial infarction, Congestive heart failure, unspecified, Intermediate coronary syndrome, Percutaneous transluminal coronary angioplasty status, Other and unspecified hyperlipidemia, Cardiac pacemaker	Yes

is not specifically identified.

Once we have identified those clusters that represent nosocomial infections versus community acquired infections, as we have done in previous chapters, we can determine which hospitals have a high proportion of patients in the nosocomial categories compared to those hospitals with more patients in the community acquired clusters. There are hospitals, too, with patients in both types of clusters, suggesting that poor infection control procedures can result in nosocomial infection acquired from those patients admitted with community acquired infection.

FUTURE TRENDS

The trend to using provider "report cards" to define reimbursements will only accelerate. Therefore, it is important to validate the risk adjustment models that are used to define these report cards. Unfortunately, validation has tended to lag behind the use of these models. As we have seen, there can be very different results generated using different measures of patient severity. Because of these problems, it will be necessary in the future to define multi-dimensional measures of quality, and to drill down into the reasons that providers have different results on these report cards.

DISCUSSION

As shown by the different examples of public reporting, there are already several states that have moved to the web display of hospital quality, some by individual hospitals and some by general region. Private companies such as healthgrades.com also have quality reports available to the public. Therefore, there has to be considerable concern that the methodology used to develop the quality rankings is adequate to the task. The more dollars that are at stake in the reimbursement formulas, the greater the incentive to "game" the system by upcoding; by taking advantage of problems with the current methodology. The only way to prevent such gaming is to use methods that do not require that we assume conditions that we know to be false.

REFERENCES

Anonymous-CMS. (2006). *Outlier Example*. Retrieved 2008, from http://www.cms.hhs.gov/AcuteIn-patientPPS/downloads/outlier_example.pdf

Anonymous-Floridareporting. (2008). *Connecting Florida With Healthcare Information*. Retrieved 2008, from http://www.floridahealthfinder.gov/CompareCare/SelectChoice.aspx

Anonymous-Missouri. (2008). *Missouri Healthcare-associated infection reporting*. Retrieved 2008, from http://www.dhss.mo.gov/HAI/index.html?target=drive_noso.php

Anonymous-Penn. (2008). *Pennsylvania Health Care Cost Containment Council*. Retrieved 2008, from http://www.phc4.org/

Anonymous-Vermont. (2008). *Act 53 Hospital Report Cards*. Retrieved from http://www.bishca.state.vt.us/HcaDiv/HRAP_Act53/HRC_BISHCAcomparison_2007/surgical_infection_prevention_2007.htm

Arias, K. M. (2008). Mandatory reporting and pay for performance: health care infections in the limelight. *AORN Journal, 87*(4), 750–758.

Bhattacharyya, T., Priyesh, M., & Freiberg, A. A. (2008). Hospital characteristics associated with success in a pay-for-performance program in orthopaedic surgery. *Journal of Bone and Joint Surgery, 90*, 1240–1243.

Bodrock, J. A., & Mion, L. C. (2008). Pay for performance in hospitals: implications for nurses and nursing care. *Quality Management in Health Care, 17*(2), 102–111.

Collier, V. U. (2007). Use of pay for performance in a community hospital private hospitalist group: a preliminary report. *Transactions of the American Clinical and Climatological Association, 118*, 263–272.

Doran, T., Fullwood, C., Reeves, D., Gravelle, H., & Roland, M. (2008). Exclusion of patients from pay-for-performance targets by English physicians. *The New England Journal of Medicine, 359*(3), 274–284.

Hayward, R. A., & Kent, D. M. (2008). EZ steps to improving your performance: (or how to make P4P pay 4U!). *Journal of the American Medical Association, 300*(3), 255–256.

Hazelwood, A., & Cook, E. D. (2008). Improving quality of healthcare through pay-for-performance programs. *The Health Care Manager, 27*(2), 104–112.

Hollingsworth, J. M., Krein, S. L., Miller, D. C., DeMonner, S., & Hollenbeck, B. K. (2007). Payer leverage and hospital compliance with a benchmark: a population-based observational study. *BMC Health Services Research, 7*, 112.

Karve, A. M., Ou, F.-S., Lytle, B. L., & Peterson, E. D. (2008). Potential unintended financial consequences of pay-for-performance on the quality of care for minority patients. *American Heart Journal, 155*, 571–576.

Lewis, J., & Friesen, S. (2006). What surgeons should know about...developments in pay for performance. *Bulletin of the American College of Surgeons, 91*(11), 8–11, 61.

Massanari, R. M., Wilkerson, K., Streed, S. A., Walter, J., & Hierholzer, J. (1987). Reliabililty of reporting nosocomial infection in the discharge abstract and implications for receipt of revenues under prospective reimbursement. *American Journal of Public Health, 77,* 561–564.

Medicare Prescription Drug, Improvement, and Modernization Act of 2003, Pub L No. 108-173, 238 C.F.R. (2003).

Thornton, T., & Hakim, R. (1997). The relationship between quality of care and financial performance in dialysis: "doing well by doing good . *Advances in Renal Replacement Therapy, 4*(4), 350–358.

Vegni, F., Panceri, M., Biffi, M., Banfi, E., Porretta, A., & Privitera, G. (2004). Three scenarios of clinical claim reimbursement for nosocomial infection: the good, the bad, and the ugly. *The Journal of Hospital Infection, 56,* 150–155.

Chapter 11
How to Check Measures for Adequacy

INTRODUCTION

Perhaps the biggest problem when checking measures for adequacy, in addition to overlooking the fact that model assumptions are invalid, is the need to examine the model for reliability, and also to generalize a reliable result to an assumption of validity. Without some test of validity, the results could be bogus because the model does not measure what it is supposed to measure. The question is, just how should a model be validated?

Reliability is much easier to show. Simply put, similar data should yield similar results. Therefore, we can compare results across hospitals and patients from one year to another to see if the results by hospital change from one year to the next, or if they are relatively the same. If the results do not really change from year to year, the measure is assumed to be reliable. Validity, however, is a much more difficult concept to demonstrate; so much so, that often validity is ignored in favor of just demonstrating reliability. As written in Donabedian, (Donabedian, 1980)

The concept of validity is itself made up of many parts; and there is no precise way of saying what belongs to it, or what belongs more appropriately under another heading....I would say that the question

DOI: 10.4018/978-1-60566-752-2.ch011

of validity covers two large domains. The first has to do with the accuracy of the data and the precision of the measures that are constructed with these data. The second has to do with the justifiability of the inferences that are drawn from the data and the measurements.

A search of Medline using the keywords "risk adjustment" and "validation" returned a total of 3 articles. It is not yet a concept that is given much consideration, which is why we have so many different measures of patient severity that can give very different results. However, as providers are more likely to be rewarded or penalized based upon the results of these measures, the measures themselves will become more heavily scrutinized.

BACKGROUND

We first look at the three papers that were found by using the key words "validation" and "risk adjustment". A recent paper compared the results of two models with a third, internally developed model to define validation. (Kunadian et al., 2008) Since the models are defined by comparing model values to each other, this does not give validation as much as it gives reliability. An earlier paper defines validation by getting similar results on new datasets. Again, this is reliability rather than validation.(Moscucci et al., 1999) A third paper used the fact that a logistic model predicted accurately, but as discussed in detail in Chapter 3, accuracy does not imply that the model is adequate or valid.(Mandeep et al., 2003)

True validation takes place when the measurement actually measures what it is supposed to measure. In other words, a patient severity index must actually measure the actual level of severity of the patient's condition. A more formal definition of validity is provided at http://www.socialresearchmethods.net/tutorial/Colosi/lcolosi2.htm. Validity is the best available approximation to the truth or falsity of a given inference, proposition or conclusion. Consideration of validity attempts to answer the question, is the severity index true? There are four major types of validity to consider:

1. **Convergent validity** examines whether there is a relationship between the program and the observed outcome. Or, in our example, is there a connection between the patient severity index and the patient's level of sickness?
2. **Internal validity** asks if there is a relationship between the measure and the outcome and whether the relationship is causal. For example, did the patient's severity level cause the outcomes in mortality, length of stay, and costs?
3. **Construct validity** asks if there is a relationship between how the concepts are operationalized in the study to the actual causal relationship. Or in our example, did the measure of severity reflect the construct of severity, and did the measured outcome reflect the construct of severity? Overall, we are trying to generalize our conceptualized measure and outcomes to broader constructs of the same concepts.
4. **External validity** refers to our ability to generalize the results of our study to other settings. In our example, could we generalize our results defined using certain providers, to all providers?

The different types of validity focus on the question of whether there is a relationship between the measure of the outcome and the outcome itself. We must consider first whether a predictive model that measures the expected mortality is a good measure of the actual mortality. As long as the r^2 value is small, and there remains considerable variability in the model, it is not a valid representation of the actual outcomes. Therefore, we need to consider the differential between the predicted and actual outcomes. An assumption is made that if the actual mortality is less than what is predicted, then the hospital must be doing something to prevent deaths that should be expected to occur. If this difference is negative so that the actual mortality is larger than predicted, then the hospital appears to be doing something wrong that increases the mortality.

Construct validity deals with an examination of the causal relationship. In our example, there should be a relationship between patient severity and mortality. There has to be a relationship to the actual patient severity. However, as we have seen, different severity measures can put the patient in the least severe category, and then a second measure can put the patient in the most severe category. Because there is such a lack of consistency across measures, the construct validity must remain in doubt.

In addition to defining severity, we must see how that severity measure relates to the outcome. There does not appear to be a cause-effect between actual and predicted mortality. Since regression and predictive models focus on predicting outcomes accurately, should we work with a measure that is defined based upon a difference in predicted and actual outcomes? Generally, these are considered to be residual or random error rather than a useful measure of difference. Yet we are using random error to define the quality of hospitals. In addition, the r^2 values tend to be small, and lift functions defined from predictive models indicate that only a portion of the population can be predicted accurately.

Unfortunately, there is no absolute standard to compare a severity index in order to make such a validation. Because validation is so difficult, reliability is often substituted. A good way to validate is to compare a severity measure to patient outcomes. However, if outcomes are used to define the severity index, they cannot then be used to validate. In the absence of such an analysis, how can validity be established?

We have been looking into the issue of validity throughout this book. When we examined the risk adjustment by mortality to find that providers with a zero mortality rate can actually rank low in terms of the differential between actual and predicted mortality (since the difference is zero), then there is a problem with validity. At the same time, it was also shown that a provider with a zero mortality rate generally does not have patients that are as severe compared to providers with higher mortality rates; for this reason, the differential between actual and predicted values is low. Therefore, there must be a better way than to compare this differential in order to assign quality. Clearly, a provider with zero mortality should rank high in a measure that uses mortality as an outcome measure.

But if there is difficulty when just comparing actual mortality to predictive mortality, just how can we define a risk adjusted method to compare provider quality, and to validate this method? Without some decisions as to how we define the quality of care, no measure will be valid. Any measure must also have some adjustment for the severity of the patient's condition since it is clear that a patient with a more severe condition will have a higher risk compared to a patient with a lower degree of severity.

The methodology cannot focus just on inputs since inputs are insufficient to compare patient outcomes. We also need to consider just what outcome we need to examine. Certainly, a high rate of patient falls is disconcerting; however, again, the patient's condition may create a higher risk of falls. Therefore, adverse events and errors also need to be risk adjusted. We still need to validate the adjusted risk.

In addition, we need to consider hospital errors and adverse outcomes. If a hospital has a high rate of resistant infection, a high rate could mean that the hospital treats a high proportion of community-acquired infections, or it has an epidemic of resistant infection because of improper infection control procedures.

Instead, consideration should be given to multi-dimensional measures of quality, with mortality and medical errors comprising just two of the dimensions. A third measure should examine outcome measures that are related to specific diagnoses or to specific procedures. For example, in bypass surgery, there is a some risk of mortality, However, there are additional risks of stroke and mental impairment that are generally ignored because they cannot be predicted so they are dismissed. There is also a risk of amputation resulting from the harvesting of veins in the leg. For this, we may have to go beyond billing data and to examine insurance claims that include follow up, or we may have to examine the electronic medical record. Again, in bypass surgery, an amputation may occur within a short time after hospital discharge because of the removal of the veins to be used in the bypass and different hospitals will have different rates of such outcomes. Therefore, outcomes should be considered with respect to different procedures, and mortality should not be the only outcome considered.

Another aspect of validity is to consider drilling down into details to determine the reasons for the difference between actual and predicted values. In particular, it should be considered whether patients have been shifted from one category into a higher severity category just by coding. If so, the ranking of quality should be modified to reflect that shifting. Severity codes should be examined regularly to determine if they need to be updated, and to determine whether they are valid. Otherwise, providers can be rewarded when they have not improved care, and providers can be penalized because of poor coding when care is of the highest quality. Therefore, in order to truly validate a measure, drill down into actual practices, and their relationship to patient outcomes should be performed. Poor performers should be compared to strong performance on the quality index.

For example, if a provider has a much higher infection rate compared to another provider, their infection control procedures and practices should be compared. Suppose the low infection provider makes greater use of prophylactic antibiotics, and has greater adherence to infection control practices compared to the provider with the higher infection rate. Then there are definite actions the provider with higher rates of infection can make to improve the quality of care. Again, this is a multi-dimensional examination of the information, but it is essential to discover why providers perform on quality measures as they do.

We must also reflect upon the statistical methodology used, and to ensure that the assumptions of the statistical models are satisfied. Otherwise, the models should be modified to reflect their actual validity of the models. Moreover, we must take into consideration just what the model outcomes represent rather than to rely on the use of surrogate markers. There is still much to be done to develop accurate models of provider quality, and accurate models of patient severity.

SUMMARY

In this text, we have examined a number of different severity indices as well as the statistical methods that are used to define the risk adjustment and quality rankings of healthcare providers. The common severity indices examined here include the Charlson Index, the APRDRG patient index, and the Medstat disease staging indices. While there are other indices available, they generally follow the same patterns: restricting attention to a specific set of diagnosis codes, using a consensus panel to define the severity level, or to use resource utilization. All of these methods depend heavily upon a basic assumption of the uniformity of data entry across healthcare providers, an assumption that is known to be false.

In addition, the tradition of using the difference between predicted and actual values of mortality makes the assumption that the predicted mortality is what can be expected and if the actual mortality is less than predicted, then it must be because the provider has better quality than if the actual mortality is greater than predicted. Another assumption using this measure is that a logistic regression model that has a high misclassification rate in the predicted mortality is useful in assessing the quality of a provider. Such an assumption tends to penalize those providers with low actual mortality because there will be little difference to the predicted mortality. However, logistic regression was never designed to be used in this way.

Also, the general use of logistic regression assumes that the underlying population is normal; as we showed in Chapter 3, this assumption is not valid. Because of the nature of healthcare outcomes, patient results tend to be skewed and to follow a gamma distribution. The use of data visualization and kernel density estimation can be used to investigate the assumption of the population distribution so that the model can be modified to accommodate the nature of that distribution.

The use of text mining to define a patient severity index does not require a number of the basic assumptions that are required for the more traditional definitions. It is more versatile in that it can be used with a variety of outcomes, including the occurrence of nosocomial infection. Since outcomes are not used to define the patient severity index with text mining, outcomes can be used to validate the results. Text mining is a little used technique in the investigation of health outcomes, but it is extremely versatile, and does not require the uniformity of data entry since it is the linkage between patient conditions that is utilized to define a patient severity index rather than just relying upon the conditions themselves. It is the only method defined in this book that accepts the assumption that patient co-morbidities are related.

If a severity index is defined using one outcome variable such as mortality, other outcomes should be used to validate the results; outcomes should be considered multi-dimensional. Instead of relying on the difference between observed and expected values in a regression that primarily take advantage of misclassification in the model (in contrast to the original definition of regression), reasons for the difference in rate should be investigated. Otherwise, providers with low actual rates will be penalized compared to providers with high rates where the deviation between actual and predicted can be much greater. Because of the concern with nosocomial infection, the likelihood and risk of acquiring such infection should be a prime component in any measure of patient quality. Another measure that is important is the occurrence of adverse events and errors, especially errors in medication dispensing and prescribing, and patient falls.

We suggest that scorecards should have diminished importance compared to a careful examination of mortality, morbidity, nosocomial problems, and errors. Patient treatment is multi-faceted, and mortality is not the only outcome that is of importance to patients. The advantage of using text clusters is that they can accommodate the multi-faceted outcomes, and are flexible enough to enable researchers to drill down into details. In combination with kernel density estimation to examine possibilities, we can examine the occurrence of nosocomial problems, which should be given considerable weight when investigating the quality of provider care. Certainly patients will be concerned if there is a considerable risk of acquiring infection because of a hospital stay. One of the biggest problems with investigating nosocomial infections is that it is under-reported, and it is difficult to extract information from the ICD9 secondary diagnoses. As we demonstrated in Chapter 10, text clusters can be used to separate community-acquired from nosocomoal infections in order to investigate hospitals that have problems with nosocomial infections. Such an examination again demonstrates the versatility of using text mining to investigate patient outcomes.

If we do not examine severity indices more carefully, their use can penalize providers that provide good quality care while rewarding those who focus their efforts on "gaming" the index. As the move to relate payer reimbursements based upon rankings of quality, it is imperative that the risk adjustment models used are validated so that the highest quality providers are the highest scoring in the models. Because of these issues, the habit of using the difference between predicted and actual outcomes should be abandoned in favor of a multi-dimensional approach.

When risk adjustment methods are used to reimburse providers based upon their ranking, the methodology needs to be scrutinized very carefully. The potential for "gaming" should be investigated, and the possibility of penalizing good quality providers is important, and should be examined carefully. Real data should be used to consider the validity of the method without just considering model reliability. Predictive modeling techniques are important when analyzing both validity and reliability, and should be used along with the more traditional regression. When large datasets are used to define and examine patient severity, the p-value is of little value and should not be used to measure the adequacy of the model. Also, the rareness of the outcome measure should be considered, and compensated for using stratified sampling. The measure of quality is a complex issue and will require some fairly complex modeling.

FUTURE TRENDS

Because patient severity and hospital quality are both multi-dimensional, the most effective measures of both will be multi-dimensional. Therefore, the use of ICD9 codes to define a patient severity should be just one dimension to define quality. Patient compliance with treatment must also be included as a dimension. Moreover, medical errors and nosocomial infections should be included as additional dimensions. If these added dimensions are not considered, there will still be a problem of validity.

Data mining techniques allow us to drill down to explore details; such drill down is not possible with standard statistical techniques. Statistical methods ultimately reflect group identity rather than to examine individual identity. Therefore, data mining can find more and better detail in the data. These techniques will certainly be used more often as more electronic data become available. While the transition to electronic records has been slow, this transition is continuing. The more electronic information available, the more knowledge that will be extracted from those electronic records.

DISCUSSION

The problem of defining a patient severity index is still not resolved. If it were, there would not be so many different measures and different attempts to create severity models. Providers should take opportunities to define their own measures of quality and to measure improvements in quality within themselves as well as in comparison to other providers.

In this text, we have discussed these additional dimensions briefly in addition to examining the current techniques available to define patient severity measures. In addition, we have demonstrated how data mining techniques, particularly data visualization, predictive modeling, and text mining can be used to define better measures of patient severity that do not require accepting false assumptions, especially the assumption of the uniformity of data entry.

REFERENCES

Donabedian, A. (1980). *Explorations in quality assessment and monitoring, Volume 1. The definition of quality and approaches to its assessment.* Chicago: Health Administration Press.

Kunadian, B., Dunning, J., Das, R., Roberts, A., Morley, R., & Turley, A. (2008). External validation of established risk adjustment models for procedural complications after percutaneous coronary intervention. *Heart (British Cardiac Society), 94*(8), 1012–1018.

Mandeep, S., Rihal, C. S., Selzer, F., Kip, K. E., Detre, K., David, R., & Holmes, J. (2003). Validation of Mayo Clinic risk adjustment model for in-hospital complications after percutaneous coronary interventions, using the national heart, lung, and blood institute dynamic registry. *Journal of the American College of Cardiology, 42,* 1722–1728.

Moscucci, M., O'Connor, G. T., Ellis, S. G., Malenka, D. J., Sievers, J., & Bates, E. R. (1999). Validation of risk adjustment models for in-hospital percutaneous transluminal coronary angioplasty mortality on an independent data set. *Journal of the American College of Cardiology, 34,* 692–697.

About the Author

Patricia Cerrito, PhD, has made considerable strides in the development of data mining techniques to investigate large, complex medical data. In particular, she has developed a method to automate the reduction of the number of levels in a nominal data field to a manageable number that can then be used in other data mining techniques. Another innovation of the PI is to combine text analysis with association rules to examine nominal data. The PI has over 30 years of experience in working with SAS software, and over 10 years of experience in data mining healthcare databases. In just the last two years, she has supervised 7 PhD students who completed dissertation research in investigating health outcomes. Dr. Cerrito has a particular research interest in the use of a patient severity index to define provider quality rankings for reimbursements. This text is the culmination of her research efforts.

Index